Imperfect Pregnancies

Imperfect Pregnancies

A History of Birth Defects
and Prenatal Diagnosis

ILANA LÖWY

Johns Hopkins University Press
Baltimore

© 2017 Johns Hopkins University Press
All rights reserved. Published 2017
Printed in the United States of America on acid-free paper
2 4 6 8 9 7 5 3 1

Johns Hopkins University Press
2715 North Charles Street
Baltimore, Maryland 21218-4363
www.press.jhu.edu

Library of Congress Cataloging-in-Publication Data

Names: Löwy, Ilana, 1948– author.
Title: Imperfect pregnancies : a history of birth defects and prenatal diagnosis
  / Ilana Löwy.
Description: Baltimore : Johns Hopkins University Press, 2017. | Includes
  bibliographical references and index.
Identifiers: LCCN 2017004270| ISBN 9781421423630 (hardcover : alk. paper) |
  ISBN 1421423634 (hardcover : alk. paper) | ISBN 9781421423647 (electronic)
  | ISBN 1421423642 (electronic)
Subjects: | MESH: Prenatal Diagnosis—history | Congenital
  Abnormalities—history
Classification: LCC RG628 | NLM WQ 11.1 | DDC 618.3/2075—dc23
  LC record available at https://lccn.loc.gov/2017004270

A catalog record for this book is available from the British Library.

*Special discounts are available for bulk purchases of this book. For more
information, please contact Special Sales at 410-516-6936 or
specialsales@press.jhu.edu.*

Johns Hopkins University Press uses environmentally friendly book materials,
including recycled text paper that is composed of at least 30 percent
post-consumer waste, whenever possible.

CONTENTS

A Biomedical Innovation

Prenatal diagnosis is a highly atypical diagnostic approach. Usually the aim of diagnosis of a pathological condition is to treat it, prevent it, or both. The main consequence—at least, for now—of the prenatal diagnosis of a major fetal anomaly is to allow the pregnant woman to choose to end the pregnancy. In that case, the "prevention" of an impairment is the prevention of the birth of a human being with that impairment, a unique and, for many, a highly problematic solution. Because of its inseparable links with selective termination of pregnancy for fetal anomaly, prenatal diagnosis is frequently perceived and studied as an unclassifiable, *sui generis* phenomenon. This book proposes a different view.

Before turning to the history of prenatal diagnosis, I investigated for many years the history of the diagnosis and prevention of cancer. My original plan was to distance myself from that frequently stressful research topic and do something entirely different. I realized rather quickly, however, that my plan had not worked. My understanding of prenatal diagnosis was strongly influenced by my earlier views on the history of the diagnosis of malignant tumors and premalignant lesions. These two diagnostic approaches share important features. Both are characterized by a gap between the sophistication of diagnostic approaches and the crudeness of the proposed solutions: surgical excision of nonvital body parts to eliminate the risk of cancer and an abortion to prevent the birth of an impaired child. In both situations, a rapid diffusion of diagnostic technologies was favored by a combination of powerful professional and commercial interests and doctors' and patients' fears of a "bad outcome," which in some cases can be very bad indeed. And in both cases, an initial focus on already-existing anomalies or the high risk of such anomalies led to the establishment of population-based screening (prenatal screening), a development that radically changed the nature of the search for irregularities.

At first I was worried that my inability to dissociate my previous and present research subjects would distort my understanding of prenatal diagnosis. At some point I decided that my inclination to compare diagnoses of fetal anomalies and malignant growths was not so bad after all. Debates on prenatal diagnosis are nearly exclusively centered on moral issues such as selective abortion, disability rights, and the long shadow of the Nazi eugenics. A comparison between prenatal diagnosis and the detection of cancer and precancerous conditions favored a focus on "diagnosis" rather than on "prenatal," that is, on traits shared by prenatal diagnosis and other diagnostic technologies. An interest in prenatal diagnosis as one biomedical technology among many others facilitated the understanding of the role of contingent historical development in the shaping of its situated uses, or, to paraphrase anthropologists Rayna Rapp and Fay Ginsburg's felicitous expression, a "stratified scrutiny of the fetus."[1] From the late 1980s on, such a stratified scrutiny has included in many industrialized countries a screening of all pregnant women for fetal risks, above all, for Down syndrome (trisomy 21). The official goal of such a screening is to reassure the great majority of pregnant women that their future child is "all right" and to inform a small minority about the existence of a well-defined fetal problem. The consequences of the screening itself are rarely discussed by professionals. Some women have a different opinion.

Poland has no organized screening for Down syndrome risk, probably because abortion for fetal indications is illegal, but many Polish health care plans include a serum test for Down syndrome risk (the PAPP test) in their provision of services for pregnant women.[2] Some Polish women bitterly regretted taking the PAPP test:

> I did the PAPP test only because it was included in my package of prenatal services, like an idiot, without thinking: why?

> I had a good result of the ultrasound, with a risk of 1:1000, but after the blood test, the risk increased to 1:25. I was obliged to undergo amniocentesis, a test I found very scary. After two weeks I got the result: a healthy girl. I'll never forgive the physicians who forced me to go through all this.

> I agreed to this PAPP test without knowing what it was about, until the physician called me to say that I had an increased risk, that he could not tell me anything more by phone, and that I should see a geneticist. It was like somebody hit me on my head. I just cried and cried, until I saw the geneticist two weeks later. Then I learned that my risk of trisomy 21 is 1 in 49—it's very high at my age.

This PAPP test is a true malediction. . . . Like all the other women I did the PAPP test, and then was furious with myself. The child was born a month earlier, because of the stress, but is healthy.

Finallyyyy! After seven weeks of stress and crying we have the result of amniocentesis, a healthy girl. All this waiting time was a true horror.[3]

Polish women may feel especially stressed when they learn that they may carry a trisomic fetus because they do not have a legal option to terminate the pregnancy.[4] However, in countries where abortion is legal, stress may be an important part of the experience of prenatal screening. US women who underwent noninvasive prenatal testing (NIPT, a test based on the study of circulating fetal DNA in the pregnant woman's blood) expressed similar distress when they were informed about a high risk of a genetic anomaly of the fetus:

I am . . . a mother going through the most terrifying experience of her life. I tested high risk for cri du chat with a 1:19 chance of having it according to Panorama. Nobody is giving any straightforward answers as to what this means. Like many, I had no idea I was being screened for this (even though I asked the office exactly what they were testing). I have been going through the worst month of my life. I had to deal with this situation while studying for my medical boards. I am waiting for my CVS [a diagnostic test] results and each day that passes, my nerves keep building. I have read many cases of this being false positives but you can't help but feel like you will be the unlucky one. I will keep praying very hard!

I too am a mother in Australia and have also had the same result as you 1:19 for cri du chat after having the Panorama NIPT and I too am a nervous wreck!! We are 15 weeks and have just completed an amnio and are impatiently awaiting our results of the microarray. RB6577, it would be great to get in contact to know how you went, I hope you got a good result.

I'm a wreck trying to figure out if I'm the unlucky one. I received a 1:19 chance for DiGeorge syndrome. Go in for my amnio in 2 weeks.

We just had a positive result with Maternity21 for 15q deletion [Angelman/Prader-Willi syndrome]. We are shocked!!! You mentioned having a referral for a NIPT positive for Angelman syndrome. Did your patient's baby end up having the syndrome? We are desperate and don't know what to do.[5]

Screening healthy individuals for the presence of a pathological trait is rarely an innocuous act. Screening future children is an especially emotionally loaded topic. A leaflet intended for pregnant women, issued by the UK National Screening Committee (NCS), warns them against the danger of initiating a medical trajectory. Agreeing to a "simple" serum test for Down syndrome risk, the NCS leaflet explains, can put pregnant women in a situation in which they do not wish to find themselves:

> If you do get a higher risk result from a screening test, your midwife or doctor will give you information and support. You will also have time to make up your mind about what to do next. If you are in this position it is important to understand that you have a difficult decision to make. You have two options. You can decide not to have the diagnostic test. This means spending the rest of your pregnancy not knowing the screening result, which might be stressful. The only other option is to have the diagnostic test, knowing that this will slightly increase the risk of miscarriage. You need to think carefully about what you would do if you found yourself in this position. Once you know the result of the screening test, you can't put the clock back. If you would not be happy with either of the above options, you need to consider very carefully whether it would be better for you not to have the screening test in the first place.[6]

In practice, it is increasingly difficult for a pregnant woman who lives in an industrialized country to avoid scrutiny of her future child. In many settings, a serum test for the risk of a fetal anomaly became part of the usual supervision of pregnancy. Such tests are quasi automatically proposed to every pregnant woman. The great majority of women accept a test that will show whether "the baby is all right."[7] Many respond to the incitation of health professionals, who may equate the acceptance of testing with being a "responsible mother." Others, such as one of the US women quoted earlier—who, despite being a health professional herself, did not initially grasp what exactly she was being screened for—might be unaware of all the ramifications of a given test. Women who actively reject prenatal screening still rarely escape the scrutiny of the fetus, because routine ultrasound examinations conducted during the pregnancy can detect numerous fetal anomalies, including an elevated probability that the fetus has Down syndrome.

The widespread diffusion of prenatal diagnosis in industrialized, and increasingly also in intermediary, countries has important professional, sociocultural, organizational, institutional, legal, and financial consequences. Parents strive to promote the well-being of their children, societies are deeply concerned about the health of future generations, and pregnant women are a sizeable marketing target. The pervasiveness of prenatal diagnosis has changed the experience of pregnancy for tens of millions of women worldwide. The aim of this book is to explain how a search for fetal anomalies was transformed into a routine component of the standard medical care of pregnant women. It is a rather complicated story because there is no single standardized way to scrutinize the fetus; rather, there is a great number of historically conditioned and situated approaches. Nevertheless, the main argument of this book is simple: prenatal diagnosis is a new biomedical technology and should be studied as such.

This book started as a collaborative project called "Prenatal Diagnosis and the Prevention of Disability: Biomedical Techniques, Clinical Practices and Public Action." This project, conducted from 2009 to 2013 at my research unit, the CERMES 3, was funded by the French Agence Nationale de la Recherche (ANR) program Sciences, Technologies and Knowledge in Society (ANR-09-SSOC-026-01). For four years, our multidisciplinary group had numerous (and often passionate) discussions on the history and present-day practice of prenatal diagnosis, which greatly enriched my understanding of this topic. Many of the ideas in this book were formed through our exchanges and reflect a collective endeavor. I'm very grateful to Isabelle Ville, who initiated this project, Emmanuelle Fillion, Lynda Lotte, Veronique Mirlesse, Benedicte Rousseau, Sophie Rosman, and Carine Vassy for their important input; they have no responsibility whatsoever for the shortcomings of this book.

Exchanges with other researchers of CERMES 3, including Isabelle Baszanger, Martine Bungener, Luc Berlivet, Soraya Boudia, Maurice Cassier, Catherine Le-Galles, Laurent Pordie, Jean-François Ravaud, and Myriam Winance, increased my awareness of the existence of multiple ways of studying prenatal diagnosis in context and helped to enrich my ideas. Special thanks to Catherine Bourgain for improving my understanding of present-day genetics, Simone Bateman for illuminating ethical dilemmas linked with the development of new diagnostic technologies, Jean-Paul Gaudillière for sharing his knowledge of the history of genetics, and Anne Lovell for clarifying my ideas and for her unfailing support of this project.

Two meetings on the history of genetics and population genetics organized by Soraya de Chadeverian and Jenny Bangham and three meetings on the history of reproduction organized by Nick Hopwood and Salim Al-Gailani allowed for fruitful exchanges with other scholars interested in prenatal diagnosis and played an important role in refining my own thinking. I'm thankful to the organizers of these meetings for favoring the development of new ways of looking at heredity, genetics, reproduction, and the unborn, and to all the participants for their input.

Academia is often described as a dog-eat-dog world. However, my experience, with very few exceptions, is just the opposite. Without the contributions of colleagues, my work would have been infinitely poorer. Over the years, I have had multiple exchanges with an extensive and geographically variable "invisible college" of scholars, many of whom I call friends, about biomedical technologies, heredity and heritability, genetics and genomics, management of health risks, and the rise of predictive medicine. A surely incomplete list of members of this "invisible college" includes Robert Aronowitz, Nathalie Bajos, Christine Brandt, Stuart Blume, Allan Brandt, Marilena Correa, Angela Creager, Adele Clarke, Nathaniel Comfort, Yael Hashiloni-Dolev, Michelle Ferrand, Evelyne Fox-Keller, Sahra Gibbon, Snait Gissis, Jeremy Greene, Cathy Herbrant, Tsipy Ivry, David Jones, Lene Koch, Joanna Latimer, Sabina Lionelli, Veronika Lipphardt, Claire Marris, Catherine Marry, Ornella Moscucci, Staffan Müller-Wille, Daniel Navon, Jesse Olszynko Gryn, Nelly Oudshoorn, Katharine Park, Naomi Pfeffer, Barbara Prainsack, Christelle Rabier, Helga Satzinger, Emilia Sanabria, María Jesús Santesmases, Lisa Schwartz, Martina Schlunder, Alexandra Stern, Elisabeth Toon, Joanna Radin, Robert Resta, Hans Joerg Rheinberger, Vololona Rhaberisoa, Charles Rosenberg, Steven Woloshin, George Weisz, and Clare Williams. Very special thanks to Rayna Rapp, who introduced me to research on prenatal diagnosis and over the years has provided a stellar example on how such research should be conducted, and to Diane Paul, who not only generously shared with me her impressive understanding of hereditary conditions but also materials she cumulated during her own research on this subject.

At Johns Hopkins University Press, Jackie Wehmueller strongly supported this project and accompanied the manuscript until its acceptance by the press (and regretfully—for me, not for her—retired before the book went into production). Catherine Goldstead then took over and followed the manuscript to press, Hilary Jacqmin dealt with the marketing, and Juliana McCarthy and Nicole Wayland did a wonderful job copyediting the manuscript. I'm very lucky to work with the JHUP team.

It is difficult to study pregnancies without thinking about the ways they produce and modify families, traditional or not. I'm grateful for my own rapidly growing family for being who they are and for teaching me what is truly important (hint: it is not writing academic books). Special thanks to Woody for being a model supporting partner in all possible ways, some of which include preparing hot meals, boosting my morale, and providing stimulating intellectual discussions; to Naomi for her input in all things medical; and to Kyan, Tania, and Esteban for being so delightful.

Scrutinized Fetuses

Live Fetuses and the Medical Gaze

In the 1960s, thanks to the development of prenatal diagnosis, medicine had found a new object of study: the living fetus. In the 1960s and 1970s, prenatal diagnosis was an exceptional approach, proposed only to women who were at a high risk of giving birth to a malformed child. In the late twentieth century, prenatal diagnosis was integrated into the routine supervision of pregnancy. With the spread of prenatal diagnosis, the majority of pregnant women are being reassured that their future child is developing well. Other women face a stressful period of waiting for results, uncertain prognosis, and difficult decisions.[1]

Until recently, pregnancy and childbirth were dangerous events, with very high rates of both maternal and child mortality.[2] From the late 1930s on, the generalization of access to health care in industrialized countries and innovations such as blood transfusions and antibiotics greatly reduced maternal mortality during childbirth.[3] In 2008, the average maternal mortality rate in Western Europe was 7 in 100,000 live births (17 in the United States; 7 in Canada).[4] The decrease in newborn mortality in industrialized countries, although impressive, was much slower, mainly because of the persistence of *birth defects*— a loose and potentially problematic term that indicates that something is wrong with the newborn child.[5] In industrialized countries, a woman's risk of having a child with a birth defect, or of losing a fetus/newborn child because of such a defect, is 2.5%–3%.[6] The juxtaposition of this number with a woman's 0.01% risk of dying during childbirth can partly explain why the focus of the oversight of pregnancy had shifted to the fetus.

In nearly all human societies, pregnant women are expected to follow specific rules in order to limit the dangers of pregnancy and childbirth, improve their future child's health, and prevent the birth of impaired, misshapen, deformed, and in extreme cases "monstrous" newborns. In the early twentieth century, obstetricians noted correlations between pregnancy outcomes and women's occupations, diets, medical problems, and lifestyles. Medical supervision of pregnant women, they proposed, would reduce the frequency of birth defects.[7] Such supervision, called antenatal or prenatal care, was intensified after the Second World War. At that time, physicians focused their attention on the pregnant woman and were only marginally interested in the unborn child. The expected well-being of the child was the statistical outcome of good maternal health. Accordingly, physicians directed their efforts to the prevention and cure of maternal pathologies known to affect fetal health, the promotion of a healthy lifestyle, and the prevention of prematurity.[8]

Careful supervision of pregnant women's health and lifestyles continues today. Pregnant women are expected to refrain from smoking, drinking alcohol, and using illegal drugs, and are strongly encouraged to maintain a certain weight, eat healthy foods, partake in the right amount of physical activity, and submit their bodies for regular supervision by health experts.[9] From the 1970s on, with the development of prenatal diagnosis, this supervision has been extended to direct observation of the live fetus. At first reserved for exceptional cases, such observation has gradually become a routine part of pregnancy management in industrialized countries.

Prenatal diagnosis was developed thanks to a partly fortuitous combination of several medical technologies: amniocentesis, the culture of fetal cells, the study of human chromosomes, and obstetrical ultrasound. The combination of these approaches made possible the development of the "prenatal diagnosis dispositif." The term *dispositif*, sometimes translated to the English term *apparatus*, was coined by the philosopher Michel Foucault to describe an entity that combines a certain "regime of truth" with the practices and institutional forms that make it a bona fide site of knowledge/power. A dispositif, Foucault explained, is "a thoroughly heterogeneous ensemble consisting of discourses, institutions, architectural forms, regulatory decisions, laws, administrative measures, scientific statements, philosophical, moral and philanthropic propositions."[10] This term captures well the essence of a heterogeneous assemblage of instruments and techniques, professional practices, and institutional and legal arrangements that, taken together, made it possible to diagnose fetal anomalies.

Some scholars argue that the development of prenatal diagnosis has led to a "discovery of the fetus." Women translated their embodied experience of pregnancy—morning sickness, swelling of the breasts, changes in digestion, fatigue, and, from the fourth month of pregnancy on, awareness of fetal move-ment ("quickening")—into a visual language of stages of pregnancy and fetal growth.[11] The rise of prenatal diagnosis undoubtedly favored the popularization of knowledge about fetal development. Conversely, images of fetuses in the 1970s did not suddenly "leap" from anatomy and embryology books into the lay culture. In the late nineteenth and twentieth centuries, such images were already present in many popular science publications and were accessible to nonprofessionals.[12] Pregnant women—or, to be more precise, educated, middle-class pregnant women—could learn about stages of fetal development from popular books about pregnancy and childbirth.[13] Lennart Nilsson's famous 1965 photo essay *Drama of Life before Birth* has often been presented as a turn-ing point in the creation of the present-day "public fetus." Nilsson's "lifelike"—in fact, heavily retouched and edited—color photographs of embryos and fetuses preceded, however, the development of prenatal diagnosis.[14] The most impor-tant difference produced by the generalization of prenatal diagnosis was not the discovery of fetal life but the possibility of following such life in real time, that is, a shift from the study of dead fetuses to the observation of living ones.[15]

The rise of prenatal diagnosis can be inscribed within a broader trend that enlarged the possibilities for investigating life processes in real time. After the Second World War, new research methods, such as radioisotopes and medical imagery, made possible dynamic studies of living bodies, both healthy and sick.[16] In the 1960s and 1970s, prenatal diagnosis extended such a possibility to the living fetus. The development of this diagnostic approach can be described as a true medical revolution; however, prenatal diagnosis did not acquire the fame of other medical feats of that period. The media widely publicized spec-tacular "medical breakthroughs" such as the first heart transplant in 1967 and the first "test tube baby" in 1978. There were no similar breakthroughs in the history of prenatal diagnosis. The dramatic increase in the level of scrutiny of the fetus in the last half-century was the result of singularly nondramatic devel-opments. Medical technologies, anthropologist Sharon Kaufman and her colleagues argued, produced a new kind of knowledge through the homogeni-zation of clinical care. The normalization of technologies and their transforma-tion into new standards of care radically shifted the perception of what counted as normal and acceptable, while the process itself was incremental and invisi-ble.[17] This is an apt description of the generalization of prenatal diagnosis. New technical developments in this domain were usually presented as an unprob-lematic extension of already-existing clinical practices or technological improve-ments. As a consequence, they escaped public scrutiny. It was not too difficult to normalize prenatal diagnosis because it had been conceived as one of the technologies of the normalization of reproduction from the very beginning.[18]

The claim that prenatal diagnosis is an unexamined domain of medical activity needs to be qualified. One consequence of the introduction of this diagnostic technology, the possibility of selectively eliminating "flawed" fetuses, is highly contentious and the topic of heated debates. The intensity of these debates may be contrasted with the paucity of discussions on the material, economic, organizational, social, and psychological consequences of this mass-diffused biomedical technology.[19] An exclusive focus on prenatal diagnosis' uniqueness makes its study as a medical innovation difficult. Or, prenatal diagnosis was shaped by the same variables as other new biomedical approaches: interactions between the laboratory and clinics, cost/profit considerations, the role of producers of instruments and reagents, division of medical labor, institutional and regulatory frameworks, public health considerations, and the recent rise of "risk medicine."[20] Successful new technologies, such as prenatal diagnosis, produce new and often unexpected effects.[21] The generalization of this diagnostic approach has transformed the understanding of pregnancy, childbirth, and human reproduction. It has also produced a technoscientific entity, "the scrutinized fetus," that shares some similarities with the fetus studied by embryologists in the late nineteenth and early twentieth centuries but is endowed with an entirely new set of properties.[22] The development of prenatal diagnosis did not lead to a "discovery of the fetus" or the discovery of the fetus by pregnant women, but it did lead to the discovery of a different fetus.

Prenatal Diagnosis: Who Is the Patient?

Prenatal diagnosis is an inseparable part of the care of pregnant women. One of the unique traits of this diagnostic approach is the difficulty to decide who the patient is. Modern democracies are founded on the principle that the main subject of law is an individual, that is, an *indivisible entity*. This term applies to all human beings with one exception: the pregnant woman. In some circumstances, a pregnant woman is seen as composed of two entities, each endowed with distinct legal rights.[23] The uncertainty regarding the legal status of a pregnant woman as an autonomous human being allowed, especially in the United States, the suspension of pregnant women's legal rights as individuals in the name of the defense of the unborn.[24] Uncertainty regarding the legal status of the fetus is at the very center of debates on the legality of abortion. Advocates of such legalization affirm that the entity that develops in the pregnant woman's womb is a part of her body, either until birth or until the fetus is considered viable outside the womb.[25] The woman therefore has the right to decide on this entity's fate. Opponents of abortion affirm that the embryo/fetus is an autonomous living human being from the moment of fertilization. They believe that although a pregnant woman hosts this new human being in her body, it does not give her any special right to "eliminate" him or her. Such an act can be fully assimilated to the killing of a baby by the baby's caretaker. The fluid status of the "divisible" pregnant woman reflects a biological reality: a fetus is genetically and biologically distinct from the maternal body and at the same time an inseparable part of it. This duality shapes the uses of prenatal diagnosis.

In routine medical practice, the term *prenatal diagnosis* covers two very different meanings. The first encompasses universally accepted tests intended to improve the health of a mother and her future child. Such tests, defined as "public health oriented," include the screening of pregnant women for the presence of infections that can harm the fetus (e.g., syphilis, rubella, cytomegalovirus, HIV, and hepatitis B), a parallel screening of women for chronic conditions that can induce fetal anomalies (e.g., diabetes and heart disease), and surveillance of pregnancy-specific pathologies (e.g., preeclampsia and Rhesus factor incompatibility). The second meaning includes more controversial tests that make fetal anomalies visible. These tests are defined as "autonomy oriented" because they allow pregnant women and their partners to make decisions about the future of the pregnancy.[26] These two definitions of prenatal diagnosis are conceptually very different but are often inseparably intertwined in practice. For example, in the 1950s physicians elaborated on a way to sample a pregnant woman's amniotic fluid in order to detect maternal-fetal Rhesus factor incompatibility and save the life of the unborn child. Later, this method made possible the scrutiny of fetal cells in the amniotic fluid and the prenatal detection of fetal anomalies, paving the way for selective abortion of affected fetuses. Pregnant women are monitored for the presence of infectious diseases to preserve their health and their future child's health, but the detection of an infection that can induce severe fetal anomalies can lead to a decision to terminate the pregnancy. Biochemical markers used in screening tests for common chromosomal anomalies can also indicate an increased risk of pregnancy complications that put a woman's health at risk, such as preeclampsia. Analysis of cell-free DNA (cfDNA) in maternal blood allows for the detection of high-risk genetic anomalies of the fetus that usually cannot be treated, but this approach is also employed to diagnose fetal-maternal Rhesus factor incompatibility, a treatable condition. Moreover, changes in the level of cfDNA in the pregnant woman's blood may reflect placental complications such as preeclampsia, growth retardation, and preterm birth and predict potentially curable complications of pregnancy.[27]

Obstetrical ultrasound is an especially important site of convergence of "public health goals" and "autonomy goals" of prenatal diagnosis. Obstetrical ultrasound is employed to verify the age of the pregnancy, the position of the fetus, and the existence of potential obstacles to safe birth, such as placenta previa (a displaced placenta that can produce a dangerous hemorrhage during childbirth). It is also used to diagnose fetal anomalies, and its best-known function is the emotionally loaded presentation of the future child to the parents. A comparison of controversies on two screening technologies—namely, mammography and obstetrical ultrasound—has shown that both are strongly shaped by institutional factors and interests of professional constituencies.[28] However, in the twenty-first century, generalized mammographic screening has become an increasingly contested technology, and it is not inconceivable that its use will be reduced in the future.[29] It seems less likely that the use of obstetrical ultrasound will diminish anytime soon. This medical imagery technology is most likely here to stay, and its use is predicted to expand, especially in middle-income countries. Additionally, in these countries the multifunctionality of obstetrical ultrasound—showing the future child to the pregnant woman and other family members, looking for possible complications of pregnancy, and scrutinizing the fetus—leads to an important increase in diagnoses of fetal anomalies and a parallel increase in difficult situations produced by such diagnoses.[30]

Women and Situated Choices

The history of the scrutiny of fetuses can be divided into four stages.[31] In the first stage, the development of biochemical and cytological methods of the study of fetal cells in the amniotic fluid make possible a prenatal diagnosis of certain hereditary conditions, such as metabolic diseases, and an abnormal number of chromosomes (aneuploidy), above all, Down syndrome (trisomy 21). In the early 1970s, prenatal diagnosis was proposed only to women who were classified as being at high risk of fetal malformations. In the second stage, the development of serum tests that detect a higher probability of fetal anomalies—first of neural tube anomalies, and then of Down syndrome—led to the extension of prenatal screening to all pregnant women independently of their risk of giving birth to an impaired child. In many industrialized countries, prenatal diagnosis of fetal malformation became prenatal screening for the risk of such malformations. In a third stage, which partly overlapped the second one, prenatal screening was refined through the combination of the results of serum tests for Down syndrome risk and an increase in "nuchal translucency" (a fluid-filled cavity behind the fetus's neck), an ultrasound marker of Down syndrome risk. At the same time, an increase in the resolution of obstetrical ultrasound and the important extension of its use favored the uncovering of numerous structural anomalies of the fetus. The supposedly benign act of "seeing the future baby" was transformed into a powerful diagnostic technique. The fourth stage, unfolding in the early twenty-first century, is driven by the use of new molecular biology technologies such as comparative genomic hybridization (CGH), which has greatly extended the possibility of studying the fetal genome. Since 2012, the study of cfDNA in maternal blood, an approach called noninvasive prenatal testing, has opened new possibilities for the enlargement of scale and scope of prenatal diagnosis.

Because of its indivisible links with selective abortion of impaired fetuses, prenatal diagnosis has been, from its inception, a contested technology, described by its opponents as a "search and destroy" mission.[32] In the early stages of prenatal diagnosis development in the 1970s and 1980s, the opposition to this diagnostic approach came mainly from two sources: opponents of abortion and feminist activists. Sociologist Kristin Luker, who studied US pro-life and pro-choice groups in the early 1980s, discovered that, according to public opinion polls, an abortion to prevent the birth of a severely impaired child was seen as acceptable by more than four-fifths of interviewed Americans and had much higher rates of acceptance than an abortion for "social reasons." However, abortion for a fetal anomaly was the least acceptable choice for pro-life individuals. For them, aborting an impaired fetus meant that human beings can be ranked on a scale of perfection and that people who fell below a certain arbitrary standard could be excluded. Prenatal diagnosis, they claimed, leads to a "selective genocide against the disabled."[33]

Feminist activists who strongly rejected prenatal diagnosis—a relatively small but highly visible group within the feminist movement—were also opposed to the medicalization of pregnancy and what they saw as an instrumentalization of motherhood and the transformation of women into machines that produce high-quality children.[34] These activists discussed the concept of "tentative pregnancy" and the possibility that in the future women would be able to choose to give birth to children with specific qualities seen as socially desirable by a utilitarian, productivist society.[35] Unlike pro-life activists, feminist opponents of prenatal diagnosis and of an abortion following a diagnosis of fetal anomaly supported abortion for social reasons. They reasoned that the decision to terminate a pregnancy because a woman does not wish to be a mother (the refusal of *a* child) and the decision to terminate a pregnancy because a fetus was diagnosed with an anomaly (the refusal of *this* child) are radically different.

Other feminists rejected this claim and argued that abortion is always a situated act.[36] Women who elect to terminate a pregnancy for fetal indications, but also those who elect to do it for social reasons, often explain that they want to "do the right thing" for their future child, themselves, and their family. In both cases, "doing the right thing" depends on their specific circumstances at the time they make decisions about the future of their pregnancy.[37] For example, two French women learned that their respective fetuses were missing a limb. One woman decided to end the pregnancy because she already had one disabled child as well as a sick partner and felt unable at that point in her life to cope with an additional challenge. The other, who had two healthy children, believed that she would be able to successfully deal with the child's moderate impairment. Both women explained that in different circumstances, they could have made the opposite decision.[38] Anthropologist Annemarie Mol decided to undergo amniocentesis: "Given where I am (I have a healthy child and work that fascinates me and it is difficult enough as it is to juggle between them) I follow the advice [to test for Down risk if the woman is over 35]."[39] The key word is *juggling*. Mol's explanation echoes the feeling of many women who may feel that they are already perniciously close to the edge of their capability to perform their numerous tasks well and will be unable to fulfill their work and family obligations if they are obliged to provide special care to an impaired child.[40]

Obstetricians, pediatricians, and experts in fetal medicine frequently explain that since future mothers/parents have the main responsibility of caring for a disabled child and, not infrequently, also an impaired adult, only they can decide if they can accept the birth of such a child in a given moment of their lives. A selective abortion for a fetal indication is always a woman's / the parents' choice.[41] Pregnant women who receive a diagnosis of fetal malformation also stress that they alone—not health professionals—should decide whether to continue with the pregnancy.[42] Conversely, the "choice" discourse often masks the paucity of real-life choices and actors' limited control over situations.[43] Women's decisions are shaped by material, institutional, and legal constraints, and are therefore strongly affected by the framing of prenatal testing in the country in which they live: the availability of specific tests, their reimbursement by the national health system or health insurance programs, health professionals' attitude toward prenatal testing, or the legal framing of women's reproductive decisions.[44] Women also have limited impact on the range and quality of public services offered to disabled children and adults in their communities. In addition, such services may also vary for different groups of disabled individuals. Some countries provide good-quality services only to certain categories of impaired people while neglecting others, a difference that, among other things, may mirror the political and communication skills of condition-specific advocacy groups.[45] The "choice" discourse often masks the importance of constraints on people's individual choices in a state or market system.[46] Only affluent women, who are able to purchase services such as a wider range of diagnostic tests and good-quality care for disabled family members outside those supported by collectivities, can escape some of these constraints.

Discourse about "choice" is linked with situated perceptions of "responsible motherhood." Pregnant women—with the exception of those who are opposed to abortion, especially due to religious beliefs—are expected to make decisions perceived as rational in a given society.[47] They are transformed, to borrow the feminist scholar Silja Samerski's apt expression, into "skilled managers of fetal risks."[48] A woman is required to understand correctly probabilistic data provided by a combination of serum test(s) and ultrasound data, to evaluate the dangers she is facing—raising a disabled child versus losing a healthy fetus— and then to decide whether she is willing to undergo amniocentesis, a sampling of amniotic fluid with fetal cells that allows these cells to be analyzed but is linked with a risk of miscarriage.[49] Some pregnant women perceive such a "choice" as a burden. Women confronted with the decision of whether to perform amniocentesis as well as those faced with the decision about whether to continue a pregnancy have expressed distress and even anger when confronted with what they perceived as an "impossible choice."[50] Women's options, once limited to decisions about a small number of prenatally detected conditions, above all, Down syndrome, have become increasingly complicated with the growing sophistication of diagnostic tests.[51] As Dutch media expert José (Johanna) van Dijck argued: "Decision-making processes concerning the continuation or termination of pregnancy are not rendered more transparent or rational when physicians have more and better imaging technologies at their disposal, and neither do they allow the patient more 'freedom to choose.' In some respects, the availability of more and more advanced prenatal tests—ultrasound figuring prominently among them—renders choices more complex and pregnant women less autonomous."[52]

The introduction of a new medical technology, anthropologist Marilyn Strathern has observed, often radically modifies the choices open to all people, including those who reject it.[53] Israeli ultraorthodox women are expected to trust in God's providence and decline medical technologies that predict the future of their child. Declining these tests, however, heightens stress in some religious women, who not only worry about the possibility of giving birth to an impaired child but that such worry indicates that their faith is not strong enough.[54] Refusal to use prenatal diagnosis is not sufficient to protect women from the consequences of the generalization of this diagnostic approach.

The Structure of the Book

This study follows the development and diffusion of the prenatal diagnosis dispositif and its transformations, with a special focus on the integration of heterogeneous technology into a coordinated pattern of scrutiny of the fetus. It focuses on developments in industrialized countries, where this diagnostic approach was initially developed, stabilized, and diffused. Few studies investigate all the aspects of prenatal diagnosis, past and present.[55] Conversely, this book could not be written—or even conceived—without the existence of numerous historical, sociological, and anthropological studies about the history of human reproduction, maternal and child health, politics of motherhood, control of women's fertility, clinical genetics, genetic counseling, disability and disability rights, and prenatal diagnosis itself. I hope this study faithfully reflects my very sizable debt to numerous scholars who investigated these topics before me.[56]

This book argues that the initial prenatal diagnosis dispositif, which came into being in the late 1960s and early 1970s, underwent two important transformations in the last part of the twentieth century: the shift to a generalized screening for Down syndrome and the transformation of obstetrical ultrasound into a major diagnostic tool.[57] These two innovations favored the transformation of prenatal diagnosis into routine medical technology, a development that, in turn, might have lowered scholars' interest in the study of this approach. Sociologists and anthropologists of medicine tend to be more interested in exceptional developments in biomedicine than in the routine use of new technologies. An interest in cutting-edge innovations in reproductive medicine, such as preimplantatory diagnosis, and their potential to produce offspring with desirable traits can be contrasted with low visibility of innovations that radically modified the management of "normal" pregnancies. The latter were often presented as unproblematic improvements of already-existing diagnostic approaches. Public debates on the predicted next major transformation of prenatal diagnosis, the switch to tests grounded in analysis of cfDNA in a pregnant woman's blood, similarly tend to focus on remote (at least for now) possibilities that this technology will enable future parents to select specific qualities of their future children and seldom examine the economic, social, cultural, and psychological ramifications predicted to be the result of the generalization of a technology that facilitates prenatal detection of numerous genetic anomalies.[58] The history of prenatal diagnosis, this study proposes, is also the history of the central importance of widely diffused "ordinary" technologies in shaping medical practices.[59]

The first chapter follows the origins of the concept of birth defects. While scientists and laypeople alike have always been fascinated by monstrous births, the term *birth defect* was developed in the nineteenth century. At that time, physicians became interested in the distinction between hereditary conditions and those acquired during pregnancy and/or childbirth but not transmitted in families. The distinction was, however, fluid: diseases such as tuberculosis or syphilis were seen as hereditary; they were linked with "degeneration" and were incorporated into the family's lineage. In the late nineteenth and early twentieth centuries, gynecologists and pediatricians such as John William Ballantyne in Edinburgh and Adolphe Pinard in Paris discovered that poor health and inadequate nutrition during pregnancy, prematurity, and accidents of childbirth were at the origin of many birth defects. Better care of pregnant and birthing women, they argued, would reduce the frequency of such defects. In contrast, other specialists proposed that improvement in the care of pregnant women could not prevent the birth of children with "true" hereditary conditions, at the origin of numerous inborn impairments. Efforts to detect and prevent inborn impairments were focused on "amentia," or "mental deficiency," a condition that was often linked with the presence of visible anomalies. This chapter investigates the central role of "visible" intellectual disabilities, above all, Down syndrome, in debates on birth defects in the nineteenth century and the first half of the twentieth century. It also examines the first prenatal/antenatal diagnosis technique: the detection of Rhesus factor incompatibility between the pregnant woman and the fetus.

The second chapter starts with the observation, made in 1959, that Down syndrome and several other inborn impairments are the consequence of aneuploidy, or the presence of an abnormal number of chromosomes in each cell. This observation favored the development of two disciplines: cytogenetics, the study of chromosomes and their anomalies, and clinical genetics, the study of human diseases produced by anomalies of the genetic material of the cell. At first, clinical geneticists studied anomalies in children and adults. In the late 1960s, the technical improvement of amniocentesis, coupled with the development of the culture of fetal cells, made possible a prenatal diagnosis of chromosomal anomalies and hereditary metabolic diseases. In the late 1960s and early 1970s, abortion became legal in many Western countries. The partly contingent coupling of biomedical innovations with social change made possible abortions for fetal indications. In the 1970s, professionals recommended prenatal diagnosis to two groups of pregnant women: those who were at high risk of giving birth to a child with a hereditary disease and those who were of an "advanced maternal age" and thus at a higher risk of giving birth to a child with Down syndrome. The diffusion of amniocentesis, in turn, favored the development of the profession of genetic counselor. This chapter investigates links between early debates on new diagnostic technologies and the study of human chromosomes and prenatal diagnosis.

The third chapter links the history of birth defects with the history of teratology (literally, the study of monsters)—a specialty that studies abnormalities that occur during embryonic and fetal development. Two events—the 1961–1962 thalidomide disaster and the 1962–1964 German measles epidemics—led to the birth of children with severe birth defects and played an important role in debates on the legalization of abortion. They promoted an interest in the effects of drugs, radiation, chemical compounds, and infectious agents on the production of birth defects. The thalidomide catastrophe also led to the development of national and international birth defect registries. Such registries increased the visibility of birth defects and favored their redefinition as a public health problem. Before the 1970s, studies of embryonic and fetal malformations were mainly the domain of biologists who worked with animal models. With a growing interest in inborn malformations in humans, scientists who investigated this issue elected to change the name of their specialty from "teratology" to "dysmorphology" (the study of atypical forms) in order to facilitate a dialogue with the parents of children born with abnormal physical traits. The study of such abnormal traits is mainly conducted by clinical geneticists and pediatricians. A typical patient in a dysmorphology clinic is a child with unexplained developmental delays suspected to be "syndromic," or linked with genetic anomalies. The study of such rare genetic anomalies opened new avenues for clinical genetics. The technical improvement of obstetrical ultrasound in the late 1970s and 1980s favored the extension of studies of abnormal morphological traits to the fetus. It linked studies of embryonic and fetal development with clinical observations of "syndromic" children and promoted the integration of fetal medicine and fetopathology with cutting-edge genetic research. This chapter focuses on the contributions of human malformation studies, including, for example, the study of specific patterns of dermatoglyphs (finger and palm prints) in people with chromosomal anomalies, to the understanding of the origins of birth defects.

The fourth chapter follows the shift from prenatal *diagnosis* (the testing of targeted groups of women at higher-than-average risk of fetal impairments) to prenatal *screening* (the testing of *all* pregnant women for such risk, above all, the risk of Down syndrome). In the 1970s, physicians and health administrators agreed that since amniocentesis was linked with a small but nonnegligible risk of spontaneous miscarriage, testing for Down syndrome should be offered only to older pregnant women, typically those older than 35. This was, however, an imperfect solution, as the majority of Down syndrome children were born to younger women. The development of serum markers of Down syndrome risk, and a parallel description of ultrasound signs of heightened probability of the presence of this condition, led to the diffusion of "screening for Down syndrome." Such screening, public health experts hoped (but rarely openly said after the 1970s), would reduce the number of children born with this condition and would lead to private management of a public health problem. The diffusion of Down syndrome screening varies greatly among different countries, as do the tests employed for such a screening and the information proposed to pregnant women. In some Western European countries (e.g., Denmark), the acceptance of Down syndrome screening is very high and is linked with the perception of being a "responsible" future mother; in other countries (e.g., Netherlands), the acceptance of this screening is low, and women are invited to enjoy their pregnancy without thinking about the small risk of giving birth to a trisomic child. In some countries (e.g., France), physicians only promote first trimester screening for Down syndrome risk; in others (e.g., the United States; as of this writing), they propose either first or second trimester screening. This chapter examines the history of screening for Down syndrome and the divergent, path-dependent patterns of dissemination of such a screening in industrialized countries.

The fifth chapter focuses on the history of two chromosomal anomalies: Turner syndrome (TS; first described in 1937) and Klinefelter syndrome (KS; first described in 1941). Both conditions were initially defined as treatable hormonal disorders. In the 1950s, the description of a "Barr body"—a cellular marker of sex—led to a redefinition of TS and KS as "sex inversion": people with TS, scientists believed at that time, are females who have a male chromosomal formula, and those with KS are males with a female chromosomal formula. Since the former always saw themselves as "normal" women and the latter nearly always as "normal" men, studies of these conditions played an important role in the birth of the concept of gender and the dissociation of gender identity and gender role from biological sex. In 1959, the development of new methods to study human chromosomes led to the redefinition of TS and KS as consequences of the presence of aneuploidy—45,Xo and 47,XXY, respectively. In the early 1960s, scientists described other sex chromosome anomalies, such as 47,XXX and 47,XYY. The latter condition became the focus of an important controversy. Some specialists claimed that XYY men were more prone to violent and deviant behavior than "normal" XY men, while other specialists strongly rejected this claim. Today, sex chromosome aneuploidies are seen as conditions with variable expression: some people with an abnormal number of sex chromosomes, especially the frequent KS, do not know that they are not "normal," while others have mild to moderate health as well as cognitive and mental health problems. This chapter traces the convoluted history of sex chromosome aneuploidies, their intersection with clinical genetics and prenatal diagnosis, and the current quandaries linked with the incidental diagnosis of these anomalies when testing for Down syndrome.

The sixth chapter follows two recent developments in the study of fetal DNA: CGH and NIPT. CGH compares tested DNA to a reference DNA sample in order to uncover possible anomalies, especially deletions and duplications of chromosome segments. CGH was employed to study DNA from fetal cells obtained through invasive methods such as amniocentesis or chorionic villus sampling. This method does not look for a specific mutation but examines the whole genome and asks whether something is wrong. Therefore, it is well adapted to a search for potential genetic problems following an observation of a structural anomaly of the fetus during an ultrasound examination. NIPT is grounded in the analysis of cfDNA in maternal blood. Initially, NIPT was destined to detect fetuses with Down syndrome but was rapidly enlarged to detect other conditions with an abnormal number of chromosomes and, since 2014, also several chromosome deletions. NIPT—especially when used to detect fetal anomalies other than major autosomal chromosomal anomalies (trisomies 21, 13, and 18)—can lead to unanticipated diagnostic dilemmas. A "simple blood test" can tell a woman that her future child is at a high risk of a genetic condition she probably has never heard about. Moreover, some of these conditions have variable expressions, increasing the difficulty of prenatal decisions. This chapter discusses the beginning of a large-scale diffusion of NIPT in Western Europe, the United States, and Brazil, and illustrates the dilemmas produced by the introduction of NIPT through the example of testing for DiGeorge syndrome, a little-known but relatively frequent chromosomal anomaly linked with a large range of physical, intellectual, and psychiatric impairments, among them a high risk of schizophrenia.

The conclusion examines the consequences of the steady expansion of scrutinizing the fetus. Debates on prenatal diagnosis are nearly exclusively focused on selective reproduction and the thorny issue of aborting "flawed" fetuses. Some prenatal diagnosis critics question the very principle of terminating a pregnancy for fetal indication, presented as a neo-eugenic approach that conveys a strong message that life with a disability is not worth living. Other critics do not object to terminating a pregnancy when the fetus is diagnosed with a lethal or severe and incurable condition but warn against an eugenic "slippery slope" that will not stop at the rejection of severely impaired fetuses but will lead to the rejection of all those who fail to meet the guidelines of "the perfect child." Other consequences of the generalization of prenatal diagnosis, such as the expansion of medicalized trajectories or proliferation of uncertain results and stress during pregnancy and sometimes beyond it, are less frequently present in discussions about prenatal diagnosis. A quasi-exclusive focus on the putative dangers of the use of prenatal diagnosis by affluent parents who wish to pursue a eugenic dream of flawless offspring detracts from the already-existent slippery slope of prenatal diagnosis: a rapid increase in the number of fetal anomalies that can be detected before birth and the shift from the search for already-existing fetal impairments to the search for increasingly small risks of health problems of the future child. Such an evolution is not fueled by narcissistic dreams of ideal progeny but by the very real fear of a bad pregnancy outcome. It can, like the expansion of other diagnostic and screening technologies do, produce iatrogenic effects that exceed the expected benefits. Interest in the potential—but for now remote—developments of prenatal diagnosis masks the presence of problems generated by already-existing uses of this diagnostic technology.

Finally, a short note on my inconsistent use of the terms *pregnant woman / mother* and *fetus/child*. Pregnant women who do not reject their pregnancy often speak about their future baby/child, especially in the context of prenatal testing. Similarly, health professionals frequently call the pregnant woman a "mother" (in France, often "la maman," or mommy), even in situations in which she is likely to decide to have an abortion. For example, the usual description of fetal DNA found in the blood of a pregnant woman is "cell-free fetal DNA in maternal circulation," despite the fact that the goal of studying cfDNA is to provide information about fetal malformations that can lead to the termination of a pregnancy.

Similarly, the entity in a woman's womb is usually called a fetus, but doctors often refer to this entity as the woman's baby/child. If the woman undergoes late miscarriage or abortion, rules on the disposal of the body will always use the term *child*, while fetopathologists who dissect the body always speak about the *fetus*. My inconsistency in the use of these terms follows the stakeholders' inconsistency. Outside the rarified sphere of philosophical and ethical debates, human reproduction is rarely simple or free from ambivalence. The uncertain and shifting status of pregnant women and the entity that develops in their bodies, and the difficulty to stabilize them, are precisely among the main themes of this book.

Prenatal diagnosis and a selective termination of a pregnancy for fetal malformation is an irreducibly contentious issue. It cannot be dissociated from political considerations and does not have a consensual "solution."[60] At the same time, prenatal diagnosis is a rapidly evolving topic as well as a moving target. It is challenging to study shifting and unstable entities and controversial questions. Scholars who investigate such questions often grapple with partial, unstable, and fragmented knowledge: their claims can only be modest.[61] Modesty is not, however, tantamount to inefficacy. Historical and comparative studies contribute to the clarification of complex issues. Current research techniques, as pioneer of social studies of science Ludwik Fleck explained, are, after all, the result of historical development. They are the way they are because of a particular history. Epistemology without historical and comparative investigations, Fleck insisted, is no more than an empty play on words, or an *epistemologia imaginabilis*.[62]

Historical and comparative perspectives denaturalize the self-evident aspect of medical practices, provide a different point of view (not from "nowhere" but from "elsewhere"), and make visible the deeply local aspect of presumably universal biomedical knowledge. They promote reflexivity and maintain a critical distance from the investigated subject ("estrangement").[63] Such a critical distance may be especially important when trying to clarify truly complicated issues—a challenging but, I hope, not entirely impossible task.

CHAPTER 1

Born Imperfect

Birth Defects before Prenatal Diagnosis

Abnormal Births

One of the main goals of prenatal diagnosis is to reduce newborn mortality. In the early twentieth century, the two main sources of such mortality were complications of pregnancy and childbirth, and "birth defects," or serious impairments.[1] The most striking examples of the latter were "monstrous births." Prenatal diagnosis' history parallels the history of attempts to differentiate birth defects that originated due to changes in the genetic material of the cell and are present from conception in the fertilized egg from those produced by external factors such as infections and exposure to environmental toxins, mechanical obstacles to fetal growth, health problems of the pregnant woman, and accidents during childbirth. Such a distinction is far from being absolute. For example, bleeding into the placenta (an external cause of fetal impairment) may be related to a genetic anomaly of the fetus (an internal cause). Nevertheless, at least since the seventeenth century physicians have attempted to distinguish truly accidental events during pregnancy from those produced by a woman's "constitutional weakness" and "morbid heredity" ("bad blood"), a danger for future generations.[2]

One of the key developments that helped to define *morbid heredity* as a distinct source of birth defects was a radical transformation of the meaning of monstrous births. In the early modern period, scientists and physicians, as well as religious authorities and laypeople, were fascinated by births of severely deformed children. Such births were given numerous, sometimes contradictory, meanings. Monstrous births were both repulsive and marvelous. They were seen as a demonstration of divine wrath and the endless power of divine creation but also as natural phenomena that displayed the playfulness of nature and its mistakes, the vagaries of chance, and the infinite creativity of the living world and might of maternal imagination.[3] Some of the "monsters" described in early modern writings, such as a boy with two bodies, born in Florence in 1317; the "two-headed monster," born at Aubervilliers near Paris in 1421; or the boy with a parasitic twin, displayed in Florence in 1513, can be translated into present-day terms as descriptions of conjoined twins.[4] Others, such as the strange "monster" born in Ravenna in 1512 and depicted in many engravings, escape current medical classifications.[5] The distinction between the birth of a "monster" (an unnatural creature) and a mutilated newborn (misshapen by an accident in the womb) was not always obvious. In 1573, anatomist Ambroise Paré classified a child born with a single hand as a "monster," while a child born with six fingers or short hands was described as being mutilated in the womb.[6]

In the seventeenth century, the investigation of monstrous births, human and animal, gradually shifted to the explanation of such births as natural phenomena. In the mid- to late eighteenth century, British and French physicians viewed "monsters" as clarifying counterexamples to normal embryological development. Dissection of abnormal children and fetuses became an important site of new medical knowledge. "Monstrous births" played an important role in eighteenth-century debates between advocates of preformationism (a view that assumed that all embryological development is predetermined from conception) and epigenesis (a view that assumed that such development was also shaped by events during pregnancy).[7] An introduction to a 1893 French textbook on abnormal births focused on the history of the shift from the perception of "monsters" as exceptions to the natural order to their integration into such an order.

This new view of monstrous births was possibly a precondition for the development of embryology, the study of normal development during pregnancy, and its twin science, teratology, the study of abnormal antenatal development. Monstrosities became birth defects: "When it became obvious that embryos develop from germs through a series of successive formation of organs, it became also evident that these notions should be applied to monsters as well as to normal beings. The only difference is that in the first, the evolution . . . does not follow precisely the same trajectory as in the second, and it leads to the formation of organs which deviate from the usual form."[8]

In the late nineteenth and early twentieth centuries, biologists who studied embryological development in the laboratory provided more precise distinctions between environmental, accidental, maternal, and hereditary causes of inborn malformation.[9] For many general practitioners, pediatricians, gynecologists, and public health experts, however, such distinctions remained imprecise and flexible.[10] A 1935 review article on the "mentally defective child" divided the causes of "idiocy" (intellectual impairment) into two categories: hereditary and acquired. The acquired causes of mental impairment included accidents of childbirth such as asphyxia, brain hemorrhage, trauma, fevers, meningitis, and poliomyelitis (seen for a long time as a possible cause of intellectual deficiency). The hereditary causes included familial traits ("like begets like") and intermarriage but also alcoholism, tuberculosis, and venereal diseases (above all, syphilis). Tuberculosis and syphilis were classified among hereditary causes because at that time the term *heredity* included all the elements that could affect the "quality of the seed." During the first half of the twentieth century, the term *pathological heredity* often continued to describe all conditions that, for whatever reason, were transmitted in families.[11]

Supervised Pregnancies

During the second half of the nineteenth century, interest in abnormal births favored the development of experimental embryology and new approaches to the study of pregnancy in humans.[12] Edinburgh gynecologist John William Ballantyne (1861–1923) began his career as a specialist in teratology. Later, he moved from the investigation of "monsters" to finding ways to prevent birth defects.[13] Ballantyne's major contributions to the subject were his books *Diseases and Deformities of the Foetus* (1892–1895) and *Manual of Antenatal Pathology and Hygiene of the Foetus* (1902–1904), which were dedicated to the study of fetal abnormalities. *Diseases and Deformities of the Foetus* focuses on the description and classification of fetal anomalies. *Manual of Antenatal Pathology and Hygiene of the Foetus* was written with the explicit goal to shed light on the advantages of preventing the birth of impaired children.[14] Before Ballantyne, embryology was seen exclusively as a domain of fundamental biology. The practitioners' interest in pregnancy was mainly limited to childbirth accidents and did not include the unborn child.[15] Thanks to Ballantyne's studies, medical practitioners became interested in life before birth. Gynecologists, Ballantyne argued, have a unique advantage as students of antenatal development. They have the ability to observe both pregnant women and their offspring, and can thus unravel correlations between events that precede birth and their consequences.

Ballantyne's *Diseases and Deformities of the Foetus* is a book on teratology with a practical twist. The book starts with a very long historical section, grounded in sources from antiquity, the middle ages, the renaissance, and the eighteenth and nineteenth centuries. It is dedicated to physician Cesare Taruffi from Bologna, the author of *Storia Della Teratologia* (published in 1889), and biologist Camille Dareste, director of the teratological laboratory at École des Hautes

Études in Paris and author of *Recherches sur la production artificielle des monstruosités* (published in 1877; a second, enlarged edition of this book was published in 1891). *Diseases and Deformities of the Foetus* is richly illustrated with line drawings and is organized according to an anatomical schema: each chapter is dedicated to the description of a specific pathological condition. Fetal anomalies, Ballantyne explained, are not mere curiosities: they are of utmost importance to the clinician. Until recently, physicians were not interested in the fetus because they attributed low value to fetal life and health. Such a view is decidedly erroneous. Fetal malformations are the main cause of high mortality in the neonatal period. Moreover, many such malformations can be prevented. Fetal problems that lead to miscarriages, stillbirths, and birth of sickly newborns are more often observed in mothers who suffer from poor physical or mental health. Certain paternal diseases, such as syphilis, tuberculosis, alcoholism, and cancer, can also diminish the quality of sperm, thereby affecting fetal health. The diffusion of the use of proper hygiene reduced mortality in adults; it is a doctor's duty to promote the application of similar rules during pregnancy.[16]

Diseases and Deformities of the Foetus was largely a treatise of teratology. In the *Manual of Antenatal Pathology and Hygiene of the Foetus*, Ballantyne's focus shifted from a description of "monstrosities" (i.e., an abnormal form) to the study of the pathologies of the fetus (i.e., an abnormal function). According to Ballantyne, we do not know the precise cause of some fetal and newborn pathologies, such as inborn malformations of the digestive and nervous systems, but we do know the cause of many other pathologies: for example, poor maternal health. Infectious diseases such as syphilis and tuberculosis, and chronic conditions such as diabetes or cancer directly hamper the development of the fetus. The same is true for poisons: lead, mercury, arsenic, alcohol, and tobacco. It is difficult to prove the direct effect of smoking tobacco on the fetus, but the high mortality rate of children born to women who work in the tobacco industry provides strong indirect evidence of this substance's harm. Ballantyne also noted that women who drink heavily during pregnancy often give birth to malformed children, probably because alcohol affects embryonic or fetal development.[17] Since the fetus is not isolated from the maternal body and is therefore strongly affected by the maternal environment, it is a doctor's responsibility to educate pregnant women about antenatal hygiene. Such an education will prevent many birth defects. Pregnant women should see a doctor on a regular basis, and those with severe health problems should be treated in "prematurity hospitals" to reduce risks for the newborn.

Ballantyne focused on preventable birth defects. He did not deny the influence of "morbid heredity" and was favorable to the encouragement of selective breeding. He had noted, however, that such breeding is very difficult to implement in practice. Conversely, Ballantyne believed that the fear of hereditary impairments was greatly exaggerated:

> The most hereditary thing in the world is the normal, not the abnormal; that health is transmitted as well as disease; that even where the past history of the family is bad, the clean livers have handed something to their children that is better than what was handed on to them. It begins to be evident that inherited diseases and anomalies are rather signs of the breaking of heredity than instances of the persistence of it. . . . Much of the harm that is done to the germ in one generation may be undone in the next; there is a constant tendency of the germ plasm to return to right physiological paths, if it be permitted.[18]

Ballantyne's prenatal care program was grounded in strict supervision of pregnant women by physicians. Ballantyne believed that such supervision was necessary for pregnant women's health, the health of their unborn children, and the future of the British nation. He was sympathetic to campaigns in favor of women's right to vote because, he argued, women are experts in maternal and child welfare, and should have a voice on these issues. Alternatively, he thought that it was, above all, the unborn infant who deserved to be heard.[19] In a 1899 lecture titled "Petition from the Unborn," written from the fetus' point of view, Ballantyne detailed the obligations and duties of the pregnant woman, the medical profession, and the state to unborn children. Every child, he argued, had the right to be engendered by self-respecting individuals, to be conceived in soberness, and to develop under healthy conditions of intrauterine life. Every young man and woman owed a sacred obligation to the unborn, who objects to springing from body cells weakened by immoral life and by toxic and pathogenic agencies such as syphilis and alcohol. Ballantyne concluded his lecture with a call for the recognition of "fetal rights."[20] As a dedicated advocate of the unborn, Ballantyne was opposed to the use of anesthesia during childbirth, because he believed that such an egoistic wish of a woman to avoid suffering could irreparably harm her child. He was also a strong opponent of "criminal abortion" and favored severe punishment of abortive practices. Ballantyne's practical goals were to protect the unborn child, reduce infant mortality, and remove the burden that the congenitally unfit imposed on the state, goals paralleled by British authorities. Ballantyne's ideas were transformed accordingly into public health recommendations in the early twentieth century.[21]

French pioneer of prenatal care Adolphe Pinard (1844–1934) was, like Ballantyne, an obstetrician interested in limiting newborn deaths and birth defects. A strong advocate of eugenics, Pinard was a founding member of the French Eugenics Society and French National League against the Venereal Danger.[22] Pinard promoted a "Latin version of eugenics," focused on interactions between heredity and environment. In a 1923 leaflet on the venereal scourge, Pinard explained that heredity had two components: ancestral and individual. He strongly criticized the view that a reduction of "bad results of conception" is an impossible task. The majority of the so-called hereditary impairments, Pinard argued, were produced by preventable causes, above all, syphilis.[23]

Pinard's claim that a majority of inborn defects could be prevented by closely monitoring pregnant women's health is similar to Ballantyne's ideas. Among other things, he invented a special stethoscope, the "Pinard's horn," that was adapted to listen to a fetal heartbeat.[24] Nevertheless, Pinard's main goal was not the elimination of fetal malformations but the reduction of neonatal mortality. He was especially interested in the prevention of premature births, one of the main causes of newborn deaths and poor health in children, and he organized campaigns to reduce pregnant women's fatigue and stress, elements that favor premature childbirth.[25] A parliament member for the Radical Party between 1919 and 1928, Pinard promoted legislation that would grant maternity leave to working women. In 1909, the French parliament voted in favor of a law that gave women the right to an unpaid maternity leave of eight weeks and secured their right to keep their jobs when they returned from this leave. In 1913, maternity leave became obligatory, and women were granted partial financial compensation during their leave; they also became entitled to free medical care.[26] Pinard also attempted to improve the survival of newborns through the development of perinatal care and the promotion of maternal breastfeeding. He is seen in France as the founder of the new discipline of "puericulture," or the care of the newborn.[27]

Ballantyne and Pinard had similar aims, namely, to promote the supervision of pregnancy in order to prevent the birth of impaired or sickly children. The methods applied to achieve this goal were, however, different on the two sides of the English Channel. Ballantyne mainly relied on medical supervision of pregnancy, while Pinard supported such supervision but was primarily interested in better medical care for newborn children and relied on social measures such as a paid maternity leave to reduce prematurity and promote breastfeeding. Pinard's interventions paved the way for state support of pronatalist policies.

Ballantyne's actions provided the foundation for the professionalization of prenatal care as well as efforts to differentiate birth defects produced by socioeconomic variables from those that stem from hereditary causes (and therefore
cannot be eliminated through medical surveillance of pregnant women).[28] The
latter category, or "irreducible" birth defects, included the majority of inborn
mental impairments.

Mental Deficiency

Mental deficiency is sometimes described as an invisible birth defect. In other
words, a child who looks perfectly "normal" at birth can later fail to reach developmental milestones or, in some cases, lose already-acquired skills. Some
mental impairments, such as untreated phenylketonuria (PKU) or autism, correspond to this image; however, many others, especially those studied during
the nineteenth and early twentieth centuries, are linked with specific "physical
stigmata." The history of inborn mental deficiency is inseparably linked with
clinical medicine.

Recent historians of mental disability are often interested in social, economic, political, and cultural aspects of dealing with intellectually impaired
people. They have studied the institutionalization and segregation of "feeble-
minded" children and adults, the attempts to deal with the influence of mental
retardation on education and the definition of citizenship, the role of efforts to
control feeble-mindedness during the rise of the eugenics movement, and the
economic and political aspects of managing people with intellectual disabilities.
Historical studies on this topic refuted many of the simplified representations
of past treatment of people with mental impairment as uniformly repressive
and displayed a great variability of attitudes regarding the treatment of intellectually impaired individuals. These historians have shown that even at the height
of the eugenic view's popularity, only a minority of the "feeble-minded" were
institutionalized in big hospitals or asylums. The majority of people with intellectual disabilities mainly relied on care provided by family members. Group
homes, special day schools, and vocational centers for children and adults with
intellectual difficulties already existed in the late nineteenth and early twentieth
centuries but were systematically underfunded and answered only to a small
fraction of parents' demands.[29]

Poor parents suffered disproportionately from the difficulties of raising an
intellectually disabled child. Thomas Cunnane, who directed a school for "mentally defective" children in California in the 1920s and 1930s, explained that it is
important for doctors to do everything they can to help the families of these

children because "there is no more distressing a problem than to be the parent of a mentally defective child." His colleague Edward Cox modulated this statement, pointing to the fact that these parents' unhappiness often has socioeconomic roots: "Not everyone who has a defective child can afford the care and training supplied by a special school, and charity institutions are full to overflowing. Public school systems in the larger cities usually have special day training schools called 'development schools.' These, also, are generally full to overflowing. So it is indeed shockingly true that 'there is no more distressing a problem than to be the parent of a mentally defective child.' "[30]

Historians' rich and nuanced picture of both private and public management of people with mental disabilities seldom includes information about the central role of the clinics in defining "mental retardation" as well as explaining how it was diagnosed, classified, and treated. It is undoubtedly true that mental retardation was presented as an educational, legal, or moral issue, but at the same time it was also presented as a major medical problem. The main difference between the "feeble-minded" and the "insane" was the presence—or the presumed presence—of a severe underlying physical problem in the former: birth malformation, degeneration, or early trauma. While the nature of the physical defect changed over time, the important role of clinical medicine in defining feeble-mindedness did not.

G. H. Howe and his colleagues studied the "causes of idiocy" in Massachusetts in the mid-nineteenth century. They concluded that the main cause of mental defects was parents' lack of care to follow the rules of producing healthy offspring. Self-abuse (masturbation), intermarriage of relatives, attempts to procure abortion, and, above all, the abuse of alcohol led to the births of children whose faulty body organization revealed their mental defect.[31] Mentally deficient people, Howe stressed, display a wide range of physical and physiological anomalies. Physicians who examine them should observe the size and shape of their head, the proportions between body parts, the condition of the nervous system, and the development of body cavities: "If any bodily particularities, however minute, always accompany peculiar mental conditions, they become important; they are the fingermarks of Creator, by which we learn to read his works."[32]

Howe and his colleagues measured the height, depth, and width of the chest as well as the dimension of the skull of the mentally deficient. They also studied their tactile sensibility, muscular contractility, recognition of musical sounds, capacity to fix sight on visible objects, and the dynamic condition of the body (agility). They discovered that "idiots" scored lower on a series of physical measures such as dynamic conditions and tactile sensibility than "normal" controls, had much higher amative feelings (i.e., sexual drive), and, predictably, were found to have less-developed language skills, capacity to count, perceptive faculties, social nature, and moral sentiments.[33] Peter Martin Duncan and William Millard, authors of an 1866 text on the education and training of imbeciles, idiots, and the feeble-minded, also insisted that there are links between physical and mental abnormality. Some feeble-minded children, they argued, look very much like "normal" children do, and their impairment is detected only when they go to school, but such cases are relatively rare. In the great majority of cases, mental and bodily deficiencies are inseparably linked. The general rule is that "the greater the body defect, the greater the idiocy."[34]

Two important textbooks on mental disabilities that shaped the thinking of generations of physicians—Shuttleworth's *Mentally Deficient Children* and Tredgold's *Mental Deficiency*—similarly presented "physical stigmata" as a key element of a differential diagnosis of feeble-mindedness.[35] Psychiatrist George Edward Shuttleworth (1842–1928) started his career as an assistant medical officer at the Earlswood Asylum, headed at that time by John Langdon Down, the psychiatrist who first described Down syndrome. (Down was later named superintendent of the Royal Albert Asylum in Lancaster, a position he held for most of his professional life.) Shuttleworth was interested in the physiology of feeble-mindedness but also in the training of people with this condition.[36] He imported into Britain methods developed by Édouard Séguin, French pioneer of the treatment of children with developmental delays, and grounded his own approach to the management of children with such delays in Séguin's humanistic principles. Shuttleworth became one of the leading UK specialists in the education of mentally defective children as well as an early advocate of their rights.[37]

In 1895, Shuttleworth published *Mentally Deficient Children: Their Treatment and Training*, a book that became the standard British textbook on mental deficiency in the late nineteenth and early twentieth centuries. The first edition of Shuttleworth's book was focused on the need to educate mentally impaired children in order to favor the best possible development of their faculties and allow them to earn a living, often in special working homes for the feeble-minded. Society, Shuttleworth argued, had a duty to help its unhappy members in the spirit of Christian charity. Unlike Howe and his colleagues, Shuttleworth believed that a majority of mental defects were inborn but not hereditary and that people with such defects were mostly the victims of unfortunate circumstances that could not be controlled.[38] In the second edition of his book, published in 1900, Shuttleworth added a chapter on the clinical aspects of mental deficiency. He proposed that a distinction be made between acquired

mental deficiency (produced in childhood by events such as trauma, febrile illness, intoxication, and emotional imbalance) and inborn mental deficiency
(produced before birth by "formative defects"). The latter category included conditions such as microcephaly (abnormally small head), hydrocephalus (accumulation of liquid in the skull), the "mongol" feeble-mindedness (today, Down syndrome), and "cretinism" (today, thyroid deficiency). It also included deficiencies
produced by diseases of the pregnant woman, such as epilepsy, syphilis, and
eclampsia (seizures during pregnancy). Mental deficiency that stems from "formative defects," Shuttleworth pointed out, is frequently associated with visible
physical defects, such as cleft lip, deficient earlobes, missing fingers, unusual
shape of face, or cranial anomalies. A trained physician should be able to recognize the physical traits of mental deficiency even in relatively mild cases; such
traits are often more exaggerated in advanced cases.[39]

The third edition of Shuttleworth's book, co-written with W. A. Potts and published in 1910, and the fourth edition, published in 1916, expanded on the chap-
ters about the classification of different forms of mental deficiency and their
etiology, diagnosis, and prognosis.[40] The fifth edition, published in 1922, incorporated new developments in the diagnosis of mental retardation, such as
the generalization of Binet-Simon intelligence tests, which evaluated the capacity of the child to improve with time. The book also included new views on the
inheritance of mental deficiency. Shuttleworth and Potts agreed with the US
eugenist Henry Goddard that feeble-mindedness was often linked with "neuropathic inheritance."[41] Nevertheless, they stressed that the environment plays an
important role in shaping outcomes, including for people with a hereditary
mental deficiency. Shuttleworth and Potts did not oppose the eugenic goal of
reducing the number of people with severe impairments but argued that this
goal should be attained through educating people about responsible reproduction, not by coercive measures such as sterilization: "In the meantime we are
responsible for those weaklings we have allowed to be born as fellow-members
of the human family."[42]

Shuttleworth promoted specialized education, vocational training, and compassionate treatment of mentally impaired individuals. His younger colleague,
psychiatrist Alfred Frank Tredgold, was, in contrast, an enthusiastic advocate of
eugenic measures. Tredgold became interested in mental deficiencies early in
his career. In 1905, he was appointed medical investigator to the Royal Commission on the Care and Control of the Feeble-Minded. After the First World War,
Tredgold divided his time among a private consultancy, a neurological practice
at the Royal Surrey County Hospital, teaching psychiatry at University College

London, and committee work. He contributed to the passing of the UK Mental Deficiency Acts of 1913 and 1927, and later was active in shaping the British government's policies for the management of mentally defective people.[43]

In 1908, Tredgold published *Textbook of Mental Deficiency*, a systematic effort to combine descriptions of mental impairments with attempts to unravel their causes. The book's numerous editions (the twelfth was published in 1980) reflect the successive shifts in the understanding of "feeble-mindedness." Tredgold's book primarily dealt with clinical aspects of *amentia*—a term he coined and propagated. He believed that mental "degeneration" was nearly always linked with "physical stigmata."[44] Approximately half of this book is dedicated to characteristic physical and mental traits of various types of amentia, as well as the different diagnoses and prognoses associated with each variety of mental impairment. It is impossible, Tredgold concluded, to cure the majority of the feeble-minded, but one can train them to be more useful to society and, above all, less prone to evil.[45] Amentia, Tredgold believed, is almost always hereditary and is a broad term that encompasses advanced parental age, alcoholism, and diseases such as syphilis and tuberculosis. He included syphilis and tuberculosis among hereditary conditions because geneticists' claim that these diseases do not affect germ plasm, he argued, is not plausible. In other words, he found it difficult to believe that a systemic pathology such as tuberculosis could not degrade the quality of sperm and egg cells.[46]

The conclusions of the first edition of *Mental Deficiency* are not very different from those of Shuttleworth's book; the main difference is Tredgold's stronger focus on hereditary feeble-mindedness and the need to control people with this condition. The second edition, published in 1914, also followed principles traced by Shuttleworth. Tredgold also concluded that sterilization of the "feeble-minded" is not an efficient way to reduce the number of people with this condition because the majority of affected individuals are not born to individuals with deficiencies but to carriers with no marks of mental abnormality. According to Tredgold, strict segregation of the "feeble-minded" would be a more efficient way to prevent them from having offspring.[47] The third and fourth editions of *Mental Deficiency*, published in 1920 and 1922, respectively, more strongly affirmed Tredgold's eugenic credo. They downplayed the role of disease in pregnant women in producing "germinal impairment" and focused on conditions transmitted in families as well as physicians' duty to limit the reproduction of the diseased and the degenerate.[48] The fifth edition, published in 1929, explained that contraception has, alas, had the opposite effect of the one sought by eugenicists. It appeals to the efficient, prudent, and thrifty, and, by consequence, its diffusion can increase the gap between the number of children born to healthy parents and those born to affected individuals.[49]

The sixth edition of *Mental Deficiency*, published in 1937, struck an alarmist tone. Society, Tredgold affirmed, is not aware of the severity of social problems produced by the uncontrolled proliferation of the mentally unfit.[50] He explained that he previously opposed the sterilization of mentally defective people but that his work as a member of the Departmental Committee on Sterilisation persuaded him that voluntary sterilization of certain defectives would be a useful measure, as would the prohibition of marriage of certain individuals.[51] Tredgold was aware of the fact that some people qualified his view as retrograde, but he was convinced that energetic measures were necessary to react to the increase in the number of mentally deficient, especially those with asocial traits: "It seems to me that to ignore portent of disaster until the storm is upon us, is neither moral nor wise—it is merely foolish."[52] He did not entirely exclude the possibility of a physical elimination of low-grade idiots (those with the most severe disability). Tredgold mentioned ancient civilizations that exposed handicapped children and explained that "it is probable that the community will one day, in self-defense, have to consider this question seriously. But it is clearly one that bristles with difficulties, and, at the present time, public opinion is so obviously unripe for any such proposal, that it may be dismissed as outside practical politics."[53]

Tredgold did not abandon his support for eugenic measures after the Second World War. In the seventh edition of his book, published in 1947, and the eighth, published in 1952 (co-written with his son, it was the last edition published in his lifetime), Tredgold reaffirmed that eugenics is the only approach able to prevent the disastrous effects produced by the excessive propagation of "defective stock." In the 1947 edition of his book, he reiterated his view that while euthanasia is not an option for high-grade (i.e., less impaired) defectives, because, among other things, public opinion will never accept such a procedure, it may be an option for low-grade defectives:

> The position is a very different one with regard to 80,000 or so more idiots and imbeciles in the country. These are not only incapable of being employed to any economic advantage, but their care and support, whether in their own homes or in institutions, absorb a large amount of time, energy, and money of the normal population which could be utilized to better purpose. Moreover, many of these defectives are utterly helpless, repulsive in appearance and revolting in manners. . . . With the present great shortage of institutional accommodations there are thousands of

mothers who are literarily worn out in caring for these persons at home. In my opinion it would have been an economical and humane procedure were their existence to be painlessly terminated and I have no doubt, from personal experience, that this would have been welcomed by a very large proportion of parents. It is doubtful if public opinion is yet ripe for this to be done compulsorily; but I am of the opinion that the time has come when euthanasia should be permitted at the request of parent or guardian. It would clearly be necessary to devise adequate safeguards, but this would not present any practical difficulty.[54]

Even after Tredgold's death, the idea of a physical elimination of the "most severe defectives" was not immediately discarded by his heirs. The 1963 edition of Tredgold's book, which had become *Tredgold's Mental Retardation*, discusses the acceptability of euthanasia for "low-grade defectives." The authors explain that "it is time for society to decide whether euthanasia will be permitted at the request of a parent or guardian." They add, nevertheless, that a decision about whether a newborn should live has to be made shortly after birth, as "every week the baby is allowed to live makes the decision more difficult."[55] Tredgold's defense of active euthanasia became socially acceptable through a shift from children and adults to babies and through debate on intensive care of severely impaired newborns. For the opponents of prenatal diagnosis, the acceptance of terminating a pregnancy for fetal indications merely moved this debate an additional step back in time: from euthanasia of "unfit" adults, to the discreet removal of "defective" newborns, to the elimination of "impaired" fetuses.

Photographs of the "Feeble-Minded"

Mental deficiency is often linked with the presence of typical physical traits.[56] The first edition of Shuttleworth's *Mentally Deficient Children: Their Treatment and Training* included several pages of photographs of individuals with conditions linked with mental deficiency: microcephaly, hydrocephalus, "mongol"-type imbecility, inherited syphilis, and sporadic cretinism. The latter illustration showed the same subject before and after treatment involving a thyroid extraction. Such a treatment dramatically modified the subject's physiognomy: a "cretin" with a dull and vacant look was transformed into a "normal"-looking, alert individual. The juxtaposition of the two photographs was a highly persuasive demonstration that "feeble-mindedness" can be a reversible condition. The same photographs were reproduced in the second, third, and fourth editions of Shuttleworth's book. The fifth edition, published in 1922, included additional photographs that displayed mentally deficient people's abnormal traits: deformations of the skull and scalp, the typical shape of the hands of a "Mongolian imbecile," and deformations observed in hereditary syphilis and inborn cerebral palsy.

One of the innovations of Tredgold's *Mental Deficiency* of 1908 was the abundance of illustrations. Each chapter was accompanied by several photographs of people with the mental impairment discussed in that chapter. Photographs displayed typical images of stable and unstable feeble-mindedness, as well as varieties of imbecility: melancholic, mischievous, docile, and destructive; idiocy and imbecility with paralysis; excitable idiocy; microcephalic amentia, and mongolian amentia. Photographs of people with "inborn amentia" are contrasted with photographs of people with "secondary amentia," induced by diseases such as epilepsy, encephalitis, sclerosis, atrophy of the brain, cretinism, and syphilis. The next five editions of Tredgold's textbook retained the photographs employed in the first edition. The sixth edition, published in 1937, included, in addition to the photographs published in previous editions, photographs of abnormal anatomical and morphological traits such as deformations of the hands, head, and palate; abnormally shaped ears; skin anomalies such as adenoma sebaceum (an anomaly linked today with tuberous sclerosis, a hereditary condition) and a proliferation of birthmarks; and hypertelorism (an abnormal distance between the eyes, a trait present in numerous genetic syndromes). The chapter on "mongolism" included photographs that prominently display morphological traits associated with this condition: enlarged and fissured tongue, abnormal eye shape, and unusual palmar and foot lines (dermatoglyphs).

The main reason for the inclusion of photographs of mentally impaired people in Tredgold's books was to assist differential diagnosis, facilitate classification, and, if applicable, demonstrate the efficacy of therapy. At the same time, visual representations of mental defectives were employed to define people with cognitive impairments as a distinct and enduring subclass of individuals. The construction of mental defectives as physically distinct, and (mainly) inborn, facilitated the identification, surveillance, and control of a presumably deviant section of the population, and furthered the attempts of medical practitioners to assert their superiority over educators in the management and control of schools and colonies for mental defectives.[57] Focus on abnormal physical traits, and thus on clinical aspects of feeble-mindedness, strengthened the jurisdiction of the physician on this group of impairments. The descriptions that accompanied the photographs were often laden with value judgments: "small, thin, and hideous"; "stunted, misshapen, hideous, and bestial specimens of morbid mankind"; "look of heavy, immobile stupidity and vacuity." Experts affirmed that in the majority of cases, they could immediately recognize the specific physiognomy of a mentally impaired individual: "As soon as the child walks into the room . . . the gait and carriage, the expression and the outlines of the features betray the feeble mind."[58]

Textbook photographs of the feeble-minded can be contrasted with photographs of people with intellectual impairments in British geneticist Lionel Penrose's collection. Penrose, known for his studies of mental deficiency, attempted to promote respect for people with mental disabilities. It has been reported that he enjoyed talking with institutionalized, intellectually impaired patients and was truly delighted to be in their company.[59] Photographs of children with mental disabilities in his archives (probably taken either by him or his collaborators) are very different from the typical photographs in medical books and articles. The latter are nearly always codified, rigid, and depersonalized, with a strong focus on the "abnormal" traits.[60] By contrast, Penrose's photographs look similar to photographs of "normal" children, taken by their parents, siblings, or friends. The children are shown in the arms of nurses, standing on cots, playing, and eating. Some look happy and playful while others look pensive, annoyed, or melancholic—as children often are. Without the presence of uniformed nurses, it would have been difficult to guess that these are institutionalized children. Such photographs, as well as those of adults with mental impairment in Penrose's collection, send a strong message that these are individuals with unique personalities, and not merely "case studies."[61]

In the twenty-first century, photographs of people with visible disabilities, especially of those who are both physically and mentally impaired, are employed to shed light on the positive aspects of their lives and their common humanity. The website Positive Exposure features striking photographs of "different" people, some of whom display physical differences that are not linked with a major functional impairment (e.g., albinism), while others are visibly impaired/ disabled. The founder of this site, photographer Rick Guidotti, explained that his goal of photographing children with inborn differences is to "get people to see those with differences not as victims, but [as] kids and people first and foremost. The pity has to disappear. The fear has to disappear. Behavior has to change. These kids need to be seen as their parents see them, as their friends see them, as valuable and positive parts of society, as beautiful."[62]

Positive Exposure provides high-quality photographs of children with inborn syndromes, some linked with severe physical and mental disabilities such as trisomy 18, Prader-Willi syndrome, Smith-Magenis syndrome, Cornelia de Lange syndrome, Costello syndrome, or Williams syndrome. Unique, a UK-based charity that helps parents of children with rare chromosomal syndromes, similarly displays on its website photographs of engaging-looking, often lively children.[63] The cover of David Wright's book *Downs: The History of a Disability* shows four broadly smiling and visibly happy teenagers with Down syndrome.[64] It is undoubtedly important to show that disabled children are just as unique as nondisabled children, to fight prejudice about disabilities, and to provide "positive exposure" to atypical (dysmorphic) features. Conversely, positive photographs of disabled children chosen to illustrate a given "deviation" are carefully selected and edited to tell a specific story. The photographs of cute, happy-looking children and adults with severe impairments convey a message that may mask other aspects of their lives.[65] In the early twentieth century, "images of deviance" relied on the viewer's belief that photographs are direct, nonmediated, and trustworthy transcriptions of reality. A similar conviction may have influenced some of the early twenty-first-century photographs of people with disabilities.[66]

"Mongoloid Idiocy"

The diffusion of prenatal diagnosis has been shaped by the wish to diagnose Down syndrome. In the nineteenth century, Down syndrome (at that time, "mongoloid idiocy," "mongoloid imbecility," or "mongolism") did not have such a privileged place among inborn mental impairments. It was seen as one of many types of "idiocy," "cretinism," and "feeble-mindedness." "Mongolism" was first designated as a distinct entity by physician John Langdon Down, a superintendent of the Earlswood Asylum for Idiots in Surrey, England. In an article published in 1866, Down described a "Mongolian type of idiocy." Ten years later, an independently published article discussed "Kalmuc idiocy." (Kalmucs—today, Kalmyk(s)—are a Mongolian tribe that migrated from central Asia to north of the Caspian Sea.) In the late nineteenth and early twentieth centuries, publications stressed the specificity of the facial traits of people with "mongoloid idiocy"; rather surprisingly, this specificity was not noted earlier, or was not seen as an essential trait.[67]

The name "mongol" referred to presumed "racial atavism" of mentally deficient individuals—a regression to a more "primitive" stage of development. The regression hypothesis was first proposed by Down. In the twentieth century, it was promoted by British doctor Francis Graham Crookshank. Crookshank argued that "Mongolian imbecility" was the result of the distant racial history of an individual's (Caucasian) parents, each of whom carried Mongol traits. "Mongolian imbeciles" represented an atavistic regression to an archaic mongoloid heritage that emerged because of their incomplete development in the womb.[68] Such a view assumed that Asian people represent a lower stage in the development of humanity but also that different racial groups share the same fundamental hereditary makeup, since one racial group can revert into another. Crookshank's theories were well received by the general public but were rejected by a majority of experts who studied mental deficiency. Nevertheless, these experts maintained the term *Mongoloid imbecility* mainly for reasons of convenience.[69]

"Mongolian imbeciles" were often born to mothers older than 40 who previously had healthy children; therefore, it was believed that this condition was likely not hereditary and was produced spontaneously. The higher percentage of "mongoloid" children born to older mothers was attributed to "uterine exhaustion" and the decline of the mother's reproductive abilities.[70] Researchers noted the contrast between the homogeneity of physical characteristics of people with this condition and the heterogeneity of their intellectual impairment. In the first edition of *Mental Deficiency*, Tredgold explained that despite the great physical similarity of people with this condition, they display a wide range of mental disabilities: "The milder members generally learn to read, write and perform simple duties with a fair amount of intelligence; the majority belong to medium grade of mental defect, a few are idiots."[71] Other specialists confirmed that people with this condition may vary greatly in their mental abilities, but the majority of individuals display a moderate mental disability that corresponds roughly to a mental age of 3–7 years (the "imbecile" grade): "they show promise as children because they are lively, notice their environment and show tendency to mimic, but they promise much and achieve little."[72] There were, nevertheless, notable exceptions to this rule. A director of a school for mentally impaired children in California attested in the 1930s that two "mongoloid types" from his school went to college; one of them graduated from Stanford University.[73]

Kate Brousseau, a professor of psychology at Mills College in California and an expert on "mongolism" in the interwar era, strongly rejected the atavist theory. She added, however, that it is reasonable to suppose that the condition is linked with impaired intrauterine development, since this defect is present at birth. The advanced age of the mother is in all probability a contributing cause, but not the only one. Other contributing factors may be alcoholism, mental strain, nutritional deficiencies, and neuropathic heredity, but the most likely explanation is an "obscure disturbance of the ductless glands. This can be either inherited, or the mother during pregnancy may develop certain endocrine disorders which may be transmitted to the child."[74] The popularity of the hormonal hypothesis of the origin of "mongolism" during the interwar era is probably related to the perceived similarities between "mongolism" and "cretinism," two conditions that combined intellectual impairment with the presence of typical facial traits. In the early twentieth century, "cretinism" was redefined as insufficiency of thyroid hormone. This observation has contradictory effects on the understanding of mongolism. One was to radically dissociate "cretinism" and "mongolism." If a feeble-minded individual improved following treatment with a thyroid extract, he or she was diagnosed as affected by "cretinism" and not "mongolism."[75] The second was to strengthen the view of "mongolism" as an inborn metabolic disorder, probably induced by hormonal disequilibrium and thus potentially treatable, a view that remained popular at least until the finding, in 1959, that "mongolism" is linked with the presence of an additional copy of the chromosome 21 (trisomy 21).

Explaining "Mongolism"

The contrasting understandings of Down syndrome before its definition as a chromosomal anomaly is displayed in the work of two leading experts on this condition in the mid-twentieth century: Lionel Penrose, who favored a protogenetic view of mongolism, and Clemens Benda, who strongly defended a metabolic-hormonal understanding of this condition. Penrose was, above all, a geneticist. He is known for his contribution to the study of genetic linkage, mutation ratios, and the heredity of blood groups, and from 1945 to 1965 he occupied the Galton Chair of Eugenics (later renamed the Chair of Human Genetics) at University College London.[76] At the same time, Penrose developed a long-standing interest in mental disability. Between 1931 and 1939, he was the research medical officer at the Royal Eastern Counties Institution in Colchester, England.[77] Penrose initiated and conducted a survey, later known as the Colchester Survey, that collected extensive information about 1,280 cases of mental impairment. The Colchester Survey was sponsored by the Medical Research Council (MRC) but also by the Darwin Trust of Edinburgh, a foundation that maintained close collaboration with the Eugenics Education Society. The aim of the Colchester Survey was a quantitative evaluation of the incidence of inherited mental deficiency. In the 1930s, data on the inheritance of mental ailments had become a highly contested issue. At that time, eugenicists circulated dramatic data about the increasing number of inherited mental disorders and advocated voluntary sterilization of the mentally deficient. Penrose, a strong opponent of eugenics, hoped that the data collected by the Colchester Survey would disprove eugenicists' claims.[78]

In the final report of the Colchester Survey, Penrose explained that the term *mental deficit* encompassed a wide range of physical and intellectual impairments. Very few mental disorders, he stressed, followed a Mendelian pattern of transmission. Huntington's disease was a clear example of such a transmission. Another example, and one that is often quoted as an important achievement of the Colchester Survey, was an investigation of a metabolic disease called phenylketonuria (PKU). PKU was first described by Norwegian physician and biochemist Ivar Asbjørn Følling in 1934.[79] Penrose coined the term *phenylketonuria* and demonstrated, thanks to the data collected by the Colchester Survey, that it was a hereditary recessive disorder.[80] PKU was presented by Penrose as a rare case of heredity mental impairment and was a strong argument against eugenicists' claims. He had calculated that about 1% of people are carriers of the PKU trait. It was pointless to try to control the reproduction of all individuals with this trait, while targeting only the affected people (assuming that they will have offspring despite their severe mental impairment) would have practically no effect on the frequency of the defective gene in a given population and thus would not prevent the birth of children with the targeted condition. Only a lunatic, Penrose concluded, would wish to sterilize 1% of the population to prevent the birth of a handful of harmless imbeciles.[81]

PKU and Huntington's disease were undoubtedly hereditary—and very rare. Penrose's main conclusion from his Colchester studies was that mental deficiency was often polygenic (dependent on multiple genes) and could be attributed to both heredity and environment.[82] Penrose viewed heredity as but one element among many others that may influence the genesis of mental deficiency. He also distinguished between the presence of hereditary elements and external circumstances that may affect their expression. Penrose's inquiry of mongolism illustrated this separation. The Colchester Survey included information about familial distribution of this condition, as part of an effort to uncover genetic markers of "mongolism." Penrose was initially convinced that the parents of "mongols" carried hereditary predisposition factors and argued that the presence of a first case of "mongolism" in a family increased the probability of finding another affected individual. He focused then on a small number of families with several cases of "mongolism," suggesting that they directly displayed the hereditary background of the disease.[83] Earlier, Penrose had shown a correlation between the age of the mother (but not of the father) and the birth of a "mongoloid" child.[84] His interpretation of this observation was that maternal age was a predisposing factor that favored the expression of an underlying genetic defect. In 1954, Penrose considered the possibility that "mongolism" was the consequence of a new mutation. He then discarded this hypothesis, because it did not explain the relative consistency of the phenotypic expression of "mongolism" (all the people with this condition look alike) and the strong influence of maternal age.[85]

Penrose, as a geneticist, was mainly interested in the study of hereditary traits, including people with mental disabilities. Clemens Benda, as a clinician, was primarily interested in the diagnosis, prevention, and treatment of mental impairment. Benda studied philosophy and medicine at the Universities of Berlin, Jena, and Heidelberg. He began his medical career in Berlin and worked as an assistant at the Heidelberg Psychiatric Clinic. He was also interested in existential philosophy and studied with philosopher Karl Jaspers, among others. Benda was forced to leave Germany in 1935, partly because of his political views and partly because his father was Jewish. He immigrated to the United States, settling in Massachusetts, where he worked at institutions for intellectually disabled children for most of his career. Benda was the director of the children's unit at the Metropolitan State Hospital in Waltham, Massachusetts; head of the Wallace Research Laboratory for the Study of Mental Deficiency at the Wrentham State School in Wrentham, Massachusetts; and, from 1947 until his retirement in 1962, the director of research and clinical psychiatry at the Walter E. Fernald State School in Waltham. He was also associated with the Harvard School of Medicine.

Benda's views on mental disability were grounded in clinical observations and numerous autopsies of people with this condition. In 1946, he explained that practically every person with a mental impairment presents physical impairments as well. As such, when working to prevent birth defects it is very important to use both medical and educational interventions that ameliorate outcomes for children with these conditions. A key element, he stressed, is the intensification of multidisciplinary research on prenatal and postnatal impairments.[86] Benda was persuaded that "mongolism," renamed "congenital acromicria" by him, originated in hormonal disequilibrium before birth. He presented this theory for the first time in an article published in 1938 and expanded it in his 1947 book *Mongolism and Cretinism: A Study of the Clinical Manifestations and the General Pathology of Pituitary and Thyroid Deficiency*. Benda further extended this argument in the second edition of his book, published in 1949.[87] Family studies, he argued, clearly refute the hypothesis that "mongolism" is linked to hereditary factors. The main cause of this birth defect was defective development of the brain during embryonic life, probably before the eighth week of pregnancy. Perturbations of the secretion of pituitary and thyroid hormones in pregnant women deprived the embryo of essential nutrients during a critical period of brain development. Benda viewed the mongoloid child as an "unfinished child," prevented from reaching intellectual maturity by nutritional deprivation in the womb. "Mongolism," he proposed, is more frequently found in the children born to older mothers, who suffer more often from insufficiency of the pituitary gland and other hormonal anomalies. It is also linked with other problems that may stem from hormonal perturbations, such as infertility and frequent spontaneous miscarriages.

Benda advised women at risk of having a "mongoloid" child—those older than 40 and those who are infertile or who have had several miscarriages—to undergo biochemical tests that could uncover latent hypothyroidism, hypogonadism, and hypopituitarism. If such tests found a hormonal anomaly, the woman should be treated with substitutive hormonal therapy. Benda also hinted that physicians who find out that a pregnant woman has a high risk of giving birth to a "mongoloid" child should be aware that the pregnant woman may be confronted with a difficult decision: "a close cooperation between endocrinologist and obstetrician in the prenatal care will provide means of differentiation of the various endocrine deficiencies and will help the obstetrician to decide which pregnancy can be safely continued."[88] The previous sentence may hint that some pregnancies can be discontinued, an indirect recommendation of abortion for a woman with a high risk of having a child with "mongolism." Then again, Benda strongly believed that children with this condition could be helped by appropriate medical interventions and educative measures. Hormonal therapy can alleviate many of the physical symptoms that make the life of a "mongoloid" child difficult, such as insufficient muscular tonus and chronic constipation. Such therapy cannot, alas, improve their intellectual capacities, but appropriate education can assist them in acquiring many useful skills. Mental handicap, Benda concluded, is an accident of nature that can happen to any family: "all civil-minded societies should take pride in helping the parents of these unfortunate children."[89]

Penrose and Benda had divergent views of the causes of "mongolism," but both believed that good physical care, affection, adapted education, and, for Benda, hormonal treatments helped children with this condition live richer and happier lives. Other experts had a more pessimistic view of the abilities of "mongoloid" children, however. In 1962, psychiatrist Mendel Schachter, the medical director of the Committee for Deficient Children (Comité de l'Enfance Deficiente) of Marseille, divided parents of children with this condition into three groups. The first group, mainly composed of uneducated people, accepted the poor outlook reserved for children with "mongolism" and did not rebel against their unhappy fate. They kept these children at home and faithfully followed the specialists' instructions. The second group, mostly made up of educated people, also had a realistic appreciation of the extent of the child's impairment, but for their own sake or the sake of their "normal" children, they placed the impaired child in an institution. These two groups were easy to manage. This was not the case, however, for the third group, composed of "rebels" who resisted the doctors' authority.[90]

The "rebel" group, Schechter explained, included parents of superior social and cultural standing, particularly those with university educations, who were painfully aware of their misfortune of having a "mongoloid" child. These parents initially seemed to accept the harsh reality of their child's mental disability but later rejected it and claimed that their child had a mild variant of this condition. The "rebel" parents (among the examples Schechter quotes are a physician, a university professor, and a judge) had a tendency to overestimate their child's mental capacities and criticized the specialists' views. Some rejected the results of intelligence tests that displayed the severity of their child's mental retardation and pretended that their daily experience was at least as valid as the results of these tests. These parents even suspected that the experts' pessimistic evaluation, transmitted to educators, hindered the child's progress. Only brutal honesty, Schechter explained, could overcome the rebellious parents' resistance: "We found it most dangerous . . . to understate the implications of mongolism out of false sympathy with the parents. We think that only complete frankness and honesty can be helpful in having a positive effect on the parents' attitude in their acceptance of a stark reality and a poor prognosis."[91]

The only "healthy" attitude of parents of a child with "mongolian retardation," Schechter concluded, is acceptance of the authority of physicians specialized in pedopsychiatry who know that this condition is invariably linked with a severe mental deficiency that cannot be alleviated by education or care.

Birth Defects, Heredity, and Environment in the Mid-Twentieth Century

In the 1940s and 1950s, pioneering efforts to provide prenatal care to women led to an increased medicalization of pregnancy. At that time, many researchers believed that while good medical care during pregnancy was important for the prevention of prematurity and birth of low-weight children, and reduced newborns' mortality and morbidity, "true" birth defects nearly always stemmed from hereditary defects in the germ plasma.[92] "Gross human congenital malformations," Philadelphia obstetrician Douglas Murphy argued in his 1940 book *Congenital Malformations*, "arise solely from influences which affect the germ cells prior to fertilization. No evidence is available to indicate that they result from factors which operate for the first time after fertilization has taken place."[93] In the second edition of his book, published in 1947, Murphy had taken into account two recent developments: the description of severe congenital malformations produced by the rubella virus (first described by Australian ophthalmologist Norman Gregg in 1941) and growing evidence that a high dose of radiation early in pregnancy (usually because the woman and her doctors were unaware that she was pregnant) can disrupt fetal development.[94] He remained nevertheless persuaded that environmental factors, acting after fertilization had taken place, played a limited role in the origin of developmental abnormalities, as compared to the role of hereditary defects.[95] The role of the latter causes is illustrated by the observation that, according to Murphy, families that had one malformed child are twenty-five times more likely to have another child with a birth defect than couples who have a "normal" child.[96]

Not all experts adopted the "all in the genes" point of view. Talks during the first international conference on congenital malformations, held in London in 1960, reflected the diversity of views on this topic.[97] Some of the speakers, such as French experts Jérôme Lejeune and Raymond Turpin, and US geneticist James Neel, focused on genetics and presented the newly described links between the presence of an abnormal number of chromosomes and birth defects, above all, "mongolism." Lejeune and Neel explained that the discovery of such a link led to a distinction between genetic causes of inborn anomalies (anomalies produced by changes in the genetic material of the cell) and hereditary causes (conditions transmitted in families). An abnormal number of chromosomes belongs to the first but usually not to the second category: it often stems from accidents in the development of egg and sperm cells. Other speakers discussed environmental factors that shaped fetal development and their intersections with genetics. Leading US teratology expert Josef Warkany affirmed that hereditary and environmental elements were inseparably linked, and that they shaped embryogenesis together.[98] Lionel Penrose similarly argued that genetics alone could not explain birth defects. It was equally important to investigate the environmental causes of genetic anomalies, for example, the reasons why older women have a higher probability of giving birth to a "mongoloid" child.[99]

The keynote speech, delivered by leading French pediatrician Robert Debré, also stressed the multifactorial origins of the majority of birth defects.[100] Only a small number of inborn malformations, Debré proposed, can be traced to a single hereditary or environmental cause. It is plausible that in the great majority of birth defects, genetic and environmental causes often act together, and it is therefore important to study both. One day, such studies would make the prevention of birth defects possible. In the meantime, however, families struggled with the difficulties of caring for severely disabled children. Better survival of these children, thanks to medical progress, paradoxically increased some families' plight: "Remarkable progress has been achieved in the treatment of congenital malformations. However, in certain cases it is only a question of extension of survival of individuals incapable of any useful physical or intellectual activity. The presence of such children is a menace to the harmony of the parents and threatens the future of normal brothers and sisters, without any advantage for the former. Therefore they must be placed in specialized institutions. The lack of appropriate facilities in this domain is flagrant."[101]

Debré was not optimistic about the possibility of a rapid development of treatments for inborn anomalies. Nevertheless, in the case of one relatively frequent inborn anomaly, hemolytic disease of the newborn, the development of a method that made possible the detection of this condition during pregnancy greatly reduced neonatal deaths and the frequency of birth defects. The oldest "prenatal diagnosis" was also one of the most successful ones.

Rhesus Incompatibility and Birth Defects in the 1950s

Incompatibility of Rhesus factor (a marker on the surface of red blood cells) between the mother and the fetus illustrates the inseparability of genetic and environmental elements in the production of severe birth defects. The management of Rhesus incompatibility is also one of the rare examples of an early success of prenatal diagnosis, or, rather, its pre-1960s variant. Rhesus factor incompatibility was first described in the early 1940s. In the 1930s, pediatricians grouped severe jaundice in newborns, coupled with severe edema (accumulation of fluids) and anemia, under a single heading: "erythroblastosis fetalis."[102] In 1940, immunologists Karl Landsteiner and Alexander Wiener described a new human blood group that could be recognized through a reaction with the blood of the rhesus monkey. They named this group "Rhesus," or Rh factor (D antigen). Approximately 85% of people are Rh positive.

In 1941, hematologist Philip Levine showed that the mysterious destruction of newborn babies' blood was produced by an immunization of an Rh-negative mother by an Rh-positive fetus. During pregnancy, and especially during childbirth, the mother produces antibodies that gradually destroy fetal red blood cells. While the first Rh-positive child was often healthy because the level of maternal anti-Rh antibodies was not high enough to produce irreversible harm, in subsequent pregnancies with a Rh-positive fetus the pregnant woman mounted a secondary, much stronger immune response to fetal red blood cells. Maternal immunization was then aggravated by each consecutive Rh-discordant pregnancy, and women therefore continued to lose babies to this condition. Pediatricians tried to save affected babies through a transfusion immediately after birth. Levine showed that if they used Rh-positive blood, red blood cells were destroyed again by maternal antibodies. Rh-negative blood was more efficient, and even more efficient was an "exchange transfusion," or a total replacement of the blood of the affected newborn by fresh blood that was free of maternal antibodies. The success of the latter method, introduced immediately after the Second World War, was facilitated by the development of thin, flexible vinyl catheters that made blood transfusions in very young babies possible.[103]

Exchange transfusion was tedious, occasionally risky, and had to be performed by skilled operators, but it greatly improved the survival of babies with hemolytic disease. Some babies were nevertheless too sick to be saved by this approach. Others did survive but suffered from irreversible effects of massive blood destruction, above all, brain damage.[104] To limit the harm produced by maternal antibodies, some pediatricians argued that in more severe cases it may be desirable to induce an early birth. Then again, prematurity, especially of already-sick babies, was also a very dangerous situation linked with high levels of mortality and inborn impairments.[105] It was important to find a way to evaluate the level of fetal harm in order to decide whether the risk of continuing the pregnancy was greater than the risk of induction of an early birth. In the 1950s, Manchester physician Douglas Bevis proposed to measure the concentration of yellow pigment, bilirubin, in the amniotic fluid to evaluate the level of destruction of fetal red blood cells. To perform this test, it was necessary to sample amniotic fluid without putting the pregnancy at risk.

In the late nineteenth century, gynecologists employed newly developed hollow hypodermic needles to siphon excess amniotic fluid, a condition called polyhydramnios. This approach was introduced into obstetrical care in the early 1920s. Severe polyhydramnios can be risky for the fetus and, in especially drastic cases, for the mother, too. Polyhydramnios is often associated with diabetes. Pregnancy in diabetic women was very rare in the early twentieth century, but it became less exceptional when, with the development of insulin, more women with diabetes survived to adulthood and decided to have children. As a result, the treatment of polyhydramnios—also called "amniotic tap"—became less rare as well.[106] This approach was then applied to the study of levels of bilirubin in the amniotic fluid. At first, the method did not yield very precise results. In 1956, however, Bevis showed that the use of a spectrometer to quantify bilirubin in the amniotic fluid improved the correlation between this measure and the severity of hemolytic disease of the fetus.[107] Thanks to the possibility of measuring the level of bilirubin in the amniotic fluid and the induction of early childbirth when such a level was dangerously high, the mortality from hemolytic disease of the newborn in the United Kingdom in the 1960s decreased from 22%–25% to 9%–10%.[108] Until the early 1970s, hemolytic disease of the newborn was a frequent pathology, and many hospitals employed Bevin's test.[109] With the diffusion of this test, more gynecologists learned to perform amniocentesis, setting the stage for the use of this technique to collect fetal cells in the late 1960s.[110]

Before the introduction of exchange transfusion and testing for the level of bilirubin in the amniotic fluid, many children with hemolytic disease died shortly after birth, and many of those who survived were severely disabled. Hemolytic disease of the newborn induced kernicterus, characterized by spasms, cerebral palsy, deafness, and mental deficiency. Until the late 1960s, hemolytic disease of the newborn was one of the main causes of inborn mental disability.[111] In his first article on the measure of bilirubin, Bevin called his approach "antenatal prediction of hemolytic disease of the newborn" (i.e., prenatal diagnosis). The term was justified: this was a true prediction of the fate of an unborn child. Bevin's test has other similarities with prenatal diagnosis developed in the late 1960s: the detection of risk; an aspiration to prevent disability, especially intellectual impairment; and the use of amniocentesis to directly scrutinize the fetus.[112] There was, however, one important difference between the diagnosis of fetal-maternal Rh factor incompatibility in the 1950s and the development of prenatal diagnosis in the late 1960s: in the former case, there was no question of abortion. Prenatal diagnosis of hemolytic disease of the newborn was a noncontroversial approach because its aim was to start efficient treatment and to limit harm, not to prevent the birth of an affected child.

CHAPTER 2

Karyotypes

Barr Bodies: Prenatal Diagnosis before Chromosomes

Prenatal diagnosis, such as it is known today, came into being in the 1960s
with the development of a cluster of technologies—the "prenatal diagnosis dispositif"—that made possible the direct study of fetal cells shed into the amniotic fluid. The term *prenatal diagnosis* is older, however. Before the 1960s, this
term was used in two distinct contexts: in the diagnosis of Rhesus disease and
in the identification of major fetal malformations using X-rays.[1] Physicians who
performed an "amniotic tap" to see whether the amniotic fluid contained bilirubin called their approach prenatal or antenatal diagnosis of hemolytic disease of
the newborn. Physicians who employed X-rays to examine pregnant women,
and occasionally uncovered major structural malformations of the fetus, also
spoke about a prenatal/antenatal diagnosis.

X-rays were introduced to obstetrics early in the history of this diagnostic
tool. In 1896, a pair of physicians in Philadelphia captured an X-ray photo of a
pregnant woman, although in that case the fetus was dead. In the early twentieth
century, the resolution of fetal X-ray images was not very good.[2] Nevertheless,
as early as 1916, Chicago physician James Thomas Case described the diagnosis
of anencephaly (the absence of a major portion of the brain) before birth using
X-ray images.[3] In the 1930s and 1940s, gynecologists and obstetricians began to
systematically employ X-rays to detect potential obstacles for childbirth, such as
a malformed pelvis. They also, although more rarely, employed this diagnostic
method to study the fetus: to detect fetal death in utero; to estimate the age of
pregnancy; to diagnose major malformations such as anencephaly, hydrocephalus (accumulation of liquid in the skull), and skeletal malformations; and even
to indicate fetal sex, since bones were usually visible earlier in a female fetus.
Obstetrical uses of X-rays were intensified in the 1950s. At that time, physicians

were aware of the risks of high doses of radiation for the fetus but believed that routine X-ray examination of a pregnant woman was not dangerous.[4] In 1956, Alice Stewart and her collaborators from the Oxford University Unit of Social and Preventive Medicine showed, however, that children whose mothers were exposed to X-rays when pregnant, including in moderate doses, suffered disproportionally from childhood cancers.[5] The growing awareness of the risks of radiation for the fetus led to a gradual abandonment of this method of visualization of the unborn.

The official history of prenatal diagnosis—as it is understood today—started in 1960, the year the first article on prenatal diagnosis of fetal sex through an analysis of fetal cells in the amniotic fluid was published. The diagnosis of fetal sex started with a chance observation. In 1949, Murray Barr and Ewart Bertram, two Canadian neuroscientists from London, Ontario, made an unexpected observation. Barr and Bertram studied the stimulation of nerve cells in cats. The aim of their investigation was to find out whether the appearance of the nuclear satellite, a small body in the nucleus of neurons described by Spanish neuroanatomist Raymond y Cajal in 1909, was related to the stimulation of the nerves of the trunk. Barr and Bertam found that the cells of some animals contained the nuclear satellite, while other animals seemed to miss it entirely, and then they realized that all the "nuclear-satellite-positive" cats were female. Intrigued by this observation, Barr and Bertram systematically looked for the presence of this structure (later renamed "sex chromatin body," or "Barr body") in other cells, and then in other animal species. They found that this structure was a universal marker of the female sex and speculated that it indicated the presence of two X chromosomes (a female chromosomal formula), while its absence indicated the presence of a single X chromosome (a male chromosomal formula).[6]

In 1956, Danish researchers Povl Riis and Fritz Fuchs described a method of diagnosing fetal sex in cells from the amniotic fluid, looking for Barr bodies in these cells. The same year, an Israeli group described a similar technique of fetal sex determination.[7] Gynecologists knew that the amniotic fluid contained fetal cells, and they also knew how to sample amniotic fluid through amniocentesis. Puncturing the amniotic membrane was much too risky to be employed simply for the purpose of satisfying the parents' curiosity about the sex of their future child, but diagnosis of fetal sex could have been very important, for example, if the mother was a carrier of a sex-linked disease such as hemophilia and knew that a boy would have a 50% chance of being affected, while a girl would be healthy.[8] In the 1950s and early 1960s, only Scandinavian countries legalized abortions for a risk of severe fetal malformation. As such, it may not be surprising that the first published case of prenatal diagnosis for sex-linked pathologies came from Denmark.

In 1960, Riis and Fuchs applied their method of fetal sex determination to diagnose the sex of the fetus of a woman who was a hemophilia carrier.[9] Her previous child, a boy, died shortly after birth from complications of hemophilia. When she had learned that she was pregnant again, she decided to terminate the pregnancy. Without testing for fetal sex, the risk of a carrier of the hemophilia gene giving birth to a child with hemophilia was 25%. This risk was seen by the Danish legislature to be high enough to justify a "eugenic" abortion.[10] When Fuchs learned about this woman's decision, he informed her that it was now possible to determine the sex of the fetus. The woman agreed to undergo amniocentesis. Riis and Fuchs examined fetal cells for the presence of Barr bodies and determined that the fetus was female. The woman continued the pregnancy and gave birth to a healthy girl. Although amniocentesis did not lead to an abortion in this case, the goal of the study of fetal cells—the elimination of a male fetus—transformed Riis and Fuchs's study into the first "official" case of prenatal diagnosis.[11]

Riis and Fuchs's second case was another woman at risk of giving birth to a hemophilic child. However, while the first patient knew that she was a hemophilia carrier, the second patient only learned that she was a carrier of this disease when she was four months pregnant. She was referred by her physician to Fuchs, agreed to amniocentesis, and found out that the fetus was female. She later miscarried the fetus, possibly as a result of a complication of the diagnostic procedure.[12] When the same woman became pregnant for the second time, she again decided to have amniocentesis, again learned that the fetus was female, and suffered a second miscarriage. Despite the two miscarriages, she elected to undergo amniocentesis in her third pregnancy. This time, she found out that the fetus was male and decided to have an abortion. Finally, in her fourth pregnancy, amniocentesis revealed that the fetus was female, and the woman successfully continued the pregnancy and gave birth to a healthy girl. Her story was probably not exceptional. Amniocentesis was known to be a risky procedure, but in the 1960s and early 1970s, pioneers of prenatal diagnosis often dealt with women determined to go to great lengths, including a serious risk of miscarrying a healthy fetus, to prevent the birth of an affected child.[13]

The frequency of complications in Riis and Fuchs's first series of women who underwent amniocentesis was indeed very high. They learned from their experience that transvaginal punctures, possible earlier on in pregnancy, produced more complications than when they waited a couple of weeks and performed transabdominal amniocentesis. This meant, however, that in the case of a "positive" diagnosis, women underwent abortion during the mid- to late second trimester of pregnancy. Between 1960 and 1970, Riis and Fuchs performed amniocentesis for sex detection on twenty pregnant hemophilia carriers. They made a correct sex diagnosis in seventeen cases, an incorrect diagnosis in one case, and in two cases they failed to make a diagnosis because the amniotic fluid did not contain sufficient fetal cells. The single incorrect diagnosis was of a fetus diagnosed as a male. The woman elected to terminate the pregnancy, and Riis and Fuchs later found out that the fetus was female; they did not report if the woman was informed of their mistake. In one case, a woman who learned that she was carrying a male fetus and initially planned to have an abortion changed her mind after amniocentesis and decided to continue with the pregnancy. Her father had died just after her "positive" diagnostic test, and she felt unable to cope at the same time with her grief as well as an abortion. This woman later gave birth to a boy with hemophilia, a result presented by Fuchs and Riis as a failure to help a patient whose capacity for rational judgment was clouded by emotional factors.[14]

Prenatal diagnosis conducted by Riis and Fuchs had explicitly eugenic aims. The Danish law of 1956 made abortion legal "if there is a close risk that the child, due to inherited qualities, may come to suffer from mental disease or deficiency, epilepsy or severe and non-curable abnormality of physical disease."[15] The law did not openly encourage abortions, and women who wished to terminate their pregnancies due to a risk of hereditary disease had to receive permission from the Danish Mothers Aid and prove the presence of a hereditary condition in the family. Conversely, the language of the Danish law was unmistakably eugenic, not only in name but in content as well, pointing to continuities between the beginnings of prenatal diagnosis and earlier eugenic practices that aimed at reducing the frequency of birth defects in populations.[16] The Danish law addressed diseases present in families. Such conditions are relatively rare. In the 1950s, the improvement of methods to investigate human chromosomes made possible the extension of prenatal diagnosis to genetic anomalies that arise during the formation of egg and sperm cells, and are therefore present in the embryo (new mutations). Such anomalies—for example, the presence of an abnormal number of chromosomes or a deletion or duplication of parts of chromosomes—are more frequent than conditions transmitted in families and, as such, became one of the main targets of prenatal diagnosis.

Chromosomes and Birth Defects

In 1956, two researchers, Indonesian-American cytogeneticist Joe Hin Tjio and Swedish geneticist Albert Levan, developed a new method of staining human chromosomes. Until that time, the study of human chromosomes was an underdeveloped domain, because the existing staining methods did not allow for adequate visualization of each chromosome and distinction between chromosome pairs. Tjio and Levan's staining method—the suspension of cells in a medium with a low concentration of salt, which favored the separation of chromosomes (hypotonic solution), their cultivation in the presence of colchicine (plant alkaloid that favors the accumulation of cells arrested in the middle of the division process), and their gentle squashing before staining—overcame these difficulties. This new technique led to the observation that humans have forty-six chromosomes, not forty-eight as was previously believed (the normal chromosomal formula, or karyotype, for humans is usually abbreviated 46,XX for women and 46,XY for men).[17] Tjio and Levan's initial studies of human cells, performed in Levan's laboratory in Lund, Sweden, were conducted with lung cells from human embryos, which were easy to cultivate in a test tube. Levan was able to obtain these cells because abortion for a fetal indication was legal in Sweden, and as such researchers had relatively easy access to fetal tissue. From the very beginning, studies of human chromosomes were linked with abortion.[18]

The development of an efficient method to visualize and count human chromosomes made possible the study of aneuploidy, or the presence of an abnormal number of chromosomes in a cell.[19] The year 1959 was the "miracle year" of human cytogenetics—a discipline that studies genetic changes on the level of cells and chromosomes.[20] That year, three researchers from Necker Hospital in Paris—Raymond Turpin, Marthe Gautier, and Jérôme Lejeune—discovered that "mongolism" was correlated with the presence of three copies of the chromosome 21 (trisomy 21). In the late 1930s, pediatrician Raymond Turpin had already evoked the possibility of a chromosomal anomaly in Down syndrome. Marthe Gautier, also a pediatrician, had learned (in the United States) how to cultivate human cells in a test tube and had probably performed the majority of the experiments with trisomic cells; however, the recognition for these experiments mainly went to her colleague, and later leading French cytogeneticist, Jérôme Lejeune.[21]

The same year, a British group composed of geneticist Charles Ford, from the Medical Research Council's Radiobiology Unit at Harwell, physician and geneticist Paul Polani, from Guy Hospital in London, and their collaborators linked Turner syndrome—a condition characterized, among other things, by the underdevelopment of sex glands in girls—with an absence of one X chromosome (chromosomal formula 45,0X), while Patricia Jacobs and her group from the MRC's Human Genetics Unit at the Western General Hospital in Edinburgh linked Klinefelter syndrome—a condition characterized, among other things, by the underdevelopment of sex glands in boys—with the presence of a supplementary X chromosome (chromosomal formula 47,XXY).[22] The following year, geneticist Paul Edwards, from the University of Birmingham, described trisomy 18 (Edwards's syndrome), and Klaus Patau, from the University of Wisconsin–Madison, described trisomy 13 (Patau's syndrome).[23]

Descriptions of links between inborn defects and the presence of an abnormal number of chromosomes provided a powerful boost for the development of medical genetics, until then a relatively marginal domain of study.[24] As Canadian geneticist Clarke Frazer explained: "Genes were interesting hypotheses but here was a cause of genetic diseases that physicians could actually *see*."[25] Similarly, geneticist Paul Polani explained that the scientific uses and practical application of studies of chromosomes revolutionized human genetics but also medicine, and physicians grasped that clinical genetics is as important to the understanding of human pathology as anatomy and physiology.[26] The notion of "revolution in medicine" was extended to anomalies of sexual development as well. Howard Jones and William Wallace Scott, authors of an authoritative study on hermaphroditism (today, disorders of sexual development), explained in 1971 that when they published the first edition of their book in 1958, they did not expect to publish a second edition of this study so quickly. However, "fantastic developments" in cytogenetics had radically modified the understanding of anomalies of sex development, causing them to publish a new, considerably rewritten, edition of their book.[27]

In the early 1960s, the new field of cytogenetics was also discussed in popular science journals, which presented this domain as the science of the future. In his article "Mongolism, a Chromosomal Disease," of 1959, Jérôme Lejeune explained that while the mechanism that produces severe mental disability in people with this condition is unknown, there are now strong hopes of unraveling it, as well as developing a cure for mongolism and other constitutive pathologies produced by chromosomal anomalies.[28] The rise of cytogenetics and the development of methods to study human chromosomes led to a better understanding of chromosomal anomalies and their consequences. Nevertheless, hopes that linked circa 1960 with studies of human chromosomes, just as hopes linked circa 2000 with the decoding of the human genome, remained, for the most part, unfulfilled. Rapid growth in understanding the links be-

tween changes in hereditary material of the cell and birth defects was not followed by an equally rapid increase in possibilities of curing these defects—
a gap that was, and continues to be, the main source of dilemmas produced by
prenatal diagnosis.[29]

Studying Chromosomal Anomalies in Wisconsin

In the early 1960s, human cytogenetics was a new field in which researchers
grappled with the difficulty of correlating chromosomal anomalies and birth
defects. At first, geneticists hoped that their investigations would rapidly lead to
a description of precise correlations between specific changes in chromosomes
and well-defined impairments.[30] Such hopes were stimulated by the 1960s finding that sometimes Down syndrome was transmitted in families.[31] Researchers
later found that hereditary Down syndrome was an exceptional condition that
occurred when a duplicated fragment of the chromosome 21 in one of the parents became attached to a different chromosome (a balanced Robertsonian
translocation). The parent with such a translocation does not have extra chromosomal material and usually is not aware of the presence of a chromosomal
anomaly. However, during cell division and the formation of gametes (egg and
sperm cells), a balanced translocation can become an imbalanced one, and a
child can receive a surplus of genetic material.[32]

The studies of Patau and his collaborators at the University of Wisconsin illustrate the dilemmas and hopes of pioneers of studies of chromosomal anomalies in humans. The main participants of the Wisconsin group were geneticists
Patau and his wife, Eeva Therman, from the Department of Pathology and
Medical Genetics at the University of Wisconsin, Madison, and pediatrician David Smith, a well-known expert on birth defects from the pediatric department
of the same university.[33] The Wisconsin group collaborated with Canadian
geneticist Irène Uchida from the Children's Hospital in Winnipeg and occasionally with other US and Canadian geneticists and pediatricians. Patau and
his colleagues collected data on suspected chromosomal anomalies in aborted
fetuses, newborns, children, and adults, and attempted to correlate pathological
manifestations with cytological findings. This task was complicated by the difficulty of distinguishing between similar pairs of chromosomes—a problem
solved only in the 1970s thanks to the development of new staining techniques—
and the absence of a standardized system of naming chromosomes.

The nomenclature of human chromosomes was first established in an international meeting of geneticists in Denver, Colorado, in 1960. The Denver agreement was that each "autosome" (non–sex chromosome) be numbered by its

relative size, with the largest being designated "chromosome 1." Sex chromosomes continued to be called X and Y.[34] The Denver agreement facilitated comparative studies of chromosomal anomalies. This, however, did not solve all the problems of identifying specific chromosomes. Geneticists present at the Denver meeting also divided human chromosomes into seven visually distinguishable groups: A (1–3), B (4, 5), C (6–12, X), D (13–15), E (16–18), F (19, 20), and G (21, 22, Y). These groupings were officially recognized during a follow-up meeting of the Denver study group held in London in 1963. Chromosomes in each lettered group looked very similar, and until the development of new staining techniques in the 1970s they were difficult to tell apart, one of the main difficulties encountered by researchers in Patau's laboratory.[35]

The Wisconsin group was primarily interested in trisomies 21, 13, and 18, conditions in which one of the autosomal (nonsex) chromosomes exists in three copies. Many fetuses with trisomy 13 and 18 do not survive until birth, and children born with these conditions usually die during the first months of life, although a small number of these children, especially with trisomy 18, can survive longer.[36] In 1960, Patau and his collaborators described the first case of a condition they named "trisomy D" (later renamed trisomy 13) in a newborn who died shortly after birth and who had multiple structural anomalies.[37] In 1960, the description of this new syndrome was tentative; Patau and his colleagues mentioned only "extra autosome" or "extra chromosome," because they were not sure which chromosome was involved. At first, they were not even certain whether they were dealing with three copies of a chromosome or with a translocation.[38] In July 1960, Patau reported to Uchida that a woman who had two "mongol" children, and thus was suspected to be a carrier of a balanced translocation, had given birth to a normal healthy boy. Patau speculated at this point that at least some partial E and D syndromes (i.e., trisomies 18 and 13) represented translocations. He also expressed a hope that an extensive study of "mongolism" may lead to the mapping of the "mongolism chromosome." To do this, Patau suggested that an exhaustive list of all the anomalies linked with "mongolism" be created, focusing on those anomalies that appeared with great frequency, coding them on IBM punch cards, and searching for correlations between chromosomal anomalies and birth defects. He asked Uchida whether she would be interested in participating in such a project.[39] She agreed.

Uchida reported that she was quite disappointed that a girl she had studied— and who, she initially suspected, was trisomic—had only forty-six chromosomes but added that the girl might have some kind of translocation. Patau agreed with her hypothesis. He had the impression that one of this girl's G chromosomes was somewhat larger than the other. Another young patient who Patau believed had a "partial D syndrome" displayed more definitive signs of translocation.[40] In November 1960, Patau reported that he and his collaborators had finally obtained a "decent slide" from a young "E trisomic" and confirmed that the triplicate chromosome was definitively the chromosome 18. At that time, they were still struggling with the manifestation of partial D syndromes. The symptoms of this condition, they noted, seemed to be quite variable, with the exception of consistent mental retardation and a severe eye defect. Patau was also worried about a case reported by Uchida of a child diagnosed with D syndrome on the basis of cytological findings because the child looked "pretty normal," did not suffer from mental retardation, and had no eye anomaly. Patau stressed the importance of clarifying whether this child had a "true D syndrome" because he and his colleagues were eager to publish an article about this syndrome grounded in an analysis of all their cases.[41] Patau questioned John Edwards's hypothesis that a child they had described earlier had three chromosome 17s. Patau was relatively certain that the anomaly involved chromosome 18, as it was the case for other children they had investigated in Wisconsin.[42]

Uchida reported to Patau that they had another E trisomic (trisomy 18) child in their clinic who was described as suffering from a "mild form of this condition": a "mongol with 48 chromosomes, and an interesting family which showed some, but not all the 'stigmata of the E syndrome', a situation that sounded 'like a beautiful translocation.'"[43] In a letter to another geneticist, James Miller, Uchida mentioned a girl with D syndrome who had problems of variable severity and added: "It is becoming clear that component anomalies of the D syndrome manifest themselves much less regularly than we originally assumed."[44] In one of his letters to Uchida, Patau discussed a clinical case in which they at first suspected a D/E translocation but then decided that it was a straightforward case of D trisomy.[45] As late as 1965, Patau spoke about a "lethal G2 trisomy" (perhaps trisomy 22), a "partial D1 trisomy" (perhaps a mosaic case of trisomy 13), and a "non-mongoloid G trisomy," for which he added, "It is impossible at the present to make a decision between two possible interpretations."[46]

Taken together, the exchanges between Uchida and Patau show how difficult it was at first to stabilize new chromosomal anomalies. The first chromosomal anomalies described in 1959—"mongolism" (trisomy 21), TS (45,Xo), and KS (47,XXY)—were relatively frequent and were known to clinicians well before the advent of cytogenetics. Geneticists could thus examine the cells of many individuals with these conditions and correlate their karyotype (the number and appearance of chromosomes) with their phenotype (the organism's observable traits). At first, D and E syndromes were described in a very small number of cases, making it difficult to determine the typical traits of each anomaly. Trisomies 13 and 18 were later found to be less rare than initially believed. Uchida was especially skilled at spotting suspected chromosomal anomalies. In a draft of an article prepared with Patau and his group in 1962, she stated that D syndrome was "relatively common." Patau answered that "this caused some hilarity here, and will not sit well with many who are still looking for their first case. You better make some allowance for the particular favor you obviously carry with the Goddess of Chance."[47]

In a letter to Lionel Penrose, Patau noted the inconsistency of manifestations of nearly all the "stigmata" in "mongoloid" patients, especially in translocation cases. Penrose answered that one of the main problems in studying "mongoloid" individuals was the difficulty of quantifying their anomalies.[48] He speculated that the great variability of pathological manifestations in "mongolism" might reflect an incomplete expression of some of the triplicate genes.[49] In a meeting on birth defects at the Pediatric Section of the Royal Medical Society on May 27, 1960, Penrose stated that "mongolism" is one of the most baffling problems in pediatrics. The symptoms of this condition are highly changeable, and while some affected children have severe cardiac defects or leukemia, others are relatively healthy. Nevertheless, he expressed his hope that scientists would soon find the mechanisms responsible for anomalies found in people with "mongolism": "the problem is now on the way of solution, but we are only at the beginning of the journey."[50]

Pioneers of chromosome studies were especially interested in cases in which a patient had several chromosomal anomalies. Penrose had a human, and not only a scientific, interest in people with such anomalies. In 1959, he and his colleagues described a patient who had three 21 chromosomes (Down syndrome) and two X chromosomes together with a Y chromosome (KS).[51] This patient, Burt, later became Penrose's favorite. In 1965, Penrose received the Joseph P. Kennedy Foundation award for his contributions to the study of mental deficiency; he used the award money to establish the Kennedy-Galton Centre for Mental Deficiency Research and Diagnosis at Harperbury Hospital. After Penrose retired from his professorship at University College London, he dedicated all of his time to this center. In her biographic sketch of Penrose, Renata Laxova recalls that all of the visitors of the Kennedy-Galton Centre were taken to discuss politics with Burt, the most famous patient of Harperbury Hospital. Burt, Laxova explained, was the only child of intellectual parents saddened by the fate of their son, who, forgotten by all, spent his entire life in an institution for the mentally retarded. He had achieved, however, a special kind of fame. In a 1972 symposium dedicated to Penrose's memory, all the participants immediately recognized Burt's photograph when it was projected on a screen. Laxova added (apparently without irony) that she regretted that Burt's parents were not present at that meeting to witness their son's unique moment of triumph.[52]

Dermatoglyphs: Fingerprints and Aneuploidy

"Mongolism" is a classic "dysmorphic" condition, linked with the presence of typical traits: flat face, slated eyes, short neck, and "furrowed" tongue. One of the traits associated with "mongolism," researchers discovered in the 1930s, is an unusual pattern of dermatoglyphs—fingerprints and ridges (lines) on the palms and soles of the feet. In the 1930s, 1940s, and 1950s, dermatoglyphs were employed to confirm the diagnosis of Down syndrome. The redefinition of this syndrome as a trisomy 21 could have put an end to interest in dermatoglyphs as a diagnostic tool. This did not happen, however. In the 1960s and 1970s, researchers who studied chromosomal anomalies continued to study dermatoglyphs. Canadian historian of medicine Alice Miller argued that the persistence of studies of dermatoglyphs in the 1960s and 1970s, like the persistence of the term *mongolism*, reflected the difficulty of replacing earlier approaches to the study of a given problem with newer ones. The study of dermatoglyphs also facilitated the integration of older clinical practices into a new genetic framework and the construction of continuities between the prechromosomal and postchromosomal era.[53] Scientists' attachment to familiar research methods, and their reluctance to adopt new approaches, does not explain, however, why studies of dermatoglyphs were intensified in the 1960s and 1970s instead of being gradually phased out. To understand this seemingly paradoxical effect, one should examine an element absent from Miller's account: the role of dermatoglyphs in studying embryonic development. From the clinical embryologist's point of view, the rise of cytogenetics enhanced researchers' interest of dermatoglyphs.

The association of fingerprints with genetics preceded their association with criminology. In the late nineteenth century, scientists discovered that each person has a unique set of fingerprints. Francis Galton, one of the pioneers of the study of fingerprints (and of eugenics), believed that, thanks to their uniqueness, fingerprints would be particularly efficient tools to study hereditability. The use of fingerprints to identify criminals (first to prevent "identity theft" and later to link people to objects they manipulated) was an ulterior, and partly unanticipated, consequence of the investigation of their singularity.[54] Thanks to detective novels, films, and TV programs, the popular image of fingerprints is linked with criminal investigations. However, scientists continued to study fingerprints as unique markers of individuality.

In 1924, Norwegian researcher Kristine Bonnevie published an important study on papillary ridges in humans. Her study included a statistical evaluation of the frequency of specific configurations of lines at the fingertips as well as a chapter on fingerprints in identical twins.[55] In 1926, Harold Cummins, an anatomist from the University of Tulane, proposed to call the scientific study of skin ridge patterns on human hands and feet and of fingerprints "dermatoglyphics."[56] In the 1930s, Cummins displayed the remarkable stability of ridge counts, which, unlike many other morphological traits, remained identical in the individual's lifetime. Cummins and his collaborator Charles Midlo proposed to divide the ridges into four main structures: simple arches, ulnar loops, radial loops, and whorls. Using this standardized system, scientists were able to count the number of specific structures on each finger and produce a unique "formula" of dermatoglyphs of a hand. At the same time, Cummins and Midlo codified the nomenclature of the creases on the palms and soles of the feet.[57] The adoption of their system facilitated the comparison and tabulation of data collected in different sites.

Cummins was especially interested in links between fetal development and the rise in unusual patterns in hand- and footprints. He and his students studied fetal fingerprints, using the important collection of several thousand normal and abnormal fetuses in the university's anatomy museum. Cummins's collaborators recalled that in the 1930s, the shelves of Cummins's office in the anatomy department of the University of Tulane were filled with hand- and footprints of fetuses and newborns sent to him by scientists all over the world.[58] In the late 1930s, Cummins investigated the fingerprints and palm prints of "mongols," a topic also studied by other researchers.[59] It was investigated by Lionel Penrose and in the early 1950s by Raymond Turpin and Jérôme Lejeune, among others. All of these researchers were interested in the unique pattern of fingerprints and palm prints of "mongols" as it related to the (postulated) heredity of this condition.[60]

The finding that "mongolism" was produced by the presence of three copies of chromosome 21 did not diminish researchers' interest in dermatoglyphs of people with this and other aneuploidies. Such studies consolidated the results of the observation of chromosomes but also, as Uchida explained, provided insights about the expression of genes: "The fact that no two human beings have identical dermal patterns might mean, in conjunction with a considerable similarity of these patterns in monozygotic twins, that the development of these systems of ridges is sensitive to genetic variation at a very large number of loci. If so, this might explain why a majority of mongoloids show a combination of dermal peculiarities that are not found in normal persons."[61]

The study of dermatoglyphs of children and adults with chromosomal anomalies was especially important in the early 1960s, when the nomenclature and techniques of chromosome staining were not yet fully stabilized. In 1960, Uchida confirmed that a girl with a "suspected partial D syndrome" investigated by Patau also had a "D type dermal pattern."[62] In 1962, she reported to Patau that she was able to predict a chromosomal anomaly on the basis of fingerprints alone: "As soon as I saw the infant, I guessed that it was a 18 trisomic, but when I looked at the fingerprints—no arches—I predicted a translocation instead."[63] The child was finally diagnosed with a ring chromosome, a rare anomaly. In 1962, Uchida was among the initiators of a Canadian project called Project Dermatoglyphics. Its goal was to collect two thousand finger and palm prints of school-age children to be used as normal controls for investigators who may need them.[64] The constitution of a reference library of normal dermatoglyphs, Uchida explained, would facilitate the use of this technique for the diagnosis of chromosomal anomalies and would also be useful for fundamental research on such anomalies.

Lionel Penrose's studies of dermatoglyphs were directly linked to his interest in genes.[65] Penrose became interested in dermatoglyphs in the early 1930s, when researchers demonstrated a great degree of similarity in the fingerprints of identical twins and found variations of fingerprints that ran in families. Penrose believed that fingerprints were uniquely qualified to become genetic markers because of their stability throughout a person's life as well as their high level of heritability. In the 1940s and 1950s, Penrose examined dermatoglyphs of "mongols" and members of their families, looking for shared hereditary traits.[66] In the 1960s, he was persuaded that the study of dermatoglyphs of people with chromosomal anomalies would provide important insights about interactions between genes and their environment, as well as the expression of genes during embryogenesis. Penrose and his collaborators intensively studied hand- and footprints of people with chromosomal anomalies. They did not see dermatoglyphs as an outdated approach but as a sophisticated tool that could promote new understanding of what genes do and how they do it.[67]

In a letter sent to Patau in 1961, Penrose explained that studies of skinfolds and ridges shared by a "mongoloid" patient and other members of his family would help to elucidate the formation of "mongoloid traits."[68] Quantitative evaluation of fingerprint patterns, Penrose affirmed two years later, indeed demonstrated familiar transmission of traits strongly influenced by heredity, such as the "density" of ridges in fingertips.[69] He studied two families in which the father carried an equilibrated form of the same translocation as his "mongoloid" child. In both cases, the father's palms exhibited similar peculiarities to those of the affected child, although in a less pronounced form. One of the most persuasive proofs of the link between chromosomal anomalies and dermatoglyphic patterns, Penrose explained in 1963, came from studies of people with mosaic forms of chromosomal anomalies (individuals with a mixture of normal and abnormal cells). These people had an intermediate dermatoglyphic pattern: an attenuated form of finger and palm prints typical for a given chromosomal anomaly, such as trisomy 21 or KS.[70]

Dermal ridges on the fingertips, Penrose argued, are formed in the early stages of fetal development and may thus provide important insight into interactions between genes and their environment. The basic fingertip pattern is an inherited trait, but the size of loops and arches is an additional and independent variable affected by embryonic and fetal development. Penrose noted that women with TS (45,0X) had substantially larger fingertip patterns than "normal" women (46,XX). He associated this difference with the observation that fetuses with TS often develop edema (accumulation of fluid between the cells). It is probable that ridge formation is affected in a TS fetus by the increased accumulation of fluid in the hands and feet. Here, a genetic cause (the absence of one X chromosome in fetuses with TS) and its possible consequences (e.g., on the chemical composition of bodily fluids) produce a physiological effect (edema) that, in turn, exercises a mechanic influence on the size, but not on the original pattern, of fingerprints. This hypothesis, Penrose proposed, can, by extension, provide clues to mechanisms responsible for normal variations in heritable traits.[71]

Patau's collaborator David Smith similarly became interested in dermatoglyphs because he believed that their study would contribute to the understanding of embryogenesis. Smith assumed that ridges and creases on the hands are formed at the same time as the formation of the hand itself and therefore provide a historical perspective of the formation of the fetal hand. He then extended this view to the study of all anomalies of fetal hands. Specific malformations, such as additional fingers (polydactyly), fused fingers (syndactyly), missing fingers (ecrodactyly), or otherwise misshapen fingers, are highly sensitive indicators of an abnormal fetal development.[72] Smith's insight was later validated by ultrasound observations. When an increase in the resolution of obstetrical ultrasound made it possible to observe the development of fetal hands in early pregnancy, anomalies of the hand became a sensitive marker for fetal malformations, including numerous genetic anomalies.[73]

The 1960s and 1970s were a period of important expansion in the study of the links between dermatoglyphs and genetics. Researchers interested in this topic formed active international networks to exchange data, while international congresses of human genetics often included special sessions on dermatoglyphics.[74] Celebrating fifty years of dermatoglyphics in 1979, Wladimir Wertelecki and Chris Plato explained that "more recently there has been an accelerating interest in the methodology of dermatoglyphics, accompanied by the need for a methodology appropriate to address dermatoglyphic traits as developmental markers. An example is the pioneering work of the late Lionel Penrose."[75] The predicted expansion of the use of dermatoglyphs, especially fingerprints, as a major tool for studies of human development did not materialize, however. In the 1980s and 1990s, the development of new techniques of molecular biology enabled researchers to directly investigate patterns of gene expression during embryogenesis. Fingers and hands continue, however, to be seen as sensitive markers of anomalies of embryonic and fetal growth. Pregnant women who sometimes half-jokingly interrogate the ultrasound expert about whether the fetus has "ten fingers and ten toes" (code for "is everything is all right?") are seldom aware of how serious a risk there is of major fetal anomaly if the answer is "maybe not."

Amniocentesis and Prenatal Diagnosis

From 1959 on, researchers were able to detect the presence of an abnormal number of chromosomes in adults and children with conditions such as Down syndrome, KS, and TS. However, the history of the prenatal diagnosis of chromosomal anomalies was more complex. At first, the description of chromosomal anomalies was not linked with clinical applications, and even less with a possibility of diagnosing these conditions before birth. In the early 1960s, cytogenetics was seen mainly as a fundamental research topic. In 1962, Dr. Sheldon Reed, from the genetics department at the University of Minnesota, advised the mother of a "mongoloid" boy to ask Patau to perform a chromosome test on the boy. Patau answered that their laboratory dealt with basic research only and added that he believed that there was no need for specialized laboratories that could perform routine chromosome analyses. The existing research laboratories were sufficient because "the cases in which there is any kind of practical need for a chromosome analysis are usually also of some research interest."[76]

The technical possibility of studying fetal chromosomes and fetal cells radically modified this view.

In 1966, researchers showed that it was possible to study the chromosomes of fetal fibroblasts present in the amniotic fluid.[77] In 1968, Henry Nadler, from the Department of Pediatrics at Northwestern University's Feinberg School of Medicine in Chicago, developed a method of cultivating such fibroblasts, a technique that facilitated the detection of chromosomal anomalies of the fetus but also, Nadler stressed, the antenatal diagnosis of hereditary metabolic disorders.[78] In the 1950s and 1960s, the development of new biochemical methods such as paper chromatography made the detection of biochemical changes possible in small samples of cells. It was thus possible to detect the accumulation of abnormal metabolites in cultured fetal fibroblasts. In the two years that followed Nadler's initial article on the culture of fetal cells from the amniotic fluid, researchers were able to detect metabolic diseases such as Niemann-Pick disease, Tay-Sachs disease, Gaucher disease, maple syrup urine disease, mucopolysaccharidoses, and amino acid disorders before birth.[79] In many cases, women who had affected children, or who had lost children to a hereditary condition, refrained from pursuing another pregnancy. These women often strongly supported the development of a method that gave them the opportunity to give birth to a healthy child.

The development of paper and liquid chromatography also made possible the detection of the presence of abnormal hemoglobin in a fetus, a method employed in prenatal diagnosis of thalassemia (a hereditary blood disease). The first attempts of prenatal diagnosis of thalassemia in the United Kingdom were made following demands of patients who did not dare to be pregnant otherwise. The main difficulty of prenatal diagnosis of this condition was the sampling of fetal blood, a procedure that was much riskier for the fetus than amniocentesis. The doctors evaluated that it carried 7%–10% risk of postprocedure miscarriage. Moreover, the sampling of fetal blood is possible only in relatively advanced pregnancy (mid- to late second trimester). If the fetus was affected, the pregnant woman faced a stressful late abortion.[80] Women at risk of giving birth to a child with severe blood disease nevertheless felt that even such a high probability of pregnancy loss was acceptable when the result was the birth of a disease-free child.[81]

The possibility of culturing fetal cells in a test tube also opened the way for the prenatal detection of chromosomal anomalies. In the early 1970s, amniocentesis was, however, a risky procedure, and gynecologists proposed it only to women who had a high probability of giving birth to an impaired child, such as women with a family history of mutation or translocation that resulted in the birth of impaired children. French pioneers of cytogenetics Joëlle and André Boué initially studied the relationships between fetal death and maternal viral infections. In the mid-1960s, Joëlle Boué became interested in chromosomal abnormalities, another cause of fetal demise and birth defects. In 1970, she studied the amniotic cells of a pregnant woman whose first child had died from multiple malformations, shown after the child's death to be linked to a chromosomal anomaly. She had heard that Kurt Hirshorn's group in London had started to study chromosomal anomalies in fetal cells. The pregnant woman was sent to London to Hirshorn's service in the company of two French obstetricians who wanted to learn how to perform amniocentesis. They came back with a flask filled with the woman's amniotic fluid. Joëlle Boué cultivated the woman's fibroblasts, showed that these cells carried the same chromosomal anomaly as those of the woman's first deceased child, and recommended a termination of the pregnancy—the first abortion performed for a chromosomal anomaly in France.[82] Some experts agreed to perform amniocentesis if a woman already had one disabled child and feared the birth of another, even when they estimated that the chance of the woman having a second disabled child was very low.[83] John Edwards's laboratory at the Institute of Child Health in Birmingham offered such "compassionate" amniocentesis to all women who had had a child with Down syndrome, independently of their risk.[84]

Researchers who had learned how to perform amniocenteses and cultivate fetal fibroblasts in a test tube became rapidly interested in the detection of Down syndrome in pregnant women of "advanced maternal age," who had a higher risk of giving birth to a child with Down syndrome. Initially, such a test, seen as an experimental procedure, was performed only in a handful of research laboratories by scientists who studied chromosomal anomalies.[85] The introduction of ultrasound technology to visualize the trajectory of the needle used to aspire the amniotic fluid reduced the risk of postamniocentesis miscarriage to 1%–2%.[86] This technical improvement favored the extension of amniocentesis to an age related to Down syndrome risk.[87] At first, gynecologists proposed this test only to women older than 40, then to those older than 38, and then to those older than 35.[88] The shift from testing women with a known and elevated risk of giving birth to a child with a hereditary disease to the testing of women of an advanced maternal age for a nonhereditary risk of Down syndrome radically changed the nature of prenatal diagnosis.[89]

Both kinds of prenatal tests—a search for hereditary diseases and a search for an abnormal number of chromosomes—were performed in the same laboratories by the same specialists. Nevertheless, they qualitatively addressed different risks.

Women who knew that they and/or their partner were carriers of a hereditary condition had either a 50% probability of giving birth to an affected child (if the condition was dominant) or a 25% probability (if the condition was recessive, or X-linked). Before the development of prenatal diagnosis many among these women elected not to have children. Later, though, a risky diagnostic procedure became preferable to its frequent alternative: remaining childless. By contrast, women of an "advanced maternal age" had a much lower risk (1%–3% according to age) of giving birth to a child with Down syndrome. Moreover, many among these women were not aware of their risk. In the 1970s, physicians had to teach women about links between maternal age and Down syndrome. According to a *Lancet* editorial from 1977, only three hundred abnormal fetuses were aborted following a diagnosis of a fetal anomaly in the previous five or six years, a very modest dent in the annual total of about 100,000 abnormal babies born in Western Europe during that period. The editorial recommended an extensive campaign to educate women about the links between maternal age and Down syndrome.[90] Such educational efforts were successful. In the early 1980s, more women became aware of age-related risks, and some explicitly asked for amniocentesis.[91]

An additional element that favored the spread of prenatal diagnosis in the 1970s and 1980s was gynecologists' and obstetricians' aspiration to acquire new skills and extend their jurisdiction—and, especially in the United States, for fear of litigation. In several high-profile cases, women sued their gynecologists for not informing them of the possibility of prenatal diagnosis, therefore depriving them of the choice to abort an affected fetus.[92] A professional's push, rather than a user's pull, coupled with the fear of being sued for malpractice, was given as the main reason for the rapid expansion of prenatal diagnosis in the United States in the late 1970s. In 1979, a US ethicist explained that gynecologists increasingly believed that they had to persuade their patients (or at least those older than 35) to undergo amniocentesis or be liable for the lifetime support of a child with a birth defect.[93] The fear of litigation probably played a less important role, if any, however, in the diffusion of prenatal diagnosis in countries with a national health care system. Nevertheless, in these countries, too, the doctors' wish to prevent the birth of an impaired child—a traumatic experience for the family but often also for the pregnant woman's obstetrician—might have been linked with a parallel aspiration to extend gynecologists' professional jurisdiction.

Amniocentesis: Balancing the Risks

In the early 1970s, amniocentesis rapidly became an accepted diagnostic approach. In 1970, ten centers in the United States performed amniocentesis for a "genetic evaluation" of the fetus. In 1972, there were thirty such centers, and in 1975, that number had grown to fifty. Moreover, each center considerably increased its diagnostic activity.[94] The rapid diffusion of amniocentesis raised the question of its safety. Henry Nadler, who first adapted amniocentesis to diagnose fetal pathologies, defended the safety of this procedure, especially in experienced hands such as his own, but did not deny the possibility of complications.[95] In 1970, James Neel, one of the pioneers of US medical genetics, explained that amniocentesis, especially before the third trimester of pregnancy, was so new that physicians did not yet have exact data on its complications. Nevertheless, it was only a matter of time before physicians who performed amniocentesis would start to report complications for the fetus or the mother: "This is not a reason to abandon the procedure, but it does suggest the need to balance risk against gain."[96]

One of the major preoccupations of physicians who performed amniocentesis was whether this procedure could harm the future child. Physicians not only feared that this test would lead to the miscarriage of a healthy fetus but also that it would induce fetal anomalies. Studies from the 1970s indicated that such fears were baseless, however. Children born to mothers who underwent amniocentesis did not suffer from a higher proportion of birth defects than those born to mothers who did not undergo this diagnostic procedure. There was only one exception reported in the literature: a child born with a depression in the right buttock that could have been interpreted as a needle impression.[97] Experts also discussed the possibility of the sensitization of a Rh-negative mother against Rh-positive fetal red blood cells, a complication that might arise if fetal tissues entered the maternal bloodstream, and the possibility that the insertion of an amniocentesis needle would produce a hemorrhage or infection. These fears were also later dismissed as exaggerated. If the gynecologist who performed the test was skilled and experienced, the specialists concluded, risks for the mother were relatively minor: the main risk of this procedure was miscarriage.[98]

In the early 1970s, the risk of miscarrying a healthy fetus was the main reason that the majority of gynecologists agreed to perform this test only if the pregnant woman agreed beforehand to undergo an abortion in the case of a "positive" result. Numerous practitioners felt that even a small risk for the fetus was unacceptable if the pregnant woman and her partner rejected the option of abortion.[99] An early text on therapeutic abortion explains that "the self-evident and practical point should be stressed that abortion should be accepted and indeed, the necessary operative permits signed, before the diagnostic studies outlines here are launched. The establishment of a diagnosis should become the basis of therapeutic action rather than a basis for further worry and aimless discussion."[100]

An agreement for an abortion in case of a "positive" result was probably not an absolute rule. Henry Nadler mentioned the case of one of his patients, a physician's wife, who refused to abort a fetus with Down syndrome. Fritz Fuchs reported a case of a hemophilia carrier who changed her mind and did not abort a male fetus, and another expert, Dr. Jacobson, told of a woman whose fetus was diagnosed with Hurler syndrome (mucopolysaccharidosis type I, a very severe metabolic disease) who elected to carry her pregnancy to term. Such cases, however, were seen as exceptional and some as reflecting the physician's failure to persuade the woman to behave in a rational manner. Participants in early discussions on prenatal diagnosis viewed the termination of pregnancy to be a normal outcome of a "positive" prenatal diagnosis. As one of the experts put it: "It seems to me that all the gentlemen agree, some more explicitly than others, that to abort is a good thing and should be encouraged."[101]

In 1975, a large-scale study conducted by the United States Department of Health, Education, and Welfare, which evaluated the results of two thousand amniocenteses, concluded that while this technique was not entirely risk free, especially for the fetus, it was safe enough to become a routine test. In October 1975, the US government officially approved the clinical use of amniocentesis, and several health insurance companies started to cover its costs, estimated at $250 per test. The 1975 report recognized, nevertheless, that amniocentesis was not a perfect technique. Many hereditary conditions could not be diagnosed before birth, physicians reported diagnostic mistakes, and the test increased the risk of spontaneous abortion. It also could not be performed safely before twenty to twenty-two weeks of pregnancy, forcing women who received a "positive" result of prenatal diagnosis to undergo a mid- to late second trimester abortion. Still, the new approach was near unanimously described by US experts as an important service for pregnant women.[102]

In the United Kingdom, the MRC's working party, which analyzed more than 4,800 cases of amniocentesis in 1978, similarly concluded that amniocentesis was a reasonably safe diagnostic approach that could be introduced into routine clinical practice. The British report was more concerned than the US report about the hazards of this technique: increased risk of miscarriage but also of Rhesus autoimmunization. To prevent the latter complication, the report advocated an administration of anti-Rh serum to Rh-negative women who underwent amniocentesis. The UK working party also reported a puzzling increase in postpartum hemorrhage in women who underwent amniocentesis as well as an increase in respiratory difficulties at birth and orthopedic postural deformities in children born to women who underwent amniocentesis. The report concluded that the reported risks, although small, could not be totally dismissed and therefore recommended the continuation of careful follow-up of the women who underwent amniocentesis.[103]

The official statement that amniocentesis was safe enough for routine use spurred a debate about what "routine use" of a risky diagnostic procedure should be. In the United States, the American College of Obstetricians and Gynecologists proposed in 1976 that all pregnant women older than 35 should be offered the option of undergoing amniocentesis for Down syndrome risk. The partly arbitrary choice for the cut-off point of 35 years was legitimated by the claim that beyond that age, the risk of losing a healthy fetus following amniocentesis was smaller than the risk of giving birth to a child with Down syndrome. Discussing the results of the 1975 US report on the safety of amniocentesis, Theodore Cooper, from the US Department of Health, Education, and Welfare, strongly defended the use of this technique: "Few advances compare with amniocentesis in their capacity of prevention of disability. . . . [W]ith this technique we can assure the older woman who is pregnant that she need not fear a birth of a child with Down's syndrome and her consequent lifetime devoted to the care of a handicapped child."[104]

The recommendation to propose amniocentesis to all pregnant women older than 35 who wished to have this test—and if the test was not covered by the woman's health insurance, who could afford to pay for it—had concrete practical consequence: an important increase in the number of women who underwent amniocentesis. One of the main problems with the test was the need for women who learned that they carried a trisomic fetus to undergo an abortion at twenty-two to twenty-four weeks of pregnancy, and sometimes later. In the early 1980s, gynecologists developed a new method to obtain access to fetal cells: chorionic villus sampling. The sampling of chorionic villi (part of the placenta that contains fetal cells) can be performed until ten to twelve weeks of pregnancy. Therefore, a woman who receives a "positive" prenatal diagnosis result using this method is able to end her pregnancy at an earlier stage.[105] CVS was first developed by Chinese scientists in the 1970s; it was mainly employed in China to detect fetal sex, and the sampling was often made by a "blind" method, or without ultrasound guidance.[106] In the 1980s, Western gynecologists improved this technique, especially through the use of advanced ultrasound equipment. At that time, many specialists believed that CVS would replace amniocentesis; however, this was not the case. Some obstetrical units shifted to the use of CVS, but others continued to favor amniocentesis. Gynecologists who learned how to do amniocentesis, and who believed that this method of sampling fetal cells was safe in their hands, were reluctant to learn a new technique, especially one that was seen to be more dangerous for the fetus and, for some, to produce less reliable results.[107] The history of invasive diagnostic methods such as amniocentesis and CVS continued to be dominated by a need to balance the risk of giving birth to an impaired child with the risk of miscarrying a healthy fetus, and by the paucity of alternative solutions.

Metabolic Hopes

In the 1960s, many researchers believed that the description of the link between an abnormal number of chromosomes and birth defects was a first step in finding efficient cures for these defects. Jérôme Lejeune's "agregation de medicine" thesis, a dissertation that is part of the requirement to be named a professor at a medical school in France, was a slim volume of thirty-one pages, composed of three parts. The introduction briefly sketched the history of "mongolism" from its description by John Langdon Down in 1866 until the late 1950s and presented earlier theories on the origin of this condition. The second part of the thesis discussed the 1959 observation of the presence of three copies of chromosome 21 in individuals with "mongolism."[108] The third and most extensive part of the thesis developed Lejeune's ideas about the reasons for nondisjunction observed in people with trisomy 21 and the biochemical nature of this disorder, and was hopeful that an understanding of the chromosomal anomaly was the first step to finding a cure for this impairment. The IQ of individuals with "mongolism," Lejeune explained, decreases with time. Young children with this condition have a greater learning capacity and are more similar to nontrisomic children than teenagers and adults with "mongolism." The curious regression of the IQ of trisomic individuals, Lejeune proposed, may indicate that the mental handicap linked with this pathology may be a consequence of the accumulation of harmful substances, a view that was probably inspired by the phenylketonuria model. It should be possible, Lejeune concluded, to correct the faulty metabolic circuits of trisomic people and allow them to restore the mental capacities that they possess in principle but are unable to use. However, in order to be successful, such a biochemical correction should start as early as possible.[109]

In the 1960s and early 1970s, many geneticists and cytogeneticists believed that the diagnosis of a genetic cause of a pathological condition (mutation, translocation, aneuploidy) would be rapidly followed by an understanding of the underlying biochemical mechanism(s) as well as the development of cures. Such hopes were influenced by the success of the use of a low-phenylalanine diet as treatment for children with PKU. Although PKU was originally described as an inborn error of metabolism, this disease became rapidly known as a "paradigmatic" genetic condition.[110] As chair of genetics at the University of Edinburgh, Allan Emery's 1968 inaugural lecture was focused on lessons from PKU treatment. For a long time, Emery explained, genetics was the "Cinderella of medicine," an exclusive province of pedigree collections and mathematicians, and a domain shunned by clinicians. However, in the past ten years, there has been phenomenal growth in this subject thanks to the development of cytogenetics, biochemical techniques, and in vitro enzyme studies. In addition, clinical genetics now had its first impressive achievement: therapy for PKU. Emery then added that geneticists predicted that scientists would identify more than twelve thousand inborn errors of metabolism before the end of the twentieth century and expressed his hope that one day it would be possible to cure the majority of these conditions. In the meantime, physicians would be able to correct many of these conditions through nutritional and metabolic interventions, an approach named euphenic engineering by US geneticist Joshua Lederberg.[111]

PKU displayed the success of euphenic engineering.[112] In the mid-1960s, many industrialized countries adopted the screening of all newborns for this condition, and PKU-positive newborns were put on a low-phenylalanine diet. Such a diet prevents the accumulation of phenylalanine in the blood and its toxic effects on the developing brain.[113] Screening for PKU was hailed as an important breakthrough in the search for a cure for mental impairment. The success of this approach was, however, less spectacular than some of its schematized descriptions led one to believe. Initially, scientists believed that a low-phenylalanine diet had to be maintained only in childhood but later discovered that the negative effect of the accumulation of phenylalanine lasted a lifetime. People with PKU are advised to adhere to this special diet for their entire lives and still face diagnostic complications, treatment challenges, and imperfect outcomes. As Jeffrey Brosco and Diane Paul explain in their history of PKU, a common analogy is between PKU and diabetes: both were presented as disabilities that could be detected by a simple blood test and corrected by an intervention (insulin injection, special diet) that enabled a person with a given condition to lead a normal life. The analogy may be accurate, but in a very different way: the therapy for both conditions involves lifelong food restrictions and permanent medical management. The diet for PKU is very difficult to maintain and interferes with a person's social life: "In this way one strand of the history of PKU follows the contours of the discovery of insulin: the famous breakthrough of scientific medicine does indeed save lives and reduce morbidity, but only through the arduous and uncertain path of living with a chronic condition."[114]

People with PKU and those with type I diabetes share a struggle with dietary restrictions, but, unlike people with diabetes, many people with PKU are also confronted with cognitive difficulties. Some people with PKU have a lower capacity of functioning in the workplace, home, or school environment, and some develop psychological or psychiatric problems.[115] The negative effects of the accumulation of phenylalanine on their cognitive capacities can affect their ability to faithfully adhere to their diet, creating a vicious cycle of higher phenylalanine levels and continued cognitive impairment. The disorder itself, some experts proposed, is the greatest obstacle in the way of efficient treatment of the problems it induces.[116] PKU carriers who are aware of their status (usually because they had one affected child) rarely seek prenatal diagnosis.[117] Nevertheless, when both partners carried the PKU gene, some couples attempted preimplantation genetic diagnosis: in vitro fertilization, the selection of mutation-free embryos, and then the implantation of these embryos. The UK Human Fertilisation and Embryology Authority (HFEA) validated this approach.[118] In 2014, the HFEA included PKU among pathologies that justified preimplantation genetic diagnosis, an indirect recognition of the difficulties of raising children with this condition.[119]

In the 1970s, the exemplary success of PKU treatment was highly visible albeit complex trade-offs. Many scientists were persuaded that PKU was the first in a long list of hereditary and metabolic diseases that would soon be cured. Lejeune's group at the Necker Hospital in Paris was one among many groups that looked for metabolic perturbation in children and adults with Down syndrome and other intellectual disabilities. A meeting held in 1971 at the CIBA Foundation in London under the auspices of the Institute for Research into Mental Retardation summed up studies on biochemical and cytological anomalies in people with diseases linked with mental impairment, above all, Down syndrome. Researchers followed numerous leads: excessive reactions of the immune system, abnormal enzymes, faulty function of the sodium pump, endocrinological defects, unusual concentrations of metabolites, and problems with RNA synthesis. All of these leads were investigated in the hope that the correction of one or several physiological anomalies in people with Down syndrome would halt the loss of intellectual abilities produced by the presence of an additional chromosome 21.[120]

Activities of the Birth Defects Group of the MRC, based at University College London and partly financed by the Rayne Foundation, illustrate the interest in correcting inborn metabolic defects. In the early 1970s, this group investigated the possibility of preventing birth defects through a creative linking of metabolic studies with pediatric research. A memorandum of the Birth Defects Group explained that one of the central axes of the group's study was a search for inborn errors of metabolism, especially among mentally retarded and physically defective children. The memorandum stressed that the work of the group "is motivated by the belief that prevention can be achieved if the problems are tackled at their beginning, by discovering and removing their causes: that research in preventing abnormalities is of even greater importance than the finding of ways to mitigate disabilities or to patch up deformed organs later in life."[121]

In 1973, Charles Dent, professor of human metabolism at University College London Hospital Medical School, submitted a grant application that proposed to investigate abnormal quantities of metabolites in premature and other infants in order to find new, inherited causes of mental defects, and then to find ways to correct these defects.[122] In 1974–1975, the Birth Defects Group still mentioned a "search for abnormal metabolites in mentally retarded children" among their activities, but then this research topic disappeared from their agenda in the mid-1970s. Members of this group began to focus on other metabolic studies in fetuses and newborns, such as the management of babies with inborn metabolic disorders, absorption of nutrients and water by the placenta, and exchange of fluids in fetal lungs. In the late 1970s, the group's researchers arrived at the conclusion that, at the present stage of knowledge, it was not possible to correct the effects of the presence of an abnormal number of chromosomes. What was seen as possible—and was vigorously pursued in London and elsewhere—was the extension of screening for treatable metabolic diseases such as thalassemia and sickle cell anemia, diffusion of newborn screening for these conditions, and their prenatal diagnosis.[123]

Jérôme Lejeune was one of the rare experts who, in the late 1970s, did not abandon the hope of curing inborn defects through the manipulation of fetal and newborn metabolism. A conservative Catholic and fervent opponent of abortion (he later became a member of the Pontifical Academy and after his death a candidate for beatification), Lejeune strongly opposed the implementation of prenatal diagnosis in France. He continued to be persuaded that research in cytogenetics should, above all, aim to produce therapies. Thanks to Lejeune's enthusiastic support of searching for a cure for Down syndrome, a research group in his laboratory, headed by Marie-Odile Réthoré, continued to study metabolic changes in Down syndrome patients long after this topic was abandoned by other laboratories.[124] Other specialists gave up the hope of quickly finding a cure for inborn anomalies. In the absence of such a cure, the best "doable" solution was to offer pregnant women the option to abort an affected fetus. Such an approach, they argued, could be legitimately seen as "prevention," because it disallowed the suffering of sick children and their families, and alleviated a heavy financial burden for society.[125]

Genetic Counseling

In the early days of prenatal diagnosis, many physicians were not aware of the distress produced by terminating a pregnancy for a fetal indication. At that time, many professionals viewed the "flawed" fetus as a problem and its removal as a solution to this problem. Specialists who developed prenatal diagnosis often encountered women who were aware of the presence of a severe hereditary disease in the family and were willing to go to great lengths to avoid the birth of an impaired child. Accordingly, many were persuaded that the majority of pregnant women wished, above all, to free themselves of an impaired fetus. Pain and discomfort linked with an induced abortion were perceived as unavoidable elements of a necessary medical treatment, not very different from the distressing side effects of a required surgical operation.

Discussing rubella in pregnancy in 1959, British geneticist Julia Bell, from the Galton Laboratory at University College London, implicitly presented abortion as an inevitable consequence of the existence of an important risk for the child, the child's family, and society: "There is no doubt that rubella in the early weeks of pregnancy is such a menace to the normal development of the fetus that it constitutes a risk one cannot allow to be taken for the unborn child."[126] Reflecting on her investigation of birth defects induced by the drug thalidomide, US pediatrician Helen Brooke Taussig defined the problem of "therapeutic abortion" as a decision to delay the birth of a child: "It does not make any difference whether your child was one year older or younger, compared to whether you had a normal child or a malformed child, or a mentally defective child. Almost anyone would much rather postpone their pregnancy a year and have a normal child than go through a pregnancy when one knew the child has been injured by German measles or injured by thalidomide."[127] Discussing the advantages and disadvantages of prenatal diagnosis, Edinburgh geneticist John Smith provided an extreme version of this argument in

1973. One of the problems of prenatal diagnosis, Smith explained, is the predicted "dilution" of its effects: it may be easy to prevent a few cases in high-risk pregnancies, but the law of diminishing returns may set in, and the cost per case prevented is likely to increase with a shift to widespread testing of pregnancies at moderate risk. One possibility of preventing such an increasing cost per case is to move from prenatal to neonatal screening: "It is salutary to note that further liberalization of legislation to allow euthanasia of defective newborns would make antenatal diagnosis largely unnecessary. However, this is unlikely for some time, so that antenatal diagnosis should remain a useful tool in the prevention of genetic disease."[128]

Physicians increasingly realized, however, that women who decided to terminate a pregnancy following a diagnosis of fetal malformation perceived the abortion as a traumatic event, not merely as a convenient solution to a problem or a delay of their childbirth project.[129] Such trauma was initially thought to be associated only with late abortions but was later found to be linked with terminations of pregnancy for a fetal indication at all stages for many women.[130] Women who considered amniocentesis, "moral pioneers" in anthropologist Rayna Rapp's felicitous expression, were aware of the possibility that they were embarking on a perilous journey.[131] The rapid institutionalization of the profession of genetic counselors in the United States and Canada was directly related to a growing demand for amniocentesis by women who were at risk of giving birth to a child with a hereditary condition as well as a parallel growth in demand for counseling about this diagnostic act and its consequences.[132]

Before the development of prenatal diagnosis, genetic counselors (at that time physicians or geneticists) had already provided nondirective advice on reproductive choices to families with an identified hereditary disorder. If a woman from such a family found herself pregnant, a genetic counselor estimated the odds that the fetus carried the hereditary disorder. Such an estimation helped the woman cope with uncertainty but also, not infrequently, decide whether she wished to continue the pregnancy. Before the official legalization of abortion in the late 1960s and early 1970s, women could not terminate a pregnancy for fetal indications; the sole exception were Scandinavian countries that had legalized "eugenic" abortion. In practice, however, affluent Western women usually had access to safe abortion. Moreover, countries such as the United Kingdom or France quietly tolerated abortions for fetal indications recommended by physicians.[133] When prenatal diagnosis became available, genetic counselors provided advice on amniocentesis, and on including it for an advanced maternal age, an intervention seen as a natural extension of their previous tasks. Such advice was especially important in the early 1970s, when amniocentesis was linked with considerable risks to the fetus.

Professional genetic counselors increasingly specialized in the management of dilemmas linked with the introduction of prenatal diagnosis and became part of the "prenatal diagnosis dispositif." Because of their central role in providing advice on invasive testing, genetic counselors became involved in decisions about fetal conditions unrelated to changes in the genetic material of the cell, such as neural tube defects, detected thanks to the presence of markers for this condition in a pregnant woman's blood or amniotic fluid. In a typical sample of fifteen Canadian women who, in 1979, consulted genetic counselors before undergoing amniocentesis, ten elected to have this test because of their age, two had children with a nonhereditary disability, and just three were carriers of a hereditary disorder.[134] With the extension of ultrasound diagnosis, genetic counselors also provided advice on structural anomalies detected by ultrasound: heart or brain malformation, absence of a limb, or skeletal deformations, for example. Occasionally, the terms *termination of pregnancy on genetic ground* or *genetic abortion* became synonyms of an abortion for a fetal impairment.[135] In this context, the "genetic" in the term *genetic counseling* became closer to "generation" than to the usual meaning of the term *genetics*.

In the 1970s, genetic counseling in the United States was often shaped by women with feminist concerns who wished to provide advice on reproductive and parental choices. Genetic counselors believed then that they should be especially attuned to the plight of women who ended a wanted pregnancy and to support them in all stages of the process, including the act of abortion itself. The professionalization of this domain, and the need for counselors to defend the specificity of their jurisdiction, favored the interest in the psychosocial aspects of counseling (since the scientific aspects remained under the control of clinical geneticists) and the rise of a distinct professional ethos of detachment and neutrality. Such an ethos led to the abandon of an earlier, more emotional involvement with clients but also of more directive approaches that may have been perceived by some women as oppressive and authoritarian.[136]

One of the elements that favored the development of an ethos of nondirective genetic counseling was a wish to deflect allegations that genetic counselors, directly involved in providing advice on the termination of pregnancy to carriers of hereditary disorders, favored a "eugenic" elimination of imperfect children. In the 1970s, such accusations were not only made by conservative opponents of abortion but also by some feminist critics. These accusations were not entirely groundless. Eugenic considerations were indeed present in the work of some of the pioneers of prenatal diagnosis, such as Cedric Carter, who headed the clinical genetic department at the Great Ormond Street Hospital in London and was one of the pioneers of clinical genetics in the United Kingdom. Moreover, there were important continuities between post–World War II eugenics and clinical genetics.[137] Prenatal diagnosis' advocates categorically rejected accusations of a "eugenic" drift. They explained that the principles that guided prenatal diagnosis were radically different from those propagated by eugenicists. Eugenicists aspired to improve the gene pool of a given population and believed that the promotion of collective well-being should take precedence over individual aspirations. Prenatal diagnosis was grounded in women's right to freely choose whether they wished to give birth to a disabled child and was totally disconnected from considerations of the frequency of "defective" genes in populations.

Prenatal diagnosis promoters also argued that prenatal diagnosis of recessive, or X-linked, hereditary conditions was dysgenic rather than eugenic. Women who previously remained childless because they were aware of the presence of a hereditary disease in the family now gave birth to children who frequently were carriers of "defective" genes: prenatal diagnosis thus increased the frequency of such genes in populations.[138] Finally, prenatal diagnosis advocates contrasted past interventions of health professionals who gave authoritative advice to carriers of "flawed" genes to refrain from having children because they aspired to limit the presence of genetic diseases in the population with the ethos of present-day genetic counselors who believe that people are free to make their own reproductive decisions, whatever they may be. The latter claim is not entirely accurate. In the twenty-first century, genetic counselors are frequently interested in the prevention of birth defects. The main difference is the advent of new ways to reach this goal. Thanks to the development of prenatal diagnosis (which makes possible a selective abortion of mutation-carrying fetuses, often early in pregnancy) and of preimplantation genetic diagnosis (which makes possible a selective implantation of embryos free of the targeted genetic anomaly), genetic counselors no longer attempt to persuade people who may give birth to impaired children to remain childless but rather provide advice on alternative ways to produce healthy children.[139]

The principle of absence of directive advice in genetic counseling, gradually adopted by the professionals in this domain, assumes that the counselors will remain entirely neutral, and if they happen to have an opinion about the desirable conduct of users of their services, they will never let it be visible.[140] In practice, counselors may oscillate between a presentation of patients' options in a way that makes their own views visible (an attitude that can hurt users who disagree with these views) and a reluctance to express any opinion (which can be read by the users of their services as abandoning them in a difficult moment of their life).[141] There are not many investigations about the ways in which genetic counselors deal with this dilemma today.[142] There is, however, one detailed study of the ways in which genetic counselors dealt with these issues in the early days of the development of prenatal diagnosis: the book *All God's Mistakes*, written by US sociologist and bioethicist Charles Bosk.[143]

In the late 1970s, Bosk was invited by genetic counselors (in his study, physicians) to observe their work, because, they explained, an external regard on the problem they faced would help them improve the quality of their services. Later, Bosk discovered that one of the reasons they asked him to study their work was that they hoped he would produce data that would confirm the need to increase funding for genetic counseling.[144] Genetic counselors, Bosk had discovered, were, in his words, "a bunch of good people involved in dirty work." They provided a "mopping-up" service, cleaning up others' messes and doing more than their share of the low-status hand-holding. Their work was "dirty" because they dealt with what they referred to as "all God's mistakes"—conditions for which no treatment existed. They were not able to offer good solutions but, at best, not-as-bad ones. The counselors described by Bosk were physicians and not, as the majority of genetic counselors in US hospitals are today, graduates of specialized MSc programs. However, they occupied a relatively low place within the "pecking order" of the hospital, and more prestigious physicians often "dumped" on them the ungrateful task of being the bearers of bad news. They also had little to offer following the announcement of a "positive" prenatal diagnosis result. Their insistence on the autonomy principle was frequently an excuse for abandoning their patients. Conversely, Bosk noted, in some cases such an abandonment of patients by professionals was not an entirely negative development because families were given a private space for making difficult decisions.[145]

Some of the dilemmas of prenatal diagnosis described by Bosk in the late 1970s were alleviated later. In the 1970s, geneticists were frequently asked by the mother of a disabled child whether the child's condition was hereditary and what the probability was that she would have another child with the same condition. Very often, they were unable to answer this question. In 2017, thanks to the rapid development of ways to diagnose genetic anomalies, genetic counselors are often able to provide more precise advice to prospective parents than the professionals studied by Bosk.[146] Nevertheless, many of the problems described in *All God's Mistakes* are present forty years later. Physicians still do not know how to treat the majority of fetal anomalies, and people with hereditary conditions still face difficult choices. Moreover, the rise of prenatal diagnosis has led, as Bosk predicted, to an increased individualization of medicine and a greater focus on personalized solutions rather than on the extension of social responsibility for the sick.[147] Genetic counselors continue to promote a discourse about prenatal testing that focuses on maximizing health and minimizing risk via responsible individual choices and adhere to the principle of an ever-expanding scope of genetic testing: "it just becomes much more complicated."[148]

CHAPTER 3

Human Malformations

Environmental Teratogens and Birth Defects

The rise of the prenatal diagnosis dispositif is linked with biomedical innovations but also with an important social change: the legalization of abortion. This statement needs to be qualified. Before the decriminalization of abortion, physicians, at least in the United Kingdom and France, often quietly offered women the option to terminate a pregnancy if it was suspected that the future child might be severely impaired. Although such interventions were illegal, they were tolerated by the authorities.[1] In these countries, the decriminalization of abortion was more important for women who aborted for "social" reasons (the great majority of all abortions) than for those who terminated a pregnancy for a fetal indication.[2] Nevertheless, changes in the status of abortion played an important role in the rapid diffusion of prenatal diagnosis. In 1960, only a handful of countries (e.g., Scandinavian countries, Japan) legalized abortion. Fifteen years later, abortion was decriminalized in numerous industrialized countries, facilitating legal and safe abortions for fetal malformations.

The liberalization of abortion is often presented as a direct consequence of the sexual revolution of the 1960s, while the advent of a (presumed) radical change in sexual mores is attributed to the development of the contraceptive pill and the rise of the women's movement.[3] The proposed chronology may be inaccurate. More liberal attitudes toward sexuality might have preceded the generalization of an efficient and reliable form of contraception in many cases.[4] Conversely, changes in sexual mores, greater access to education and prestigious segments of the labor market for women, and an increase in women's political influence and power did not automatically lead to a liberalization of abortion. In Ireland, Poland, and nearly all of the Latin American countries, women also greatly increased their sexual freedom, achieved legal equality, became the majority of university students, increasingly entered the workforce, and, today, occupy important economic and political positions but as of the time of this writing do not have the right to terminate an unwanted pregnancy. Moreover, in some countries, especially the United States, this right is increasingly contested and threatened. Inversely, Japan legalized abortion in 1948 under the Eugenic Protection Law, a development that was primarily the result of the government's aspiration to reduce the nation's birth rate and was not linked with a fight for women's rights.[5] Changes in sexual mores and in women's legal and professional status undoubtedly played a role in the modification of abortion laws in Western Europe and North America. In addition, however, two dramatic and widely publicized events—the thalidomide scandal of 1961 and the German measles epidemic of 1962–1964—brought to the fore the role of environmental teratogens (agents that produce fetal malformations) and contributed to an important shift in the perception of abortion.[6]

In 1962, thalidomide, a popular tranquilizer developed in 1957 and often used by pregnant women to alleviate morning sickness, was found to be responsible for the birth of deformed children. The link between the uptake of this drug and an epidemic of malformations, especially the absence of limbs (phocomelia), was first proposed by an Australian physician, William McBride, in a 1961 letter to *The Lancet*.[7] Other researchers confirmed McBride's findings.[8] Well-known US pioneer of pediatric heart surgery Helen Brooke Taussig heard about the suspicion that thalidomide induced fetal and neonatal malformations from a German doctor, Alois Beuren. In the summer of 1961, Taussig decided to travel to Germany to find out more about this issue. After interviewing several German doctors, she was convinced that the drug (named Contregan in Germany) was indeed responsible for the observed malformations, but only when taken at a precise moment during early pregnancy. The short time during pregnancy in which thalidomide induces teratogenic effects explained why many women who took the drug gave birth to normal babies. Taussig wrote an article about the drug for the popular journal *Scientific American* and insisted that it should be illustrated with photographs of malformed children. Her views helped block the marketing of thalidomide in the United States.[9] The thalidomide disaster led to a modification of the surveillance of drugs in the United States. According to the new rules, industrialists were obliged to test all new drugs for their capacity to induce birth defects (teratogenesis), while doctors were warned that they should be especially careful when prescribing medication to pregnant women.[10]

In 1962, Sherri Finkbine, a TV presenter from Arizona, discovered that she had taken thalidomide early in her pregnancy. The medical board in Arizona at first granted her the right to an abortion on medical grounds, but when she went public with her story in order to warn other women about the danger of taking thalidomide, the hospital in which she was expected to have her abortion refused to perform the procedure, fearing negative publicity. Finkbine sued the hospital and spoke publically about her predicament but finally was forced to travel to Sweden to terminate her pregnancy.[11] Twenty other women who took thalidomide were encouraged by Finkbine's highly publicized example to do the same, but the Swedish medical board gave permission to only one among them, claiming that they did not want to transform Sweden into the abortion capital of the world.[12] Finkbine's dramatic story was an ideal vehicle for the claim that abortion may be justified in certain cases. Finkbine was a white, middle-class, educated, devoted mother of four children and the animator of a popular children's TV show (later, she lost her job over the abortion controversy). She was thus very different from the stereotypical image of an immoral and irresponsible lower-class woman who seeks an illegal abortion.[13]

In 1962–1964, outbreaks of rubella again caused many women to fear that they would give birth to deformed children. From the 1940s on, doctors were aware of the link between rubella (German measles) and fetal malformations.[14] The increased visibility of such malformations during the 1962–1964 epidemic might have reflected the heightened sensitivity of the problem produced by the thalidomide scandal. Physicians estimated that a rubella infection produced major fetal malformation in 15%–20% of affected pregnant women and probably early pregnancy loss in many others.[15] In the 1960s, doctors could confirm a rubella infection in a pregnant woman by measuring the rise in the titer of specific antiviral antibodies in her blood, but they were not able to verify if her fetus would be affected by this infection.[16] Experts were divided on whether a woman should be able to request an abortion when she knew she was infected by the rubella virus early in pregnancy.[17] Some physicians believed that the risk of birth defects produced by such an infection was not high enough to legitimate abortion in each case, since such an act would eliminate many healthy fetuses as well. Others, such as Julia Bell from the Galton Laboratory at University College London, believed that such risk was considerable and fully justified abortion.

In 1959, Bell explained in a widely debated text that "the facts of the situation have accumulated so that one can state without doubt that rubella in the early weeks of pregnancy is such a menace to the normal development of the foetus that it constitutes a risk one cannot allow to be taken for the unborn child."[18] Answering critical comments on her paper, Bell added that the problem of birth defects induced by infection by the rubella virus are both individual and collective: "There are three main aspects of this problem concerned with (a) the risks of severe handicap to the unborn child, (b) the risks of acute distress and difficulty for the potential parent, perhaps for the rest of her life, (c) the burden likely to rest upon the Welfare State. I appreciate the difficulty in reaching a decision in certain cases, but these must be very rare and do not touch the main problem."[19] According to British obstetrician Bevis H. Brock of St. Bartholomew's Hospital, there was widespread agreement that "when a pregnant mother, having had rubella, is aware of the risks and is prepared to face them, then no one would try to persuade her to accept termination. But if she feels unable to face the appalling anxiety of a pregnancy overshadowed by fear of a blind or deaf child, then it requires strong convictions to refuse this request."[20] Abortion, geneticist Julia Bell proposed, had become the generally recognized treatment for the risk of fetal malformation induced by a rubella virus infection: "To such an extent has this become routine treatment that maybe we can no longer hope to get measure of the risk involved or discover what proportion of such occurrences can be expected to result in a normally developed child."[21]

The thalidomide disaster and rubella epidemic led to an important change in lay and professional attitudes toward abortion. Doctors who previously were not very interested in the abortion question suddenly faced numerous demands for pregnancy terminations, many among them from middle-class women, and were obliged to rethink their position on this issue. At the same time, many physicians realized that upper-class women who feared for the fate of their child, but also those confronted with an unwanted pregnancy, frequently found a way to obtain a safe termination of their pregnancy, while lower-class women disproportionably suffered from the consequences of risky abortions. For example, in New York, the great majority of women able to obtain a legal abortion on medical grounds in the 1960s were white; the great majority of those who died as a result of a botched back-alley abortion were black.[22] Change in doctors' attitudes toward the termination of pregnancy favored the decriminalization of abortion in numerous Western countries.[23]

In the United States, in 1967 Colorado and California legalized abortion for pregnancies that resulted from rape or incest, for pregnancies that threatened the life of the mother, or for pregnancies of severely handicapped children. Over the next three years, Alaska, Arkansas, Delaware, Georgia, Hawaii, Kansas, Maryland, Mississippi, New Mexico, North Carolina, Oregon, South Carolina, and Virginia passed similar legislation. In 1970, New York became the first state to offer unrestricted abortion during the first twenty-four weeks of pregnancy. Hawaii, Alaska, and Washington soon followed. The wave of legalizations changed the attitudes of doctors in states where abortion was still criminalized. For example, female students at Yale University were informed in 1970 that if they got pregnant, the university would help them get a safe abortion, despite the fact that abortion was still illegal in Connecticut at that time.[24] In 1973, the US Supreme Court, in the *Roe v. Wade* case, made "abortion on demand" the law in the United States. Abortion was made legal in the United Kingdom in 1967, and in France in 1975.

The US law did not initially put time limits on abortion on demand; later, such limits were established by state legislations. In the United Kingdom, such a limit was fixed at twenty-four weeks, defined as the limit of fetal viability. Other countries produced more restrictive abortion laws. Until 2001, an abortion on demand was possible in France only up to ten weeks of pregnancy; this period was extended to twelve weeks in 2001, and then to fourteen weeks in 2008. The French law distinguished abortion for "personal" reasons (interruption volontaire de la grossesse, or IVG) from abortion for "medical" reasons. The latter, initially named "therapeutic interruption of pregnancy," included risks for the mother but also fetal malformations that would result in severe and incurable disease or disability of the future child. Fetal indications rapidly became the main reason for a "therapeutic" abortion, later renamed "medical termination of pregnancy" to avoid the impression that the elimination of a fetus is a "therapy" (interruption médicale de la grossesse, or IMG).

With the legalization of abortion for fetal indications, laws in many industrialized countries created a new legal entity: the "unacceptable" fetus.[25] The refusal of such a fetus—unlike the rejection of a fetus by a woman who found herself pregnant and who did not wish to become a mother—is produced by the "prenatal diagnosis dispositif": the application of new diagnostic technologies (amniocentesis and obstetrical ultrasound) and experts' interpretations of the data produced by these techniques. Public debates on prenatal diagnosis are frequently focused on hereditary diseases and genetic anomalies such as Down syndrome, but a significant proportion of abortions for fetal indications are justified by a direct observation of major fetal malformations. For example, in 2012, 45.2% of abortions for fetal indications in France were legitimated by structural malformations, 40.6% by chromosomal indications, and 6.0% by the presence of known hereditary conditions.[26] The "unacceptable fetus" is frequently a visibly malformed one.

From Teratology to Dysmorphology

Clinicians observe. One of the main elements in the differentiation between the normal and the pathological in modern scientific medicine is the central place of the clinical gaze. Before the nineteenth century, physicians relied not only on sight but also on other senses: smell, hearing, touch, taste. Touch retained some of its importance in modern medicine, too, especially in surgery and pathology, but from the nineteenth century on the main analytical sense of the physician was sight. The birth of clinical medicine, Michel Foucault argued, was directly linked with physicians' capacity to correlate disease symptoms in living patients with changes in organs and tissues observed during a dissection. A central trait of the modern clinic is "the care with which it silently lets things surface to the observing gaze without disturbing them with discourse."[27] Clinicians learned through training and experience to decipher traces left by disease in patients' bodies. Images in anatomical atlases favored the circulation of knowledge about visible signs of disease and facilitated the homogenization of classifications of pathological conditions.[28] Pioneer of the sociology of science Ludwik Fleck drew on his experience as a bacteriologist and immunologist to study how scientists and doctors learned to perceive specific elements of observed entities as "signals" and to eliminate others as "noise." Thanks to the acquisition of specialized knowledge and skills, especially the training of the eye, bacteriologists acquired an ability to perceive typical images of bacteria at a glance under a microscope, dermatologists learned how to read subtle changes in the skin, and general practitioners became increasingly able to grasp changes in a patient's behavior.[29]

The art of clinical medicine often relies on the reading of subtle signs of pathological change; however, sometimes the signs are extreme rather than subtle. John Ballantyne's involvement in prenatal care was rooted in his earlier interest in teratology—the study of monstrous births.[30] For a long time, teratology was mainly a subdivision of embryology and a branch of experimental biology. Scientists who investigated the development of embryos and fetuses in laboratory animals knew that such development can be disrupted by numerous physical, chemical, and infectious agents. They also knew that substances given to a pregnant female affected fetal development. Physicians who treated pregnant women had, however, limited contact with the scientists who investigated fetuses in the laboratory. Moreover, many believed that the human placenta acted as a "filter," able to reject substances that might harm the fetus.[31] The thalidomide disaster of 1961–1962 disproved this belief. Physicians found out that a seemingly innocuous drug taken by pregnant women in the early stages of pregnancy induced severe malformations of the newborn child, and that the placenta did not protect the fetus from the effects of harmful substances in maternal circulation. The thalidomide scandal coincided with the rise of the ecologist movement. Rachel Carson's *Silent Spring*, the book that played a key role in the development of this movement, was published in the fall of 1962, at the height of the revelation on the disastrous effects of thalidomide on fetal development.[32] The wave of birth defects induced by thalidomide provided a dramatic illustration of the claim that toxic chemicals literarily produced monsters and endangered the future of humanity. The combined effect of the thalidomide disaster and the rapidly growing interest in environmental risks, in turn, favored the growth of teratology and an application of research in this area to clinical medicine.

Before the 1970s, only a handful of experts were interested in the study of birth defects in humans. One of the leading US experts on this subject was pediatrician Josef Warkany.[33] Born and educated in Vienna, Austria, in 1932 Warkany moved to Cincinnati, Ohio, where he worked at the Children's Hospital Medical Center for the remainder of his life. Warkany had become interested in inborn malformations in the 1940s. This interest was rooted in his earlier studies on the effects of vitamin D deficiency and in his familiarity with cretinism (inborn deficiency of thyroid hormones), a condition frequently found in the Austrian Alps. Warkany's experimental studies on rats persuaded him that nutritional deficiency during pregnancy could produce inborn malformations. At that time, the majority of experts, especially in the United States, believed that all such malformations were hereditary. The description, in 1941, of the severe birth defects produced by an infection with the rubella virus attracted scientists' attention to maternal causes of fetal pathologies. After World War II, the observation of the consequences of the atomic bomb explosion in Japan and of tests of atomic weapons in the Pacific stimulated studies of links between birth defects and exposure to radiation. However, until the 1960s, Warkany's specialty—teratology—was perceived as a marginalized area of medicine.[34] For example, until the 1960s, obstetricians and pediatricians automatically assumed that all babies born small were premature. Warkany and his colleagues demonstrated that this was not the case: a small size of a newborn baby is often the consequence of an "intrauterine growth delay," a frequent fetal malformation that may be linked to a maternal pathology or an anomaly of the placenta.[35]

In 1948, Warkany showed that pink disease (acrodynia) in children, a condition linked with a painful rash, hair and tooth loss, perspiration, hypertension, and failure to thrive, was produced by intoxication with mercury. At that time, calomel (mercurous chloride) was a frequent component of teething powders, pomades employed to treat diaper rash, and drugs used to treat worms and diarrhea in children. Warkany's demonstration of the dangers of calomel led to a federal ban of the compound's use in medication and greatly reduced the incidence of acrodynia. The pink disease study increased Warkany's scientific prestige and his capacity to influence health policy decisions.[36] In 1957, he was instrumental in persuading the directors of the US charity March of Dimes to finance research on birth defects. March of Dimes' original goal, to fight polio, became obsolete in the mid-1950s, when polio became a rare disease in the United States following the introduction of an efficient anti-polio vaccine. Warkany convincingly argued that birth defects were the new frontier in the effort to reduce disability in children. In the 1970s and 1980s, March of Dimes was at the forefront of funding and research coordination on this topic.

In the 1950s, thanks to the efforts of Warkany and his colleagues, teratology became a recognized, although modest, medical subspecialty. Warkany organized four small conferences on inborn malformations but was not in favor of the institutionalization of this subspecialty.[37] The thalidomide disaster suddenly attracted attention to nonhereditary causes of inborn defects, and therefore to teratology. The US Teratology Society was founded in 1961, and Warkany became its first president.[38] The society's intense activity in the 1960s was directly related to a growing interest in the environmental causes of fetal malformations. The focus on such malformations also led to a growing interest in studies of other events that might affect embryological development.

In 1966, pediatrician David Smith coined the term *dysmorphology* (the study of the abnormal form) to replace the ominous-sounding *teratology*.[39] The new name, Smith hoped, would put an end to the labeling of birth defects as "monstrosities" and facilitate communication with parents of children with such defects.[40] In the late 1950s and early 1960s, Smith closely collaborated with the Patau's and Therman's pioneering studies of trisomy 13 and trisomy 18.[41] However, his research mainly focused on the anomalies of embryogenesis and fetal development. Genetic anomalies were but one among many causes of "human malformation." Down syndrome and "D trisomy syndrome" (trisomy 13) were, Smith explained, "internal dysmorphogenic influences," while infections such as rubella and maternal factors such as severe diabetes or a malformation of the uterus were "external dysmorphogenic influences." Both external and internal influences produce multiple fetal malformations. In some cases, a malformation produced by an external cause is similar to the one produced by an internal one. For example, cleft palate can be the result of a genetic anomaly or the faulty growth of an embryo produced by maternal factors. Moreover, the distinction between external "maternal factors" (e.g., infection, diabetes, heart disease) and internal "genetic factors" is far from absolute. Maternal factors can modulate gene expression and contribute to the variability of impairments produced by a mutation. Smith's understanding of dysmorphology was decidedly oriented toward a multifactorial understanding of developmental delays and an integrated view of human embryogenesis that did not privilege genetic factors over others.[42]

Dysmorphologists who study fetal development classify fetal anomalies according to the nature of the event at the origin of a given anomaly. Experts distinguish between: (a) malformation, a basic alteration of structure, usually occurring before ten weeks of gestation (e.g., deformation of the skull, anencephaly, agenesis of a limb or part of a limb); (b) malformation sequence, when multiple malformations are the consequence of a single primary event (e.g., hydrocephalus, or accumulation of liquid in the fetal skull, is often a secondary result of an original neural tube defect); (c) association, a group of anomalies that occur more frequently than would be expected by chance alone but that do not have a predictable pattern or unified etiology, or such an etiology is not known; (d) disruption, the destruction of tissue that was previously normal by disruptive events, such as amniotic bands (protein "ropes" in the amniotic fluid that constrain fetal growth), local destruction of tissue (which may be related to the faulty development of blood vessels and an insufficient supply of nutritive substances, or to hemorrhage, especially to the brain); and (e) dysplasia, abnormal cellular organization within tissue resulting in structural changes (e.g., changes in skeletal tissues that lead to small stature, or achondroplasia). Only dysplasia is a progressive defect, frequently produced by a mutation. All the other aforementioned anomalies are seen as accidents of embryological or placental development, which, in absence of similar cases in the family, have a low chance of recurrence. In 1966, Smith presented dysmorphology as a subspecialty of pediatrics. In 1977, he extended the jurisdiction of dysmorphology to prenatal events. When the cause of a malformation is hereditary, Smith explained, "early amniocentesis and chromosomal studies can obviate the birth of subsequent affected fetuses," and, thanks to the use of obstetrical ultrasound, "early fetal recognition and termination of pregnancy is now practical for the majority of the anencephaly-meningomyelocele anomalads."[43]

Smith's approach to morphogenesis is illustrated by what is probably his best-known study: the description of fetal alcohol syndrome (FAS). In 1973, Smith and his collaborator Kenneth Jones reported an association between typical "dysmorphic" traits and behavioral and cognitive disorders in children of mothers who consumed significant quantities of alcohol during pregnancy. A similar phenomenon was reported in 1968 by French physician Pierre Lemoine and his colleagues, but their article, published in French in a regional medical journal, remained virtually unknown until the description of the same phenomenon by Smith and Jones.[44] FAS had become one of the main models of dysmorphology studies in the United States. It combined an observation of "typical facial traits," a successful correlation of these traits with physiological anomalies and cognitive delays, the elucidation of the primary cause of these anomalies, and recommendations for how to prevent it—mainly by persuading pregnant women to limit their alcohol intake. FAS is also seen as dysmorphology's exemplary success story—an inborn syndrome that, once identified, can be prevented, in principle at least.[45]

Human Malformations

In 1970, Smith published a textbook titled *Recognizable Patterns of Human Malformation: Genetic, Embryologic, and Clinical Aspects*. The book's title summarized its topic, "recognizable" malformations, that is, those malformations that a clinician can spot by direct observation of a child, an adult, or a fetus. The art of clinical gaze is at the very center of Smith's book. *Recognizable Patterns of Human Malformation* rapidly became a reference volume for pediatricians, clinical geneticists, and ultrasound experts who dealt with the expression of inborn defects.[46] The book was published in a series titled Major Problems in Clinical Pediatrics. In the foreword to the first edition, the series editor states: "We have long wanted a volume in this series on the subject of the 'odd looking' baby."[47] In a review of Smith's book, leading US clinical geneticist Victor McKusick explained that *dysmorphogenesis*, a term coined by Smith, creatively combined nosology (the classification of diseases) with embryopathogenesis (errors in an embryo's development). There were very few books that dealt with the practical aspects of the diagnosis of inborn malformations. The only comprehensive study on this topic was John Ballantyne's book on inborn malformations, published in the early twentieth century. Smith's book therefore fills an important gap. McKusick added that one of the main innovations of Smith's book was the coupling of each description of an inborn malformation with photographs of affected children. Such visual evidence would be especially useful for clinicians.[48]

The focus on visual recognition of birth defects was indeed one of the main elements that differentiated Smith's work from books on related topics, such as McKusick's own *Mendelian Inheritance in Man* (published in 1966), Robert Gorlin and Jens Pindborg's *Syndromes of the Head and Neck* (published in 1964), or Warkany's study of inborn malformations, *Congenital Malformations: Notes and Comments* (published one year after *Recognizable Patterns of Human Malformation*).[49] Consecutive editions of Smith's *Recognizable Patterns of Human Malformation* (the seventh edition was published in 2013) have maintained the book's basic structure and its strong focus on visually "recognizable" malformations. The starting point of an investigation is always an "odd looking" baby, child, adult, or fetus. Experts sometimes say that a child looks "syndromic," that is, displays a cluster of anomalies that may have a shared origin in a single genetic cause (a localized mutation, a missing or duplicated segment of a chromosome) or a single developmental error that may have occurred during embryonic or fetal life. Each chapter of *Recognizable Patterns of Human Malformation* is focused on a major dysmorphic trait or group of traits: anomalies of the face, cranium, limbs, bones, genital organs, and so forth. The only exceptions are the chapter on environmental agents such as infections or pharmaceuticals and the chapter on syndromes induced by chromosomal abnormalities.

Successive editions of *Recognizable Patterns of Human Malformation* illustrate the evolution of dysmorphology. Such evolution is reflected in the steady growth in the book's size (the first edition has 368 pages and the seventh has 989 pages) and, above all, the rapid increase in the number of inborn syndromes linked to changes in the genetic material of the cell. The first two editions discussed only genetic syndromes produced by an abnormal number of chromosomes, such as Down, Patau, Edwards, KS, and TS. The third edition (published in 1982, after Smith's death) also included the description of anomalies produced by the deletion of part of a chromosome, because at that time the introduction of new methods of staining chromosomes (banding) made the detection of such chromosomal anomalies possible.[50] The number of chromosomal anomalies linked with inborn impairments increased in each subsequent edition of *Recognizable Patterns of Human Malformation*.[51] The seventh edition of this book included a separate chapter on "molecular syndromes," diagnosed thanks to the development of new molecular biology methods such as fluorescent hybridization in situ and DNA microarrays. In addition, nearly every description of a "visible malformation" in this edition (with the exception of those produced by environmental teratogens) included a subsection on genetics that listed mutations linked with a given syndrome or a group of syndromes.[52] The seventh edition of *Smith's Recognizable Patterns of Human Malformation* continues nevertheless to be first and foremost a textbook intended for pediatricians who observe children with atypical traits to compare their patients with photographs of affected individuals.[53] Such photographs, especially in the later editions of the book, do not present individuals with a black band that masks their eyes but are images of children and adults who look directly at the reader. The photographed individuals express a wide range of emotions, from distress through indifference, to happiness and pride. The latter expression also may be found in photographs of children with severe deformations. Human malformation, the book's indirect message seems to be, is at the same time "malformation" and "human."[54]

Recognizable Patterns of Human Malformation deals with "malformations"— anomalies produced by a major physiological obstacle to the development of tissues and organs before birth. In 1981, just before his death, Smith produced a smaller sister volume, *Recognizable Patterns of Human Deformation*, dedicated to "deformations"—anomalies induced by purely mechanical causes, such as a premature rupture of membranes, lack of amniotic fluid, amniotic bands, or an abnormal structure of the uterus.[55] The multiple editions of *Recognizable Patterns of Human Malformation* reflect a growing interest in intersections between morphological and genetic studies. *Recognizable Patterns of Human Deformation* was reedited only once, in 2007, twenty-five years after the publication of Smith's original volume. The preface of the new edition stated that purely mechanical explanations were no longer sufficient. Today, experts look beyond purely mechanistic approaches and seek out biochemical, molecular, or physiological explanations for observed anomalies.[56] In the new edition of *Recognizable Patterns of Human Deformations*, purely mechanical "deformations" were integrated accordingly with those on other causes that lead to the birth of a child with visible impairments. For example, a chapter on clubfoot explains that this birth defect can result from numerous causes, among them a mechanical intra-uterine compression, abnormal development of muscles, neurological abnormalities, vascular insufficiency, and genetic factors.[57]

Birth defects are often rare. In some cases, the description of a given anomaly is grounded in a study of fewer than one hundred cases. However, as McKusick explained in his 1964 preface to Gorlin and Pindborg's *Syndromes of Head and Neck*, studies of such rare conditions are important for two distinct reasons.[58] First, they favor the understanding of fundamental biological mechanisms: the pathological illuminates the normal. McKusick quoted seventeenth-century physician William Harvey, who first described the circulation of blood and who wrote in 1657 that "nature is nowhere accustomed more openly to display her secret mysteries than in cases where she shows tracings of her workings apart from the beaten paths; nor is there any better way to advance the proper practice of medicine than to give our minds to the discovery of the usual law of nature, by careful investigation of cases of rarer forms of disease."[59] Second, while isolated inborn syndromes are indeed rare, taken together they account for a significant proportion of physicians' activity. This is especially true in pediatrics and fetal medicine, where birth defects replaced infectious and nutritional diseases as the main cause of child mortality and severe morbidity.[60] On the public health level, "human malformations" are far from being a rare problem.

Birth Defects Registries

The thalidomide disaster sharply increased the awareness of the risks of environmental teratogens. One important consequence of this disaster was a striving to monitor such risks through the development of regional, national, and international registries of birth defects.[61] Some registries were founded before the thalidomide scandal. One of the first observations made by the scientists in charge of the Liverpool Congenital Anomalies Registry, founded circa 1960, was a curious epidemic of limb defects in newborn babies. This epidemic was later identified as the effect of maternal intake of thalidomide.[62] In the early 1960s, the thalidomide disaster promoted rapid development of already-existing birth defects registries, the founding of new registries, and the transformation of such registries into a powerful tool of epidemiological investigations. It also favored the development of a distinct branch of epidemiology dedicated to the surveillance of reproductive outcomes.[63]

The original goal of registries of newborn malformations was the surveillance of environmental teratogens, above all, drugs. According to Ian Leck, one of the pioneers of birth defects registries in the United Kingdom, malformations produced by thalidomide and rubella were unnoticed for a long time, until they became frequent enough to impress clinicians. It is clearly desirable to recognize epidemics of malformations before they reach catastrophic proportions. It is thus important to examine trends in large populations of births, a tedious but nevertheless essential task.[64] In the 1960s and 1970s, many countries organized a national and regional system of surveillance of birth defects. In the 1970s, the US Centers for Disease Control and Prevention (CDC) in Atlanta opened a birth defects branch as part of the Chronic Diseases Division of its Center for Environmental Health. In 2003, this branch became an autonomous division: the National Center on Birth Defects and Developmental Disabilities. Researchers of this division held a leading role in teratology and the study of birth defects, a domain that remained closely related to environmental health in the United States.[65] The CDC promoted two systems for registering birth defects. The Metropolitan Atlanta Congenital Defects Program, active in the Atlanta area, collected very detailed data on inborn defects and made the observation of fine-grained trends possible. The Birth Defects Monitoring Program had nationwide implementation but collected a much more restrained range of data.[66]

Other countries organized similar national and regional services. In 1972, the World Health Organization (WHO) started international consultations on congenital malformation reporting. In 1973, four countries submitted data on birth defects on a computer tape, but WHO's experts discovered that important differences in the ways in which these data were collected made common tabulations difficult. In 1974, the March of Dimes organized an informal working session, later called the First Working Conference on Birth Defects Monitoring. The conference, held in Helsinki, Finland, in June 1974, gathered representatives of ten birth defects registries in Europe and the Americas. Participants of the Helsinki conference decided to create a common registry, the International Clearinghouse for Birth Defects. They also established rules of harmonization for coding malformations in the participating registries.[67] In 1994, the European community decided to transform a small organization founded in 1979, the European Concerted Action on Congenital Anomalies and Twins, into a much broader coalition of European registries of birth defects, the European Surveillance of Congenital Anomalies (EUROCAT), an additional step toward the standardization of definitions, diagnoses, and systems of notification in this area.[68]

Many national birth defects registries continued to focus on the surveillance of potential teratogens. Thus, the Swedish registry followed links between women's occupations and birth defects. Such data revealed that the frequency of birth defects among children of women who came into contact with strongly teratogenic substances in their workplace was lower than the frequency of such defects among children of women who were in contact with less teratogenic substances. This paradoxical effect was attributed to the fact that strong teratogens induce lethal malformations of the fetus, sometimes very early in pregnancy: they caused more miscarriages but fewer birth defects.[69] Surveillance of teratogens uncovered numerous associations between chemical substances or drugs and inborn malformations but had only modest effects on the prevention of such malformations. Efficient preventive interventions such as the administration of folic acid to pregnant women to prevent neural tube defects, advice to women to limit consumption of alcohol during pregnancy, and the vaccination of girls against rubella were not related to the identification of causes of birth defects through epidemiological surveillance.[70] Such surveillance had, however, a different effect: the identification of rare hereditary conditions.

The accumulation of epidemiological data on birth defects opened new opportunities for fundamental genetic studies. For example, data from UK birth defects registries indicated that while neural tube defects were affected mainly by environmental factors, the majority of cases of cleft palate had a genetic background and were therefore less receptive to intervention during pregnancy.[71] Accumulation of epidemiological data facilitated the identification of families with rare genetic conditions and coordination between researchers who studied these conditions. The International Clearinghouse for Birth Defects continued to monitor congenital anomalies associated with known and suspected environmental teratogens and first trimester exposure to medication but increasingly organized databases on inborn anomalies linked with genetic anomalies. It also promoted the development of databases on specific aspects of human genome epidemiology destined to promote research on the etiology of birth defects with new molecular tools.[72] In 2005, the International Clearinghouse for Birth Defects, which, in the meantime, had become a federation of forty national registries, changed its name to the International Clearinghouse for Birth Defects Surveillance and Research.[73]

The Latino American birth defect registry followed a similar trajectory. This registry, the Latin American Collaborative Study of Congenital Malformations (ECLAMC, or Estudio Colaborativo Latinoamericano de Malformações Congênitas), was founded in the late 1960s, an outgrowth of a small, earlier registry based in Buenos Aires. ECLAMC collected its data through a voluntary adhesion of Latin American hospitals. Physicians who participated in the ECLAMC network traced unusual clusters of anomalies and occasionally were able to link such clusters with the presence of an infectious agent or an environmental teratogen such as a pesticide. At the same time, because many of the hospitals who adhered to ECLAMC were situated in regions that served isolated populations with high levels of inbreeding, doctors affiliated with ECLAMC uncovered families or groups of families with rare and "interesting" hereditary syndromes.[74] Latin American physicians who first described a new genetic syndrome, especially if such a syndrome was found at a remote and isolated site, seldom had the technical means to continue to study affected families using advanced molecular biology methods. Thanks to their collaboration with ECLAMC, they could supply research materials to geneticists who studied new genetic syndromes in cutting-edge laboratories, and who became co-authors of publications in prestigious scientific journals.[75]

Registries of birth defects, originally created to supervise the environmental causes of fetal malformations, gradually became a key tool for research on rare genetic conditions. Registries made possible the identification of clusters of such conditions and, if the condition was hereditary, genealogical investigation and tracing of migration patterns. Accumulation of rare cases also favored fundamental research on genetic anomalies. Studies of environmental teratogens were less "productive" from a scientific point of view than research on rare genetic conditions, because the rapid development of molecular biology was not matched by a similarly rapid development of the epidemiology of environmental teratogenesis. Strong environmental teratogens are relatively rare. The majority of suspected environmental teratogens produce much weaker and sometimes contradictory effects. Moreover, such substances often act in combination with other, often unidentified factors: it is difficult to prove causation and not only correlation. By contrast, it is often much easier to identify mutations linked with a genetic anomaly, study the expression of these mutations, and obtain results that lead to prestigious publications.[76] The disparity in the capacity to study environmental teratogens and genetic syndromes favored the transformation of an administrative device originally destined to prevent environmental damage to the fetus into a data-collecting mechanism that strengthened the geneticization of inborn defects.

Obstetrical Ultrasound and Diagnosis
of Morphological Anomalies

Debates on prenatal diagnosis focus on genetic defects: the relatively rare hereditary conditions transmitted in families and the much more frequent chromosomal and genetic anomalies, such as Down syndrome, that arise as accidents of the formation of sperm and egg cells (de novo mutations). Sociologists and bioethicists seldom discuss ultrasound detection of structural fetal malformations. Social scientists who have studied obstetrical ultrasound from the 1980s on often focus on the transformation of the intimate experience of pregnancy by the production of fetal images, and on the social, political, economic, and cultural roles of such images, and rarely discuss the diagnostic uses of this medical imagery technique.[77] One reason for the relative invisibility of obstetrical ultrasound as a major diagnostic tool might have been the incremental increase in the capacity of this technology to visualize fetal malformations; another reason might have been the late integration of ultrasound diagnoses into the "prenatal diagnosis dispositif." In the 1980s, when this approach began to be systematically applied to the study of structural malformations of the fetus, the term *prenatal diagnosis* was already firmly linked with the study of fetal cells in the amniotic fluid and the search for genetic anomalies.

The history of obstetrical ultrasound began in 1950, when a Glasgow group led by Ian Donald employed this technology—originated in the military—to visualize gynecological pathologies such as ovarian cysts and tumors.[78] Ultrasound was introduced into obstetrics in the late 1950s. At that time, obstetrical uses of ultrasound paralleled the main use of X-rays in obstetrics: the detection of potential problems during childbirth, such as a malformed pelvis or an unusual position of the fetus, and, occasionally, a display of major fetal malformations. In the 1960s, obstetrical ultrasound was also employed to visualize multiple pregnancies before the obstetrician was able to hear more than one heartbeat, indicate whether a woman was at high risk of miscarriage because the fetus was situated too low in the womb, diagnose a pregnancy outside the womb (ectopic pregnancy), establish the age of pregnancy in women who were not sure when their last period was, check whether the growth of the fetus was too slow (intrauterine growth delay), and visualize an abnormal position of the placenta that put a woman at risk of hemorrhage during childbirth (placenta previa). In the 1970s, this medical imagery technology was also employed to make amniocentesis safer by allowing the operator to follow the trajectory of the amniocentesis needle and, in some cases, to check whether an induced abortion or a spontaneous miscarriage were completed and no residual fetal tissue remained in the uterus.[79]

In the late 1960s, Donald described the machines he used as "crude."[80] In the early 1970s, the resolution of obstetrical ultrasound images was not good enough to diagnose the majority of fetal problems. The only exceptions were major malformations such as anencephaly. The resolution of ultrasound machines improved rapidly in the 1970s, thanks to two technical innovations: the introduction in the mid-1970s to linear array scanning and in the late 1970s to transvaginal ultrasound. The latter innovation was linked with the development of in vitro fertilization, a technique that officially came into being with the announcement of the birth of the first "test tube baby," Louise Brown, in 1978. Ultrasound was essential for the collection of eggs that were then fertilized in a test tube. Transvaginal ultrasound was then employed to visualize the implantation of the fertilized egg.[81] The increase in ultrasound's resolution made it possible to scrutinize the fetus and detect structural malformations. At the same time, the routine use of ultrasound increased the frequency of uncovering fetal anomalies. The inclusion of obstetrical ultrasound into the supervision of all pregnancies was not supported by proof that systematic use of this technology improved a pregnancy's outcome. The only—belated—attempt to evaluate the contribution of routine use of ultrasound to pregnancy management was the US clinical trial RADIUS. The results of this trial, published in 1993, indicated that routine use of obstetrical ultrasound did not reduce complications during childbirth or diminish fetal deaths. Organizers of the RADIUS trial concluded that obstetrical ultrasound should be used in the same manner as other medical imagery technologies—only when it is suspected that something is wrong. This conclusion might have reflected, among other things, the impossibility of "correcting" the great majority of severe fetal malformations visible on the ultrasound screen, or, as the authors of this study put it: "the ultrasonical detection of congenital anomalies has no effect on perinatal outcome."[82]

The RADIUS trial's conclusion had practically no effect on obstetrical practice.[83] In the 1990s, ultrasound examinations were already firmly incorporated into the routine care of pregnant women in industrialized, and increasingly also intermediary, countries. Obstetrical ultrasound became an inseparably medical and social technology. Women and health professionals learned to rely on this technology, including for emotional reasons. Pregnant women and their partners were pleased to "meet" their future child, learned about the fetus' "real age" and stage of development, and were often reassured that their child would be "normal."[84] Sometimes, however, the expected joyful encounter with the future child did not happen as predicted. Dramatic stories of the detection of a severe fetal malformation often started with the shock felt by a pregnant woman and her partner when a routine appointment for an ultrasound examination was suddenly transformed into an announcement of a disaster.[85]

"Must Be a Syndrome—but Which?" Abnormal Form and Abnormal Genes

Morphological abnormalities diagnosed by ultrasound are at the origin of about half of all pregnancy terminations for fetal indications. The story of prenatal diagnosis is, to an important extent, the story of the convergence of studies of abnormal form and of abnormal heredity. The clinical discipline of dysmorphology combines both. In the late twentieth and early twenty-first centuries, investigation of malformations in children and adults was extended to their investigation in fetuses as well, and were combined with increasingly powerful methods of investigation of the genome.

Dysmorphologists who study children with inborn impairments often have strong identities as clinical geneticists. Two of the three UK experts who became the first UK trainees in clinical genetics, Dian Donnai and Robin Winter, also became leading British dysmorphologists and the founders of a "dysmorphology club" that met at the Great Ormond Street Hospital in London to study diagnostic puzzles. The two later became the nucleus of the British association of dysmorphology.[86] The club started with informal exchanges between Donnai, Winter, and another pediatrician, Michael Baraitser: the three swapped photos and information during conferences of the British Clinical Genetic Society. Such informal encounters became, in the late 1970s, lunch meetings, and then half-day meetings during which the participants reviewed difficult cases. The dysmorphology club followed the well-established model of pathology clubs: reunions during which expert pathologists reviewed microscopic slides of difficult cases and attempted to reach an agreement about a diagnosis.[87] The main difference was that in the dysmorphology club meetings, the participants looked at projections of photographs of the investigated children, that is, entities that corresponded to the original meaning of the term *slide*: a projection on a screen.[88]

The sessions of the London dysmorphology club were focused on solving diagnostic puzzles. A report from a session of May 1981—in the early days of the club—exemplified a typical session. Each participant was asked to bring a typed or clearly written description of an inborn condition, up to fifty words. If they knew the diagnosis, they were asked not to include it. The organizer of the club then duplicated the slips and distributed them to all the participants. Participants who did not produce a slip with a case description were still allowed to present their cases at the end of the day, if there was enough time to do it.[89] Typical descriptions were, for example:

Patient I.C. 2 years, developmental delay, rather coarse face, depressed nasal bridge, bulbous tip of nose, thickish lips, multiple café au lait spots on trunk. No family history. No fits or nodular lesions. Diagnosis, probably neurofibromatosis [an autosomal dominant condition with highly variable expression; approximately half of the cases are new mutations].

Patient J.P. Neonate (newborn). Ashkenazi Jewish extraction. Delivery by caesarian section at 37 weeks for maternal hypertension. Hypotonia and poor feeding in neonatal period. Odd looking face. Micrognathia [small jaw], prominent occiput, very dry skin. Did not cry at circumcision. Diagnosis Riley Day Syndrome [an autosomal recessive condition, today usually called familial dysautonomia, a condition prevalent among Ashkenazi Jews].

Fetus B.A. Consanguineous parents. One previous normal child. Fetal death in utero at 29 weeks. Male infant with gross hydrocephalus. Low seated simple ears. Membranous strand attached to the globe of right eye, wide spaced eyes. Marked shortening of fingers. Left talipes [clubfoot]. Tentative diagnosis, recessive hydrocephalus syndrome [a hereditary condition linked today to several genetic anomalies, the most frequent mutations are in CCDCC8C and MPDZ genes].

Patient L.W. male, age 4 years. Developmental retardation. At 3 months hypotonic, strabismus, lens opacity. Slow growth. High myopia, non-progressive lens opacities [eye anomaly]. Prominent mid-forehead, flared alar nasea [bottom of the nose looks wider than normal], posteriorly rotated ears, rather simple, wide spaced small teeth. Broad fingertips. Father and paternal uncles have myopia, father has squints and "clicking ankle." Diagnosis unknown.

Patient N.B. 4 and [a] half years. Height less than 3rd centile [i.e., pronounced delay of growth] moderate retardation, more severe in speech. Face prominent frontal region, broad nasal bridge, prominent epicanthus [fold of skin in corner of the eye], anteriorly facing nostrils, long philtrum [vertical grove on the surface of the upper lip], limbs and genitalia are normal. Chromosomes normal. Must be a syndrome—but which?[90]

The last statement ("must be a syndrome—but which?"), probably written by Winter, who submitted this case, aptly summarizes many past and present debates in dysmorphology.

In the 1990s, dysmorphology became a more codified domain of study. In 1992, Donnai and Winter founded the first journal exclusively dedicated to this specialty—*Clinical Dysmorphology*. The US journal *Teratology*, founded in 1968 and renamed *Birth Defects* in 2003, also published numerous texts dealing with dysmorphology but maintained a strong allegiance to embryonic development.[91] By contrast, *Clinical Dysmorphology* has a strong genetic orientation. In the United States, dysmorphologists are less exclusively focused on changes in the genetic material of the cell and tend to pay more attention to environmental causes of inborn anomalies. Divergences between US and European traditions of dysmorphology are, however, far from being absolute. They may reflect differences in training, in institutional settings and locally allocated tasks, but also in personal preferences and allegiances. Moreover, the boundaries between "hereditary," "genetic," and "environmental" causes of inborn impairments are often fluid.[92] Some inborn conditions—diseases such as hemophilia, Tay-Sachs, or cystic fibrosis and syndromes such as Marfan syndrome, CHARGE syndrome, or retinitis pigmentosa—run in families. Other inborn conditions—such as Down, Klinefelter, Noonan, Costello, or Prader-Willi syndromes—are produced nearly always by new mutations. Others still—for example, neurofibromatosis, Cornelia de Lange syndrome, or DiGeorge syndrome—have hereditary and nonhereditary forms. Finally, in some cases the same anomaly, such as clubfoot or cleft palate, can be produced by a new mutation or by environmental factors.[93] It is not surprising that dysmorphology clinics became one of the key sites of the integration of morphological and genetic data, first through the study of children with visible structural malformations, and then, especially with the increase in the resolution power of obstetrical ultrasound, through studies of malformed fetuses.

One of the important goals of the genetic diagnosis of a "dysmorphic syndrome" in a fetus is to provide genetic counseling. Parents who have one affected child frequently want to know their chances of having a second affected child. If the parents do not wish to have more children, information about the hereditability of the child's condition may still be important to other family members.[94] Not infrequently, a diagnosis of a hereditary anomaly in a child/fetus leads to the diagnosis of the same condition in parents and other family members with a milder variant of this anomaly. Such diagnosis may affect the way these people see themselves and may shape their reproductive strategies. Dysmorphology clinics are one of the sites of the production of responsible mothers/parents.[95] This task may be complicated by an uncertainty about the consequences of specific mutations. When a given hereditary condition is rare and has a variable expression, specialists may be unable to tell the couple precisely what their risk of giving birth to a severely affected child is. The predicted growing role of prenatal diagnosis in the—frequently incidental—detection of rare hereditary conditions may increase the number of people facing challenging reproductive decisions.

The Final Verification: Fetal Pathology

In the twenty-first century, fetopathologists made key contributions to the understanding of new genetic syndromes. In a nonnegligible number of cases, their input was at least as important as the input of clinical geneticists. This may sound surprising. Pathology, and especially the dissection of cadavers, is a very conservative branch of medicine.[96] A pathologist trained in the 1860s in the laboratory of the "father of modern pathology," Rudolf Virchow, at the Charité hospital in Berlin would have probably felt at home with many aspects of the work of his twenty-first-century colleagues: detailed observation of intact dead bodies, a rigorously codified order of dissection, a macroscopic observation of organs and their arrangements, sampling of tissues and their fixation in a paraffin block, cutting these blocks with a microtome, and staining the thin slices of tissue for study under the microscope. Pathologists observe bodies, organs, and cells, and then compare the elements they see with pictures in pathology atlases and textbooks—and today often with photographs on specialized websites and in internet-based databases. They also use other senses such as touch (e.g., to assess whether the tissue is soft or hard, how it reacts to cutting) and, occasionally, smell. Despite the importance of instruments and techniques, their work relies primarily on embodied expertise acquired through experience.

The development of modern clinical science, at least its French version, was the result of an opportunity to closely observe hospitalized patients, and then, if they died (a very frequent event), to immediately dissect their bodies.[97] Physicians were able to correlate their clinical data, including those obtained by the use of instruments such as the stethoscope, with a study of changes produced by the disease in organs and tissues. This process favored the refinement of diagnostic procedures and the sharpening of doctors' perceptions. As a consequence, doctors were able to affirm with increasing confidence that, for example, a specific sound they heard when auscultating the chest was produced by the accumulation of liquid in the chest cavity. This key role of pathology in the production of medical knowledge was summarized in early nineteenth-century French anatomist Xavier Bichat's famous injunction: "Open a few cadavers: you will immediately witness the disappearance of the obscurity that observation alone could not eliminate."[98]

Pathologists who dissect human bodies are often invisible medical experts, with the notable exception of those who participate in high-profile criminal investigations and the heroes, or more often heroines, of popular detective novels and TV shows. Fetopathogists do not reach this kind of fame: dead fetuses are rarely at the center of a publicized criminal investigation and are seldom visible in television programs.[99] To follow French physiologist Claude Bernard's 1865 image of the physiology laboratory, a pathology department can also be described as a "long ghastly kitchen" where researchers produce advanced knowledge about healthy and sick bodies that then reaches the superbly lighted hall of cutting-edge science.[100] In fetal medicine, the "kitchen" is often the fetal pathology service, frequently situated in a basement or a hospital annex in small and cramped rooms full of antiquated furniture and equipment, and the "hall" is frequently a gleaming new department of molecular genetics with spacious rooms, bright lights, and ultramodern machines, which relies nevertheless on knowledge produced by fetopathologists.[101]

Until the second half of the twentieth century, the dissection of cadavers was the main site of new medical knowledge. This is no longer the case. In the second half of the twentieth century, the number of autopsies conducted in hospitals drastically decreased. Autopsies continue to be conducted systematically in cases of violent, sudden, or unexpected deaths but are less frequently used to understand why a given patient has died. The main exceptions are diagnostic puzzles and suspected cases of medical mismanagement.[102] Technologies of biomedicine, and intensive studies of cells, bodily fluids, molecules, and macro-molecules to an important extent, have replaced the "light" provided by the opening of cadavers. Fetal pathology is different. Despite the important pro-gress of prenatal diagnosis, opportunities to observe and study the fetus are much more limited than those to study a patient. Patients are physically present and usually either able to tell their own story or are surrounded by people who can inform the physician(s) about the patient's history and health status. Since there are no similar sources of information about the unborn child, autopsy continues to be one of the key sources of knowledge about fetal malformations. In some aspects at least, fetal medicine experts who rely on ultrasound images can be likened to the nineteenth-century doctors who tried to correlate sounds they heard during the auscultation of the patient with changes in heart, lungs, and blood vessels.[103] Another, perhaps more accurate, comparison may be with the pioneers of medical uses of X-rays, who attempted to understand how X-ray im-ages related to pathological modifications of organs and tissues by comparing X-ray images with clinical data but also, in the early stages of the development of this technology, by juxtaposing X-ray images of cadavers with results of the dissection of these cadavers.[104]

Pathological approaches employed to study fetuses are akin to those employed to study children and adults. Conversely, while organs and tissues of babies, young children, adults, and the elderly are often similar, those of fetuses, especially in the early stages of fetal development, may look dramatically different. The detection of fetal malformations is closely connected with the understanding of fetal growth. From the nineteenth century on, embryologists intensively stud-ied animal embryos, and occasionally human embryos as well. fetuses, includ-ing human ones.[105] Physicians frequently dissected fetuses and stillborn children.[106] These studies were, however, more often fueled by curiosity about rare anomalies than by a wish to investigate the cause of fetal demise. The latter approach—systematic studies of all the causes of fetal and neonatal deaths—is linked with the pioneering work of American pathologist Edith Potter.[107] In the mid-twentieth century, thanks to the studies of Potter and her colleagues, the pathological investigation of fetuses became part of mainstream research in obstetrics and pediatrics.

Potter's interest in fetuses originated from her aspiration to reduce newborn mortality. In the 1930s, stillbirths and newborn deaths were no longer seen as unavoidable, and physicians attempted to evaluate what proportion of such deaths could be prevented by adequate interventions. Systematic autopsies of fetuses, stillborn children, and those who died immediately after birth were essential for such an evaluation. Potter's first book, *Fetal and Neonatal Death*, written together with Fred Adair and published in 1939, investigated the causes of fetal and newborn demise. The book, grounded in Potter's and Adair's practices as pathologists in Chicago, was focused on the main causes of newborn deaths at that time: infections, maternal pathologies, hemolytic disease, and accidents of childbirth. Potter and Adair also discussed structural malformations of fetuses and stillborn babies, such as hydrocephalus, anomalies of the central nerve, and malignant tumors. However, as Potter and Adair explained, structural anomalies of the fetus were relatively rare. The main causes of stillbirths and newborn mortality were maternal diseases and accidents of childbirth, that is, in principle at least, preventable events.[108]

The second edition of Potter and Adair's book, published in 1948, reported a substantial decrease in newborn deaths. The authors attributed this decrease to the improvement of obstetrical techniques, the generalization of blood transfusion, and an efficient treatment of infectious diseases such as syphilis.[109] The impressive progress of the prevention of newborn deaths invalidated, they argued, earlier estimates of a presumably irreducible proportion of newborn deaths: in certain obstetric hospitals today, newborns' mortality is well below the hypothetical irreducible minimum of such deaths established in the 1940s. A better understanding of the causes of newborn deaths is essential to the continuation of this positive trend. One of the important innovations of the second edition of *Fetal and Neonatal Deaths* was the description of a standardized method to conduct a fetal autopsy that delineated all the steps of such an autopsy: a careful observation of the intact body of the fetus/stillborn child, weighing and measuring the body, opening it according to a standardized protocol, and performing a systematic examination of the internal organs, the skeleton, the head and the brain, and the spine and spinal cord. A dissection of a fetus should always include the placenta and the umbilical cord. If doctors suspect that the cause of the death is infection, autopsy protocol should also include bacteriological and serological studies of body fluids.[110]

Potter's best-known book, *Pathology of the Fetus and the Newborn*, published in 1952, was grounded in her eighteen-year experience at the Chicago Lying-In

Hospital, where she performed more than six thousand fetal and newborn autopsies.[111] Potter distinguished between maternal/birth-related causes of fetal and newborn demise (prematurity, anoxia [lack of oxygen], birth trauma, and infections) and fetal causes (hereditary and environmental malformation of the fetus). The second part of *Pathology of the Fetus and the Newborn* describes anomalies of specific organs or groups of organs, such as the digestive and central nervous systems. Potter's book contained numerous black-and-white photographs of dissections that displayed the discussed pathological changes. The inclusion of these photographs greatly increased the book's utility as a training tool for pathologists.

The introduction of *Pathology of the Fetus and the Newborn* stresses that fetal pathology is a neglected but very important domain that should be integrated with studies of heredity, conception, intrauterine development, extrauterine environment, and women's health. The death of a fetus or a newborn child, Potter explains, is too often still seen as an unavoidable "act of God." This is an erroneous view. Each death is always produced by a specific cause, even if, especially when dealing with very young fetuses, the cause of fetal demise may be very difficult to discover.[112] Potter's experience taught her that the most frequent reasons for fetal mortality were accidents of fetal development, above all, interference with oxygenation. Other important causes of fetal death are infectious diseases, Rhesus factor incompatibility, placental anomalies, and hormonal problems. Heredity, Potter argued, is an important, but relatively less frequent, reason for fetal demise. Of the 132 pages of the first part of *Pathology of the Fetus and the Newborn* dedicated to causes of fetal/newborn demise, only seven describe malformations induced by hereditary conditions such as hemophilia or achondroplastic dwarfism. She added that physicians should pay attention to interactions between heredity and environment. Even in a pair of identical (monozygotic) twins, one may be severely malformed while the other is not affected. Moreover, the same anomaly can be produced by multiple causes. Thus, microcephaly (an abnormally small brain volume) can be induced by X-rays, toxoplasmosis (a parasitic infection), and hereditary factors.[113]

British pathologist Edgar Morrison, author of *Fetal and Neonatal Pathology*, another textbook on fetal pathology also published in 1952, agreed with Potter's main conclusions. Morrison also focused mainly on external causes of birth defects, such as infections, maternal diseases, placental anomalies, and problems of childbirth, and he, too, argued that similar malformations may result from the operation of totally different genetic or environmental influences, or, not infrequently, a combination of both.[114] The difficulty to understand the causes of such impairments, and an even greater difficulty to prevent them, does not leave much room for optimism. Fetal malformations are, and in all probability will remain, "one of the greatest and most difficult problems in biology."[115] Fetopathology, Morrison added, can nevertheless make important contributions to the understanding of this problem.

The main goal of fetal dissections, Potter argued, is to prevent pregnancy loss and newborn deaths. From the early 1960s on, studies of miscarried and aborted fetuses became closely associated with the investigation of chromosomal anomalies and mutations, and also became a key site of the production of cutting-edge genetic knowledge.[116] In his introduction to Enid Gilbert-Barness and Diane Debich-Spicer's book *Embryo and Fetal Pathology*, John Opitz, a leading US specialist in clinical genetics, explained that in 1961, as a young medical resident interested in embryology and human development, he applied simultaneously for training in teratology in Cincinnati with Josef Warkany and in clinical genetics in Madison, Wisconsin, with David Smith and Klaus Patau. The Madison department answered first, and Opitz went there, a chance event that radically changed the direction of his professional life. One of the most productive aspects of his training in Madison was the study of trisomy 13 and trisomy 18 with Patau and Smith. When Enid Gilbert arrived at the University of Wisconsin, she initiated Opitz to developmental pathology. Thanks to her teachings, Opitz was able to enrich his understanding of embryology and genetics with data from the dissection of fetuses and stillborn children. Far from being a "backward" and conservative branch of medicine, Opitz stressed, fetal pathology continues to make crucial contributions to cutting-edge domains of biomedical investigation.[117]

CHAPTER 4

From Prenatal Diagnosis to Prenatal Screening

Prevention of Mental Disability as a Public Health Issue

In the early 1970s, only a small number of women of an "advanced maternal age," mostly from privileged social strata, had access to prenatal diagnosis of Down syndrome. In 1971, two epidemiologists from the Columbia University Mailman School of Public Health, Zena Stein and Mervyn Susser, discussed the prevention of Down syndrome in an article titled "The Preventability of Down's Syndrome." The number of people with trisomy 21, they explained, is increasing rapidly because new therapies, especially the use of antibiotics to treat respiratory diseases and surgery for heart defects, allowed them to survive beyond childhood. Between 1940 and 1960, Stein and Susser noted that life expectancy at birth for people with Down syndrome had risen from twelve to sixteen years, and more recent studies indicate that half among them survive until adulthood. New educational methods lessen their degree of social dependency, "but whatever is done, the survivors continue in a state of permanent dependence that imposes a severe burden on their families and on existing forms of social organization."[1] This *burden*, to use Stein and Susser's term, can be alleviated. The key element in Stein and Susser's argument was that we know which population is at higher risk of giving birth to a trisomic child: older mothers, especially those older than 40: "These older mothers are a salient target group for a preventive program. Such a program is made feasible by the changing attitude and laws about contraception and abortion and advances in prenatal diagnosis."[2]

Two years later, Stein and Susser (with Andrea Guterman) radicalized their proposal. Many couples and doctors, they claimed, already employed amniocentesis for a prenatal diagnosis of Down syndrome. However, the existing programs focused exclusively on women at genetic risk of this condition (a very small fraction, estimated at less than 2% of all Down syndrome births) and, above all, older pregnant women, while the majority of children with Down syndrome are born to younger mothers. Programs that exclusively target older women will not significantly reduce the number of trisomic children: "The key to transforming the diagnostic procedure from a clinical measure for sporadic use into a public health measure for systematic use is to adapt it as a screening device."[3] Stein, Susser, and Guterman added that an almost complete prevention of Down syndrome could be achieved by screening all pregnant women. They did not calculate a precise cost of such screening but asked, "Is a detailed estimate of money costs required? The lifelong care of severely retarded persons is so burdensome in almost every human dimension that no preventive program is likely to overweigh the burden."[4]

Stein, Susser, and Guterman were concerned about inequality in access to amniocentesis. In some countries, they explained, all abortions were illegal and could only be obtained by those who could afford to circumvent the law or travel. The prevention of Down syndrome in such countries is the privilege of the rich and powerful, a situation that other people may or may not choose to bear with patience. Countries where abortion is legal can, however, institute a prenatal screening program for Down syndrome: "The effects of policy advocated here will bring relief to the community and new assurance to prospective parents. These benefits are already available to a privileged few. Societies can choose to offer them to everyone."[5] For Stein, Susser, and Guterman, screening for Down syndrome was most importantly a question of social justice. Their argument— that such screening will provide "assurance for prospective parents" and, at the same time, "benefits for the community"—nevertheless blurred the boundary between individual and societal choices. This ambivalence about the goals of prenatal screening shaped the history of this intervention.

Stein and Susser's interest in the prevention of Down syndrome stemmed from their earlier studies of mentally handicapped children. In the 1950s, Stein and Susser, who at that time worked in the United Kingdom at an institution for children with intellectual disabilities, noticed that lower-class children were much more frequently labeled as suffering from "mental retardation" than upper-class children. Stein and Susser's working hypothesis was that cognitive problems of lower-class children might reflect a nutritional deficiency during pregnancy. They investigated a "natural experiment"—the great Dutch famine of 1944–1945—and compared cognitive capacities of children born during the famine with those born later. This study disproved their original hypothesis: children born to undernourished mothers had similar mental capacities as those born after the famine ended.[6]

The Dutch famine study and similar investigations led Susser and Stein to the conclusion that mental impairment was often linked with hereditary change and therefore could be prevented through environmental intervention. They distinguished between so-called mild mental retardation, more often found in children from a modest social background, and severe mental retardation, which was not linked with social class. Mild mental retardation often reflected the child's difficulties at school and reflected social variables such as insufficient intellectual stimulation at home or growing up in a chaotic or harsh environment. It was also linked to the fact that poor children were more frequently labeled "mentally retarded" than children from more affluent families. By contrast, severe intellectual difficulties were found in similar proportion in all social classes.[7] The description of "mongolism" as trisomy 21 vindicated Stein and Susser's view that severe intellectual deficiency was inborn, and not produced by environmental variables. It also opened the way to the prenatal diagnosis of this condition.

Stein and Susser grounded their advocacy of screening for Down syndrome in their analysis of an already-existing screening program for a disease linked with mental retardation: phenylketonuria (PKU). The generalization of screening for Down syndrome, Stein, Susser, and Guterman proposed, would have a much more favorable cost-effectiveness ratio than screening for PKU. The prevention of PKU through newborn screening was expected to reduce the prevalence of severe mental retardation in populations by about 1%, while the prevention of Down syndrome could reduce the prevalence of such severe retardation by 30%.[8] They did not mention the important difference between these two interventions, however. The goal of screening for PKU was to cure already-existing children, while testing for Down syndrome was suggested to prevent the birth of children with this condition. Another important difference was that testing for PKU in a drop of blood from a newborn's heel was risk free, while amniocentesis endangered the tested fetus. Stein, Susser, and Guterman's proposal to generalize the detection of trisomic fetuses was not feasible in the 1970s, because, among other things, this diagnostic test was too risky to offer it to all pregnant women. This proposal, however, became practicable twenty years later with the development of serum tests for Down syndrome, a risk-free screening method for this condition.

The Price Tag of Testing for Down Syndrome

Stein, Susser, and Guterman's 1973 paper affirmed that testing for Down syndrome would reassure prospective parents and bring "relief to the community." The latter aspect was omnipresent in early debates among experts on cost-effectiveness of amniocentesis.[9] The sampling of amniotic fluid was performed by gynecologists; later, laboratory technicians cultivated fetal cells and cytogeneticists or cytogenetics technicians counted the number of chromosomes. Unlike later developments in prenatal diagnosis, diagnostic ultrasound, and serum tests, the development of amniocentesis was not linked with industrial interests.[10] Conversely, the new approach was labor intensive, and thus relatively expensive. Because of this, health administrators were concerned about its cost-effectiveness.

In 1970, shortly after the beginning of prenatal testing for Down syndrome, Terrance Swanson argued that approximately 7,500 to 8,000 children with Down syndrome were born every year in the United States. A reasonable estimate of the average cost of care and maintenance of a "mongoloid" is $5,000 per year, while the life expectancy of people with this condition is more than 50 years. Swanson, unlike other writers on this topic in the 1970s, did not present children with Down syndrome exclusively as a "burden" for their families and spoke also about the positive effects of raising a child with this condition: "No one can put a dollar value on anguish, broken families, destroyed careers, and other attendant emotional problems triggered by the trial of giving birth to a mongoloid child in some families. No one can put a dollar value on the love and brightness a child can bring into a home, even if the child is mentally retarded."[11] Nevertheless, Swanson added, on the collective level, human and economic resources that a society spends on the care and maintenance of "mongoloids" yield very small dividends: "Efforts to reduce the incidence of mongolism have the potential to be extremely cost-effective in terms of economic value." Swanson calculated that voluntary genetic counseling and a liberal abortion practice would cut the incidence of "mongolism" in half. The monetary benefit for society would be 18 billion dollars over the next twenty years. These funds could be channeled into other urgent social programs.[12]

Philip Welch evaluated the cost of testing all pregnant women in Nova Scotia for the risk of Down syndrome and concluded, as Swanson did, that detection would cost approximately $10,000 per case, while the cost of care of an individual with Down syndrome was approximately $60,000.[13] Ronald Conley and Aubrey Milunsky proposed a different way of calculating the monetary value of testing for Down syndrome. On one side of the equation, they put the cost of amniocentesis, and on the other side, they put the cost of caring for people with Down syndrome, but also the loss of income from the birth of a unimpaired child who might have contributed to society. The latter calculation was based on the assumption that a woman who terminated a pregnancy with a Down fetus would "replace" the lost future child with a healthy child who would be able to generate income when he or she came of age. Despite their inclusion of income generated by a "replacement child" after the termination of a pregnancy with a Down fetus, they concluded that from a purely economic point of view, amniocentesis for the risk of Down syndrome was cost-effective, but only when the test was proposed to women who have a high risk of giving birth to a child with this condition. Proposing this test to all pregnant women would lead to an excessive increase in the cost of detection of each case of Down syndrome.[14] Danish experts also argued that testing for Down syndrome was especially cost-effective in women older than 40; this effect was partly diluted if the testing was proposed to women older than 35.[15]

Ernest Hook and Geraldine Chambers explained that the cost–benefit ratio of amniocentesis varied greatly according to the mother's age. They proposed to either fix an age above which the procedure would be reimbursed by health insurance or, alternatively, to reimburse amniocentesis only when the woman's risk of giving birth to a child with Down syndrome was greater than 1%.[16] Insurers, such as Blue Shield of Massachusetts, adopted the first solution and elected to cover some of the costs of prenatal diagnosis for women older than 35. Nonetheless, Blue Shield of Massachusetts did not cover the costs of genetic counseling. Private health insurers in New York City adapted a similar approach. Medicaid decided in 1979 to cover not only the costs of amniocentesis but also those of genetic counseling, hoping that this move would put pressure on third-party health insurers to provide similar coverage.[17] Obstetricians in the United States, like the insurance companies, recommended 35 years as the cutoff point beyond which women could undergo amniocentesis (if they wished to). This was, however, a recommendation, not a binding guideline. Women could elect to have amniocentesis at an earlier age, and many did. One of the reasons obstetricians agreed to perform amniocentesis on women in their early thirties was their growing realization that the age of 35 did not represent a significant jump in the risk of giving birth to a child with Down syndrome. The curve of increase in the risk of giving birth to a child with Down syndrome is continuous rather than abrupt, so there was no strong justification to agree to amniocentesis for a 35-year-old woman while refusing to perform this test on a 33- or 34-year-old woman.[18]

The decision to recommend amniocentesis to women older than 35 was legitimated by the statement that at the age of 35, the risk of having a Down syndrome fetus is greater than the risk of losing a healthy fetus following amniocentesis. The first risk was well documented, but the second was not. Researchers who studied birth defects registries produced solid epidemiological data on the correlation between maternal age and the risk of Down syndrome.[19]

However, it was quasi-impossible to obtain reliable data about the risk of miscarriage following amniocentesis. Such a risk varied according to the skill and experience of doctors who performed this test, and the quality of the ultrasound equipment they used. Unsurprisingly, data on the risk of miscarriage following amniocentesis were highly variable. The logical explanation that the cutoff point of 35 years was carefully chosen to balance the risk of Down syndrome and the risk of amniocentesis masked a partly arbitrary decision motivated primarily by an aspiration to control health expenses.[20]

Experts who analyzed the cost–benefit ratio of testing for Down syndrome explained that offering this procedure to all pregnant women older than 35 would generate a "net" benefit even if only 30% to 40% of concerned women took this test, a level of "compliance" seen as realistic.[21] In practice, however, women's "compliance" was often much lower. A 1981 survey in Ohio found that in different counties of that state, between 7% and 17% of pregnant women older than 35 underwent amniocentesis. The main reasons that pregnant women did not test for Down syndrome risk were that they did not think of themselves as being at risk or they had never heard of this test. Only 21% among "eligible" women declared that they were not interested in amniocentesis because they were opposed to abortion. Nearly half of the women who did not undergo amniocentesis claimed that they would have used the test if they had been informed by their obstetrician that such a test was available. Women in that sample did not mention the risk of miscarriage following amniocentesis or the test's cost as a reason why they did not participate.[22] In 1995, 3.2% of US pregnant women underwent amniocentesis; this percentage was much lower than the percentage of women who underwent amniocentesis in Western Europe. White women took this test twice as often as black women; the use of amniocentesis was especially low among poor rural populations.[23] In the early 1990s, as in the early 1970s, testing for Down syndrome in the United States was mainly limited to middle-class women.

Serum Markers and the Shift to Prenatal Screening

In the mid-1970s, amniocentesis for Down syndrome risk was proposed only to pregnant women older than 35. Stein, Susser, and Guterman had already pointed out that this was a very imperfect solution, as the majority of children with Down syndrome were born to mothers younger than 35. Public health experts strove to find a way to increase the efficacy of prenatal detection of trisomic fetuses. In the early 1990s, the parallel description of serum and ultrasound markers for the risk of Down syndrome made it possible to screen all pregnant women for this condition.[24] The detection of fetal malformations became a population-based approach.

The discovery of serum markers in maternal blood originated in biochemical investigations of the amniotic fluid. Geneticists studied fetal cells that had shed into the amniotic fluid, but at the same time biochemists examined the amniotic fluid itself, looking for possible correlations between its composition and inborn defects. The diffusion of amniocentesis in the 1970s provided them with an ample supply of research material. One of the first results of their research was the observation that women who gave birth to children with major neural tube defects (anencephaly, spina bifida) had abnormally high levels of alpha-fetoprotein (AFP, one of the proteins secreted by the fetus) in the amniotic fluid. Scientists had then found out that in such cases the pregnant woman's serum also contained higher than average levels of this protein. This finding led the way to a simple and risk-free method of looking for an increased risk of neural tube defects.[25] At first, obstetricians measured the level of AFP in the serum of women who already had affected children, but later experts proposed to measure AFP in the serum of all pregnant women.[26]

In the United Kingdom, the introduction of testing for AFP into a routine obstetrical practice was stimulated by concerns about elevated rates of neural tube defects, especially in the northern parts of Britain. Some specialists were also preoccupied by the dilemmas produced by the improved survival of people with spina bifida (or myelomeningocele, an incomplete closure of the neural tube). These interrogations may be compared to those produced in the post–World War II era by important progress in the survival of individuals with Down syndrome. Conversely, experts who discussed the survival of people with severe neural tube defects focused on their quality of life, rather than on the cost of their care. An article published in 1972 in the *British Medical Journal* explained that up until the time of the article, about 85% of children born with myelomeningocele died in infancy or early childhood. With advances in surgery, in 1972 about 60% survived until school-age or later, but "half of these survivors are grossly disabled, incontinent of urine, and [walk] with great difficulty or [are] not able to walk at all. Medicine in making some sort of life possible for these unfortunate children has presented their families and the society in which they live with the sometimes intractable problem of making that life tolerable."[27] Prenatal detection of these conditions, epidemiologists assumed, would in the majority of cases be followed by pregnancy termination. It could therefore provide a solution to this "intractable problem." Screening is acceptable when the tests are

valid and health professionals can offer effective treatment. Screening for neural tube anomalies fulfilled, as some specialists argued, all of these conditions:
the efficacy of the proposed "treatment" was demonstrated by the reduction in
the number of children born with spinal cord anomalies.[28]

A 1977 report of a UK collaborative study recommended the introduction of
AFP screening.[29] The following year, a report of the Working Party of the Clinical Genetic Society (United Kingdom), headed by geneticist Malcolm Ferguson-
Smith, arrived at a similar conclusion. Such a screening, the consulted experts
agreed, was only an indication of risk, not a sufficient reason to terminate a pregnancy: the serum measures needed to be confirmed by testing the amniotic
fluid.[30] British gynecologists quickly adopted screening for maternal AFP. In
1978, approximately half of pregnant women in the United Kingdom underwent
such a screening.[31] US physicians were initially more reluctant to introduce this
test. The generalization of this test in the United States was prompted by the
American Medical Association's concerns about legal liability of obstetricians for
undetected neural tube defects. In 1978 and 1979, several women sued their obstetricians for failure to propose prenatal testing, claiming that such a failure
had deprived them of the opportunity to abort an affected fetus.[32] In 1983, the US
Food and Drug Administration approved the first kit for screening for AFP.[33]
The first mass screening program for the level of AFP in the amniotic fluid of
pregnant women was proposed in California in 1986.[34] French obstetricians
were less preoccupied by the detection of neural tube defects because of their
relative rarity in France; however, they became interested in AFP when this
marker was linked with an increased risk of a more frequent fetal anomaly: Down
syndrome.

In the early 1980s, the accumulation of the results of routine testing for AFP
led to the unexpected observation that women who carried Down syndrome fetuses had an unusually low level of this protein in their bodies. The latter observation was rapidly translated into a proposal to screen all pregnant women for
Down syndrome risk.[35] The sensitivity of serum tests for Down syndrome risk
was increased through the addition of two new markers: human chorionic go-
nadotropin (a protein secreted by the placenta; especially high in women who
carry a Down fetus) and unconjugated estriol (a fetal protein; lower in Down
pregnancies). The combination of these three markers became a standard test
for Down syndrome risk (the so-called triple test).[36] Later, researchers described
two additional markers of Down risk—inhibin A and pregnancy-associated
plasma protein A (PAPP-A)—and these markers were added to some screening

kits.[37] In the twenty-first century, some tests are grounded in the search for abnormal levels of PAPP-A only, seen as an especially efficient indicator of Down syndrome risk.

In the late 1990s, gynecologists increasingly proposed serums tests to screen for Down syndrome risk in all pregnant women, independently of their age. UK experts who advocated a switch to generalized screening for Down syndrome explained that "the prevalence of Down syndrome has major resource implications as it is the third most important cause of mental handicap. In addition more than 80% of the 1976–1985 birth cohort survived to 5 years compared with only around 40% of the 1940–1960 cohort, owing to improved treatment, particularly of cardiac defects. . . . The current residential and community services for young mentally handicapped adults are facing a twofold increase in the number of clients with Down syndrome."[38]

In France, gynecologists and fetal medicine experts did not openly discuss the cost of care for people with Down syndrome, but economic considerations, experts explained later, played a significant role in the generalization of screening for Down syndrome.[39] Another important element was the experts' convictions that such a screening would benefit the concerned families. In France, as in the United Kingdom, serum tests for the risk of fetal malformations became generalized in the quasi-absence of public debate or input from the tests' users.[40] In the United States, public debates on the cost-effectiveness of screening for Down syndrome became more difficult in the 1990s when disability movement activists started to oppose selective abortion for this indication, but individual gynecologists usually proposed serum tests for Down syndrome risk. Many of these tests were covered by insurance companies.[41]

The generalization of screening for serum markers for Down syndrome risk created an important market for products and instruments used in prenatal screening: monoclonal antibodies against serum markers linked with fetal anomalies and automated immunoassay platforms for the analysis of serum samples.[42] Multinational firms, such as Abbott Diagnostics, Beckman Coulter, Bayer Diagnostic, bioMérieux, PerkinElmer, or Dade Behring, produced instruments and reagents used in serum tests, and sometimes worked directly with the experts who calibrated these tests and participated in the elaboration of guidelines of good clinical practice.[43] In the 1990s, "serum markers" for Down syndrome were coupled with a different kind of test: ultrasound markers of this condition. This development led to the involvement of an additional group of industrial partners in prenatal screening: companies such as Toshiba, General Electric, Chison, Philips, or Siemens, which produced ultrasound equipment.

Screening for Down syndrome was often seen as an ethical issue and, although less frequently, as a question related to health policies, institutional and legal variables, and the organization of medical labor. It was seldom investigated as a domain of important industrial development.

The Combined Screening for Down Syndrome Risk

In the early 1980s, obstetrical ultrasound was gradually transformed into an important tool for the detection of fetal anomalies. At that time, ultrasound experts developed an approach that analyzed all the internal organs of early second trimester fetuses. Such an examination was, however, labor intensive and expensive. It was therefore employed only to confirm an already-existing suspicion of a fetal malformation.[44] At that time, not all experts saw ultrasound diagnosis as trustworthy. Ferguson-Smith explained in 1983 that when biochemical tests for a high level of AFP in the blood and in the amniotic fluid indicated a high probability of a neural tube defect but the ultrasound examination failed to reveal any fetal abnormality, the latter result should not be trusted: "Most patients will not risk continuing their pregnancy and will opt for termination. In many such cases an obvious fetal anomaly is found, for example a low lumbar spina bifida defect or a small anterior abdominal wall defect. . . . Unfortunately, in a few cases no lesion can be found in the abortus to account for the clearly abnormal biochemical results."[45]

In the early 1980s, Ferguson-Smith and his colleagues in Glasgow believed that an ultrasound diagnosis of neural tube defects (or, rather, an absence of such a diagnosis) was less reliable than a result of a biochemical test. Stuart Campbell's group at King's College London held the opposite view. They systematically proposed ultrasound examination to all pregnant women diagnosed with high levels of AFP in their amniotic fluid, and if such an examination did not reveal any problems, they assumed that the fetus was normal.[46] In the early 1990s, obstetricians accepted this view, and ultrasound examination came to be seen as more dependable evidence of neural tube defects than biochemical data. In 1991, some British specialists affirmed that screening for neural tube defects by measuring the level of AFP in maternal blood was no longer necessary because an ultrasound examination could safely identify such malformations.[47] One of the reasons France never introduced AFP screening for neural tube defects might have been the rapid diffusion of diagnostic ultrasound in France. In the late 1980s, French obstetricians were confident that thanks to the generalization of ultrasound examinations they were able to identify neural tube defects before birth.[48] One important consequence of the transformation of obstetrical ultrasound into a powerful diagnostic tool was the rise of a distinct specialty, fetal medicine, and the transformation of a fetus into a patient.[49] Another consequence was a firm integration of this approach into the routine surveillance of pregnancy, despite initial doubts about its safety.[50] The systematic search for fetal anomalies during routine ultrasound examination was in turn one of the elements that favored the view that all pregnancies are "at risk" and all women should undergo some form of scrutiny of the fetus.

In the 1980s and 1990s, ultrasound experts who studied hundreds of normal and abnormal fetuses acquired the capacity to observe even minimal structural changes in the fetus. Such changes were then correlated with observations made in newborn children and, if the fetus was miscarried or aborted, with autopsy results. Thanks to such studies, experts were able to show a higher frequency of specific traits in ultrasound images of Down fetuses. Such traits, which indicated an increased risk that the fetus was trisomic, were called "soft ultrasound markers," in order to distinguish them from "hard ultrasound markers": a direct observation of a structural defect such as spina bifida or the absence of a limb. In the late 1980s, ultrasound experts started to propose "genetic sonograms," a detailed ultrasound examination of the fetus aimed specifically at the detection of signs of trisomy 21. The search for "soft markers" of Down syndrome, first seen as a diagnostic approach, later became part of the screening for this condition.

The term *genetic sonogram* originated from the work of ultrasonographer Beryl Benacerraf and her colleagues at the Harvard School of Medicine. In the mid-1980s, this group described "sonographic signs" of Down syndrome such as an excessive thickness of the fold of skin at the fetal neck (nuchal skinfold) during the second trimester of pregnancy (fourteen to twenty-eight weeks).[51] Taking into account several independent soft markers of Down syndrome, Benacerraf and her colleagues argued, a genetic sonogram can identify the majority (up to 87%) of Down syndrome fetuses.[52] One of the important conclusions of their work was that ultrasound diagnosis could greatly reduce the need for amniocentesis. When a woman's serum tests point to an increased risk of Down syndrome, instead of immediately proposing an invasive test, her doctor can recommend a diagnostic ultrasound. In many cases, the woman will then learn that her risk of carrying a trisomic fetus is well below the risk of having a miscarriage following an invasive test.[53] However, to be reliable, a genetic sonogram has to be performed by a competent specialist with training in both gynecology and radiology.[54]

While Benacerraf and her colleagues improved the second trimester genetic sonogram, Kypros Nicolaides and his group at King's College London identified a different "soft ultrasound marker" of Down syndrome: the increase in nuchal translucency, or the accumulation of fluid behind the fetus' neck during the first trimester of pregnancy (eleven to thirteen weeks).[55] Despite their apparent similarity, increased nuchal translucency and the thickening of the nuchal skinfold are seen as independent indications of Down syndrome risk and can be measured sequentially.[56] An important advantage of Nicolaides's approach was the possibility of identifying women who were at a higher risk of carrying a Down syndrome fetus much earlier. These women could then elect to have chorionic villus sampling, and if they received a "positive" result they could undergo an earlier and physically less traumatic abortion. Another important difference between Benacerraf's and Nicolaides's approaches was the perceived use of their respective "Down markers." Benacerraf developed a test adapted to use in private practice and insisted on the key importance of the ultrasound expert's embodied skills. Nicolaides was looking for a way to develop a screening method that could be used by all public maternity services in the United Kingdom. He therefore paid special attention to the standardization and simplification of measures of nuchal translucency.

Ultrasound "soft markers" for Down syndrome denote a higher than average probability of a woman carrying a trisomic fetus, as abnormal levels of serum markers do. Hence, the idea that combining these two probabilistic measures would provide a more accurate idea of a woman's risk of carrying a Down syndrome fetus.[57] The majority of Western countries that introduced systematic screening for Down syndrome adopted such a combined approach. Typically, data obtained from ultrasonogram findings and from serum tests are entered into a computer program, together with additional data such as the pregnant woman's age, in order to calculate her risk of giving birth to a trisomic child. If such risk is perceived to be higher than the average risk of miscarriage following an invasive test—usually estimated as 1/200 to 1/300—physicians recommend amniocentesis or CVS.[58] The introduction of the combined screening for Down fetuses modified the timing of tests for serological markers of this condition. Such tests were initially performed during the second trimester of pregnancy (sixteen to twenty weeks), since at that time serum markers for Down syndrome have better predictive power. Alternatively, nuchal translucency and several other ultrasound markers of Down syndrome are best visible at ten to twelve weeks. While biochemists advocated a second trimester screening, in Europe the opinion of ultrasound experts had prevailed: screening for Down syndrome gradually shifted to the first trimester of pregnancy, because, among other things, it enabled a woman who has been diagnosed with a Down fetus to have an abortion earlier in pregnancy.[59]

In all countries that introduced screening for Down syndrome, pregnant women are invited to sign a consent form for serum tests. Women who sign such a form rely, one may assume, on the expert knowledge of their health providers. Physicians' understanding of prenatal testing may, however, be far from perfect. A 2007 bioethics thesis written by a specialist of fetal medicine revealed that the great majority of French physicians (91% of the studied sample) were strongly in favor of prenatal screening for Down syndrome, but many had an imperfect understanding of the tests they offered. Among the 226 gynecologists and 46 general practitioners who answered a detailed questionnaire about prenatal screening, 35.5% had a fair understanding of its methods and results (a correct answer for at least half of the twenty questions asked), and 64.5% had a more limited understanding (less than half of correct answers). The majority of the interrogated physicians knew which tests and measures should be proposed to pregnant women. Few, however, correctly estimated the positive predictive value of a specific result (what the chances are that a given positive result means that the fetus indeed has Down syndrome), and less than half were aware of the high (more than 50%) proportion of spontaneous abortion of trisomic fetuses.[60] Facing the imperfect knowledge of health providers, and the even less perfect knowledge of users of health services, signing a consent form for prenatal screening may be seen as a quasi-ritual act. Such an act, according to anthropologists Klaus Hoeyer and Linda Hogle, projects a stable image of a recognizable and manageable procedure with a particular moral appeal and at the same time is an empty signifier: "The consent requirement has become entrenched in practices through insistence on particular morally sanctioned intentions, regardless of whether these intentions are ever realized."[61]

US sociologists Aliza Kolker and Meredith Burke, who surveyed the conditions in which pregnant women gave consent for prenatal screening, found that in the United States signing a consent form for Down syndrome screening was closer to a ritual than an effort to provide useful information. Women who signed these forms often had stereotyped and inaccurate views of Down syndrome, and such views were seldom corrected by health professionals. Some interviewed women believed that all people with Down syndrome are unable to achieve even modest personal autonomy, while other women were persuaded that all people with this condition are similar to the high-functioning and very likable star with Down syndrome who appeared on the television show *Life Goes On*.[62] To overcome this difficulty, Kolker and Burke proposed to show pregnant women educational videos that presented children and adults with Down syndrome of different degrees of severity and provide these pregnant women with accurate data on the frequency of each level of impairment. Such information, Kolker and Burke added, should be completed by presenting interviews with two equally sympathetic women who, upon learning that they had fetuses with the same diagnosis, reached opposite reproductive decisions.[63] I'm not aware of any country or institution that provides pregnant women with even a simplified version of such a presentation.

Local Fetal Risks

Combined screening for Down syndrome risk was introduced in many Western European countries, but the implementation of such screening was highly variable.[64] As a consequence, women did not have the same opportunity (or, for some, misfortune) to learn whether they carried a trisomic fetus and, since the screening for Down syndrome contributed to the uncovering of additional fetal problems, whether the fetus had other anomalies. Differences in the diffusion of screening for Down syndrome produced "local fetal biology" and "local fetal risk."[65]

The adoption of generalized screening for Down syndrome in France illustrates the switch from testing "at-risk" women to the testing of all pregnant women. Prospective trials of predictive validity of a combination of diagnostic ultrasonogram and serum tests started in the late 1980s.[66] In the late 1990s, many French obstetricians were persuaded that a combined approach to screening for Down syndrome was indeed efficient and suggested this approach to the quasi-totality of their patients. Experts complained, however, that the implantation of screening for Down syndrome was incoherent and sometimes chaotic, and led to too many amniocenteses: 13% of pregnant women in the Parisian region underwent amniocentesis in 2005. French specialists' goal was to bring the level of amniocenteses down to 5% and to detect 70% of trisomic fetuses at that level.[67] Public health specialists were especially concerned by the important regional and socioeconomic disparities in the uptake of screening.[68] To improve the efficacy of screening and put an end to such disparities, in 2009 the French health ministry issued official rules that recommended first trimester screening and fixed its norms.[69]

The great majority of pregnant French women (about 85%, although regional estimates vary), undergo screening for Down syndrome. The screening is voluntary, and women have to sign an informed consent form for a serum test. Refusals are relatively rare. French women who reject testing may be motivated by an opposition to abortion for a fetal indication, an unwillingness to start a medicalized trajectory that may lead them to difficult decisions about amniocentesis and termination of pregnancy, insufficient information about their options, a mistrust of testing, or a combination of the aforementioned reasons. French gynecologists and public health specialists assumed that the great majority of women diagnosed with a trisomic fetus would elect to have an abortion.[70] This is indeed the case. According to data from the French Agence du Médicament, in 2010 less than 10% of women who learned that the fetus was diagnosed with autosomal chromosomal anomalies confirmed by amniocentesis decided to pursue the pregnancy (other sources give a somewhat higher evaluation).[71]

French public health experts perceive the generalization of screening for Down syndrome as a problem of social justice. They stress that while the overall incidence of Down syndrome does not vary according to socioeconomic status, access to testing produced important differences in the incidence of this condition in France.[72] Women of lower socioeconomic status have a higher chance of giving birth to a child with Down syndrome than women in upper socioeconomic strata, despite a higher proportion of older pregnant women in the latter socioeconomic category. Families with fewer resources therefore become disproportionately responsible for the care of impaired infants.[73] French advocates of the generalization of screening for Down syndrome argued that thanks to such screening, choices previously available mainly to middle-class women became available to all women, while specialists who opposed prenatal screening pointed to the dangers of its transformation into a "moral obligation" for pregnant women, pressures on women who refuse testing, and implicit condemnation of women who give birth to a child with Down syndrome.[74]

The United Kingdom implemented pioneering programs for first trimester screening, funded by the National Health Service circa 2000.[75] These programs were gradually extended in the following years.[76] The overall level of screening for Down syndrome in the United Kingdom is, however, lower than in France, as is the (official) number of abortions for fetal indications. In 2013, the UK Department of Health reported 2,921 abortions for fetal indications in England and Wales, while in 2012 France reported 7,134 abortions for such indications.[77] The French and the UK data are not entirely comparable, however, since in the United Kingdom women can abort until twenty-four weeks of pregnancy without providing a medical reason, and in France this time frame is only until fourteen weeks. Down syndrome and numerous other fetal malformations are usually diagnosed before twenty-four weeks of pregnancy. It is not excluded that some British women and some physicians report abortions for fetal malformations (indication E) as abortions for the refusal of a pregnancy. Then again, it is also reasonable to assume that the number of abortions for fetal indications is indeed higher in France because more health professionals actively support screening for fetal anomalies.

Differences between the uptake of screening for fetal anomalies in France and in the United Kingdom might have been affected by high-profile court cases. In 2000, the French Court of Cassation (the equivalent of the US Supreme Court) accorded Nicolas Perruche, who was born severely handicapped because his mother had undiagnosed rubella early in pregnancy, the right to individual compensation for "wrongful life" (the disadvantage of being born) in addition to compensation won by his parents for prejudice they had suffered. Disability rights activists strongly contested this verdict, as did physicians and legislators. In 2001, the French parliament passed a law that would make it impossible to sue doctors for "wrongful life."[78] However, doctors continued to be liable for diagnostic mistakes that caused prejudice to families. The Perruche affair attracted attention to the consequences of errors of prenatal diagnosis. It might have persuaded French doctors that, when in doubt, it is safer to recommend abortion. In the United Kingdom, a parallel affair might have had the opposite effect on the medical profession. In 2001, Joanna Jepson, a Church of England priest, contested the abortion of a 28-week-old fetus with cleft lip and palate. Such malformations, Jepson argued, did not constitute a serious handicap under the terms of the 1967 UK abortion act; the abortion was therefore an unlawful killing. Jepson, today a strikingly good-looking woman, was born with a congenital jaw defect that was surgically corrected when she was a teenager. Such defects, she argued, are fully curable.[79] Jepson lost her lawsuit, but the publicity surrounding the case and the intervention of disability rights advocates might have persuaded British doctors to be more cautious when recommending a termination of pregnancy for a fetal indication, or, alternatively, that it is safer for them to present such a termination as an abortion for a refusal of pregnancy.

There are important regional and local differences in the diffusion of screening for Down syndrome in the United Kingdom.[80] The overall detection rates of Down syndrome in the United Kingdom (57%) are lower than in France (estimated at 80%). In socially deprived areas, the rate of Down syndrome detection is markedly lower, and the rate of the birth of children with serious inborn impairments is, accordingly, higher. Such disparities were attributed to class-dependent and regional inequality of access to screening for Down syndrome rather than to differences in attitudes toward abortion for a fetal indication, because regional and class disparities in the number of children born with severe structural anomalies detected by routine ultrasound examinations are much lower.[81] A leaflet titled "Screening Programmes: Antenatal and Newborn," produced by the National Screening Committee (NSC) of the British National Health Service, presents problems that may arise in the context of screening for Down syndrome, including the risk of embarking on an irreversible medicalized trajectory; it also mentions the variability of manifestations of Down syndrome.[82] Sociologists who observed prenatal consultations in the United Kingdom concluded, however, that the NSC leaflet, while well balanced, is long and complicated, and pregnant women have difficulties extracting from it information they consider relevant.[83] Sociologists also discovered that the view of Down syndrome conveyed to pregnant women during prenatal consultations can be schematic and inaccurate.[84] The distribution of a leaflet may not be enough to promote efficient transmission of knowledge on a complex topic.

Denmark was the first country to introduce generalized screening for Down syndrome. From 2004 on, screening for this condition has been offered to all pregnant women in Denmark, independently of their age. The acceptance rate of the screening is at least 90%. One study, conducted in 2005, revealed that only 2% of the surveyed women refused screening for Down syndrome, while another study established that the acceptance of screening in Copenhagen was 95%. The Danish government, perhaps wishing to neutralize accusations that it promotes eugenic measures, especially in light of Denmark's eugenic past, stressed that the goal of prenatal testing was not to prevent children with serious diseases from being born but to assist pregnant women in making their own choices. Danish women were reported to have recognized the explanations they received from health professionals and the possibility given to them to elect whether to undergo prenatal screening and testing as a form of care.[85] Finland's model is similar to the Danish one. Certain Finnish regions and municipalities started to offer systematic serum testing for Down syndrome risk to all pregnant women in the mid-1990s. A 2006 decree generalized such screening in the whole country. All pregnant women are offered first trimester serum tests coupled with measurements of nuchal translucency. Although some disability activists protested the generalization of prenatal screening, such a protest was short-lived and had limited visibility. Policymakers explained that the Finnish public's largely noncritical acceptance of prenatal screening reflects a high level of trust in the country's public health system.[86]

In Norway, screening for Down syndrome is offered only to women older than 38 and to those known to have an increased risk of giving birth to a disabled child. The approval of such screening is relatively low. In 2007, the Swedish Medical Ethics Board recommended that all pregnant women be offered information about the assessment of their risk of carrying a Down fetus as well as access to relevant tests. Before the introduction of this measure, experts primarily discussed the costs and reliability of serum tests. Public debates in Sweden had quickly shifted to ethical considerations, with a special focus on the need to take into account different cultural sensibilities, especially among immigrant populations.[87] In Iceland, every pregnant woman receives detailed information about the possibility of testing for Down syndrome risk, but if she elects to undergo such testing, she has to pay for it herself.[88] This is the case in the Netherlands, too: women who wish to be screened for Down syndrome risk have to pay for this expense from their own pocket.

Important differences in the uptake of Down syndrome screening in Western European countries may be affected by distinct attitudes toward women's "right not to know." The right not to know is not present in debates on screening for Down syndrome in the United Kingdom or in France. In the Netherlands, health professionals, but also pregnant women, are very concerned about women's right to ignore the health status of the fetus. In Denmark, the right not to know has an official legal standing, but the implementation of this principle is less compelling than in the Netherlands. Danish professionals have a more positive view of prenatal screening than their Dutch or British peers. They recognize women's right to opt out of screening but are mainly interested in providing women the opportunity to undergo such screening and are concerned by the lack of opportunity to make informed reproductive choices. Attitudes toward prenatal screening affect the organization of health services. In Denmark, such screening is seen as a routine intervention and a part of services provided to all pregnant women by the National Health Service, while in the Netherlands it is seen as an exceptional approach that is not covered by the National Health Service. Such framing of prenatal screening may send Dutch women a message that this is an unnecessary test and may partly explain its low uptake.[89]

Another explanation for the low acceptance of screening for Down syndrome in the Netherlands (26% of pregnant women undergo such screening) is the structure of prenatal consultations. In France, pregnant women see a gynecologist in a fully medicalized setting. Screening for Down syndrome is embedded in a local tradition of intensive medicalization of pregnancy: pregnant women have an important number of tests that are fully covered by the national social security system. Screening is often presented as a self-evident part of the medical supervision of pregnancy, and its refusal, if not motivated by religious or "cultural" reasons (the latter is a code name for beliefs of migrant women), is often presented as irrational behavior. French consultations that present screening for Down syndrome are very brief, and women do not receive detailed information

on the goals and pitfalls of screening. Prenatal consultations in the United Kingdom, often but not exclusively conducted by midwives, are longer and less medicalized than those in France, but women only receive partial information on testing for Down syndrome risk. In the Netherlands, pregnant women always meet
with a midwife in a nonmedicalized setting. Information about screening for
Down syndrome is embedded in a long consultation focused on the pregnant
woman's health and well-being.[90] Dutch midwives' interactions with pregnant
women reflect their professional commitment to the understanding of pregnancy
as a natural process that should be protected from overmedicalization and during which women should focus on the positive aspects of becoming mothers.
Their counseling style can also be seen as midwives' strategy to protect their
professional autonomy and their "ownership" of the jurisdiction of pregnancy
supervision.[91] "Risk of a fetal malformation," comparative studies indicate, is a
situated entity produced through complex interactions between legal, economic,
material, and professional considerations.

Screening and Emotions

Screening for Down syndrome, according to its advocates, reassures women
that their future child is all right. Not all women are reassured, however. A Polish study displays, probably to an extreme degree, problems faced by women
who embark on a bumpy medicalized trajectory. Poland has no organized
screening for Down syndrome risk, probably because abortion is illegal in Poland with the exception of a handful of well-defined cases such as rape or immediate danger to a woman's life. Nevertheless, Polish health plans frequently
offer women a "package" of prenatal tests, which includes a serum test for
Down syndrome risk (PAPP-A). Several women bitterly regretted taking this
test. They unthinkingly agreed to be tested for Down syndrome risk, and then
found themselves in a stressful and unhappy situation.[92] The Polish study is
grounded in a small number of interviews and in the analysis of text posted on
internet sites dedicated to pregnancy. It is very difficult to know how representative they are. Moreover, in the absence of a legal possibility to terminate a
pregnancy for a fetal indication, Polish women may be especially distressed
upon learning that they are at a higher than average risk of giving birth to a
trisomic child.[93] Practically all the stories reported in this study have a "happy
ending"—meaning that the fetus was found to be nontrisomic. Polish women
who received a "positive" amniocentesis result may be less willing to share
their experience, especially if the diagnosis of Down syndrome led to an illegal
abortion.

Danish women's reactions to prenatal screening seem to be at the opposite end of the emotional spectrum from those exhibited by Polish women. Sociologists report that for many women in Denmark, screening for Down syndrome seems to be an opportunity to exercise a right for rational, although constrained, choices. Danish women often accept the view that prenatal screening and testing is the right path toward having a healthy baby, and that health professionals who help them in the process of decision making are offering individualized care. Such care may include information on what the majority of Danish women do in a given case but also, according to ultrasound experts, allows pregnant women to act in unexpected ways. The existence of atypical behavior patterns is presented as sufficient proof that Danish women have a true reproductive choice.[94]

Israel is often presented as a specific case because of the high level of enthusiasm for prenatal testing and screening, and an especially high rate of termination of pregnancies for fetal indications. The latter statement needs to be qualified. The overall rate of termination of pregnancy for fetal indications in Israel is not different from the rates in other industrialized countries; however, statewide statistics are misleading because they lump together two very different populations: religious and secular. Judaism and Islam do not categorically forbid abortion, but this intervention is seen by religious Jewish and Muslim women as a last resort.[95] In contrast, secular Israeli-Jewish women and to some extent, at least, "modern" segments of Israeli-Palestinian women are interested in prenatal diagnosis and were described as strongly committed to the termination of pregnancy for a fetal indication. In Israel, rates of abortion for sex chromosome anomalies such as Klinefelter and triple X syndromes were reported to be higher than in Western Europe. Such high rates of termination for conditions often labeled as "mild" might have been affected by the attitudes of genetic counselors. Despite counselors' affirmation that they provided neutral advice, the majority of Israeli women reported that they felt as if the counselor encouraged them to have an abortion. This impression cannot be simply attributed to women's efforts to attenuate guilt about the decision to have an abortion, because women who chose to continue with the pregnancy following a diagnosis of a sex chromosome anomaly also frequently reported that they had the impression that the counselor favored a termination of pregnancy.[96]

Anthropologist Yael Hashiloni-Dolev's interviews with Israeli and German genetic counselors confirm this impression. Israeli genetic counselors often openly supported the termination of "flawed" pregnancies. They explained that their main allegiance is to the pregnant woman and her family, not to the unborn child.[97]

Israeli genetic counselors explained:

I have nothing against abortion. I think it can reduce suffering. In any case I respect the parents' wishes, and if they want to abort, I see it as their full right. Generally I trust the parents that when it's a wanted pregnancy, as is usually the case when people reach me, they will not rush into abortion for stupid reasons. And I am also not to decide what a major or a minor problem is. Abortion is very hard for women; it involves a lot of grief, and I sympathise with the mother's pain. But the fetus? It is really nothing to me. Only a potential life, with no rights.

The fetus belongs to the mother. It is her business, and she is allowed to do with it things that I might dislike. I am always there primarily for her. After all, she is the one who would have to raise this child. For me, the fetus is part of the woman's body, until very late. Of course in the 30th week of pregnancy it is harder to see it that way, but I would hardly see the fetus as independent.

Israeli genetic counselors claimed that they are aware of pregnant women's feelings and are sensitive to their suffering. They also differentiated early and late abortion, and were decidedly less at ease with the latter. Nevertheless, the bottom line seems to be a sharp differentiation between already-existing people and potential human beings, as well as the conviction that the fetus does not have distinct rights: "I think that until the moment of birth the mothers' rights override those of the fetus in every sense. The fetus has an obvious legal guardian, its mother, and she should decide about its fate. As long as there is no self-consciousness, and I am sure the fetus does not have any, to my mind it can be killed without any problem. I think using the different weeks of pregnancy as the criterion is superficial. The last line is crossed at birth."

By contrast, German genetic counselors tend to see themselves as advocates of the unborn child and identify with this child. They often see the fetus and even the embryo as an autonomous being endowed with rights of its own. As one counselor explains: "The embryo must be protected. Within the family situation it has rights, like anyone else. Not more or less, but like the others."[98]

German genetic counselors who see themselves as protectors of the rights of the unborn child sometimes view a woman who elects to terminate a "flawed" pregnancy as "selfish," because she is placing her own needs before those of her future child.[99] Israeli genetic counselors, who strongly identify with the family and the community, may hold an opposite point of view and may see a woman who decides to continue a pregnancy with an affected fetus as "selfish" because, unwilling to undergo the trauma of abortion, she refuses to take into consideration the risk of the negative effects of the birth of a disabled child on her living children and other family members.[100]

One of the key elements that shapes the approval of prenatal diagnosis in Israel, according to anthropologist Tsipy Ivry, is the belief that pregnancy is always fraught with danger.[101] Pregnant Israeli women are warned about all the misfortunes that can befall them if they give birth to an impaired child. In prenatal events organized by hospitals, medical experts discuss in detail fetal deformations such as cleft lip, hernia, distorted sexual organs, extra fingers, and fetuses with two heads (a form of conjoined twins), and show images of these malformations on a large screen. Experts convey the message that nature is bound to make serious mistakes. Prenatal diagnosis, they explain, can detect some, but not all, such mistakes, a discourse that both encourages consumption of new technologies and increases pregnant women's anxiety. Instead of adhering to a rational discourse about risk, many Israeli women react to the worst-case scenario. A story told by an Israeli fetal medicine expert at a "prenatal event" illustrates this tendency. A 27-year-old woman who had no indication of a fetal problem insisted nevertheless to undergo amniocentesis, because, she explained, if she had a miscarriage following the test she might be angry, but since she was young she could conceive again. If she had a child with Down syndrome, this would be, she claimed, the end of her life. Amniocentesis indeed revealed that this woman was carrying a Down syndrome fetus.[102]

In Israel, Ivry proposes, all pregnancies, regardless of their medical categorization as low or high risk, are perceived by doctors and women to be a potential source of a reproductive misfortune. In many industrialized countries, medical discourse about "risky pregnancies" often refers to risks for the fetus. In Israel, such discourse often refers to risks represented by the fetus to the pregnant woman and her family. The fear that shapes the experience of pregnancy of many Israeli women, Ivry believes, is rooted in other aspects of Israeli life. The idea that a catastrophe—physical, spiritual, or both—lies around the corner is omnipresent in Jewish collective memory and is permanently consolidated through the commemoration of traumatic events in Jewish history. Such a "catastrophic" view also dominates the understanding of pregnancy. Fetal images in Israel have become entangled in a "politics of threatened life," where "life" typically stands for the pregnant woman and "threat" stands for the unborn child.[103]

Significant disparities in the use of prenatal screening among industrialized countries can be explained by differences in health care structures, especially access to tests and the level of reimbursement of screening; the organization of medical labor, for example, whether information about "Down syndrome risk" is provided by midwives, general practitioners, gynecologists, or genetic counselors; and "cultural variables." The latter term usually refers to elements such as history, religion, tradition, and customs. It also includes a situated perception of maternal obligations and duties as well as women's status in the labor market. It is probably not by chance that the approval of Down syndrome screening tends to be lower in countries in which a higher percentage of mothers of young children leave full-time work and dedicate themselves mainly to childcare.[104] Kristin Luker's important insight that the debate on abortion rights cannot be dissociated from the debate on women's role in society and a broader understanding of women's tasks as mothers and caretakers can be extended to selective reproduction as well.[105]

To follow Luker, people who believe that it is a woman's prime duty and vocation to give and sustain life can occasionally justify an abortion for a fetal indication because of a desire to prevent severe suffering of the future child but not because of the claim that the care of an impaired child will limit the life options of the mother. If being a caretaker, including a caretaker of a "special needs" child and a disabled adult, is seen as more important and rewarding than any other female activity, then there is no need to promote screening for Down syndrome.[106] People who believe that a woman should not be defined by motherhood and should be free at each moment of her life to decide whether she wishes to dedicate herself to care tasks or to other life plans often support abortion for refusal of motherhood and selective abortion for fetal impairment. They also frequently favor a generalized screening for Down syndrome in the name of social justice: it is unfair that only middle-class women are able to decide whether they wish to give birth to a trisomic child. Debates on screening for fetal anomalies may be, again echoing Luker, less about disability rights or human diversity and more about a contrast between two worldviews: one that sees women, above all, as mothers and caretakers, and therefore radically different from (but by no means inferior to) men, and another that stresses the equality between the sexes and a woman's right to reject maternity and care tasks or to decide what priority she is willing to give to these tasks. The term *cultural variables* also contains a value judgment about the place of women in society.

CHAPTER 5

Sex Chromosome Aneuploidies

Hormonal Disorders: Infantile Women and Underdeveloped Men

The history of prenatal diagnosis of sex chromosome anomalies is an especially telling illustration of dilemmas produced by detecting a fetal anomaly before birth. Prenatal diagnosis of sex chromosome anomalies is inseparably intertwined with the search for Down syndrome fetuses. Such a search led, in some cases, to an unexpected result: a diagnosis of the presence of an abnormal number of sex chromosomes, especially Turner syndrome (45,Xo) and Klinefelter syndrome (47,XXY). Many pregnant women have at least an approximate idea of the impairments linked with the presence of a supplementary chromosome 21, but very few are informed about problems linked with an abnormal number of sex chromosomes. Pregnant women are also frequently unaware of the existence of other autosomal aneuploidies (an abnormal number of non–sex chromosomes) besides trisomy 21, especially trisomy 13 (Patau syndrome) and trisomy 18 (Edwards syndrome), but the severity of the symptoms produced by the latter anomalies often facilitates reproductive decisions. Just the opposite is true for sex chromosome anomalies. The majority of these anomalies are linked with relatively minor but not insignificant developmental problems. Moreover, the expression of such problems is highly variable. Prenatal diagnosis of sex chromosome anomalies is an especially revealing object of study, or, following anthropologist Claude Lévi Strauss's expression, a "bon à penser" (good for thinking) topic, which reveals the unstable and shifting definitions of the normal fetus and the pathological fetus and their shaping by technoscientific developments.

TS was named after the researcher who described it in 1938, endocrinologist Henry Turner from the University of Oklahoma.[1] Turner had observed among his patients several women with a cluster of similar anatomical and physiological manifestations: a short stature, a thick (webbed) neck, a low hairline, a tendency to develop edema, an increased carrying angle at the elbow, and, above all, "infantilism": the absence of secondary sexual development. Women studied by Turner did not menstruate, lacked breast development, and maintained a childlike body after puberty. In addition, Turner was unable to palpate their ovaries. The syndrome was therefore described as an arrested sexual development in girls. Turner's first idea was that his patients' symptoms reflected an anomaly of the pituitary gland, but he and other endocrinologists quickly decided that these women suffered from "ovarian agenesis" (insufficient development of the ovaries), and that many of their symptoms reflected the absence of female sex hormones secreted by the ovaries.

In the 1920s and 1930s, scientists learned to isolate and then to synthetize sex hormones.[2] One of the potential uses of such hormones was the treatment of sexual development anomalies. Surgeons elaborated new techniques of "correcting" inborn malformations of sexual organs.[3] In the same period, scientists purified male and female sex hormones, and pharmaceutical companies commercialized hormone preparation. As leading US endocrinologist Fuller Albright put it in the 1930s, "sex was weighed, bottled and put on the market."[4] Scientists believed that patients with other anomalies of sexual organ development and secondary manifestation of sex would benefit from sex hormone therapy. Turner treated women diagnosed with ovarian agenesis with estrogen and discovered that they indeed responded well to this treatment. The patients developed breasts, the size of their uterus increased, and they acquired a more feminine silhouette. The administration of female hormones brought them, Turner explained, "up to a point where they [could] get married and lead a normal life as a female." The therapy could not, alas, cure their sterility, but, "still, they can be partners in marriages and successfully bring up the children. They can rear them."[5]

In the 1930s and 1940s, experts usually agreed with Turner and classified ovarian agenesis among hormonal disorders.[6] This was, for example, the view that guided the studies of sex development disorders in Albright's laboratory at Massachusetts General Hospital in Boston. Albright and his colleagues became very interested in the syndrome described by Turner, because they saw it as a "nature experiment" that would enable them to study the physiological consequences of the absence of hormones secreted by the ovaries.[7] They investigated, among other things, effects of hormones on pilosity. The presence of some axillary and pubic hair in girls with TS was interpreted as additional proof that they were not suffering from pituitary insufficiency but only from a lack of sex hormones.[8] Patients with ovarian agenesis who were treated by Albright and his colleagues were submitted to batteries of tests, and then treated with numerous hormonal preparations. For example, one of their "star patients," "Kay" (patient no. 6), first seen in Albright's laboratory in 1938, participated in an extended study of the effects of diet on her condition and was treated with several hormones: adrenocorticotropic hormone (or corticotrophin), thyrotropin, and ethyltestosterone. As one of her doctors explained, "There are very few things in our repertory that she hasn't received."[9]

For Turner and Albright, TS was a typical endocrine disorder. German researcher Otto Ullrich, however, proposed a different explanation of the syndrome described by Harry Turner. Ullrich saw the lack of development of the ovaries as a secondary manifestation of an error of early embryonic development. Ullrich claimed that in 1930, eight years before the publication of Turner's paper, he had described an 8-year-old girl with a webbed neck and generalized edema. In 1932, Norwegian biologist Kristine Bonnevie (known for her pioneering studies of dermatoglyphs, among other studies) described similar manifestations (webbed neck and edema) in a strain of mutant mice: the my/my strain, developed by Bagg and Little at Jackson Laboratories in Bar Harbor, Maine.[10] Ullrich proposed to call the phenomenon he described Status Bonnevie-Ullrich (SBU), a suggestion adopted in the 1940s and 1950s by researchers in continental Europe. Conversely, as Ullrich himself stressed, it was not certain that TS and SBU were identical, because they were described in different types of studies. Turner and Albright investigated endocrine disorders in girls, while Ullrich and Bonnevie focused on the effects of mutations on embryogenesis, mainly in laboratory animals (and their possible parallels in humans). Ullrich also knew that similar anatomical and physiological manifestations could be produced by very different mechanisms: "To be sure, we need to forewarn ourselves against the dangers of inferring homologous genetic events for single characteristics. For we have learned from general genetics that phenotypically very similar traits can not only be due to different genes, but can also result from entirely different epigenetic events."[11] Nevertheless, Ullrich believed that the majority of cases described as TS in the literature did represent a subset of SBU and might have their origins in embryological development.

The controversy on the priority of the discovery of ovarian agenesis ended with a compromise: in the 1950s, many authors called this syndrome Turner-Ullrich syndrome (TUS).[12] It was more difficult to agree on precisely what the manifestations of this syndrome were, and on how to classify the cases that only showed some of these manifestations. Most experts agreed that the main traits of TS/TUS are a webbed neck and edema of extremities, and, in older girls/women, "streak ovaries" (small, degenerated glands) and the absence of puberty.

In the early 1950s, scientists were not sure whether TS/TUS (and, for some continental experts, SBU) was a condition present only in women, or whether it could be found in men, too. They were also not sure whether this syndrome was primarily a hormonal disorder or a consequence of faulty embryogenesis, and possibly a mutation. Many researchers agreed with the latter statement because TS/TUS was linked with a large spectrum of symptoms; moreover, some of these symptoms (edema, webbed neck) were found in female newborns who later developed ovarian agenesis. Other researchers believed that the cluster of physiological manifestations gathered under the heading TS/TUS might reflect the aggregation of several independent causes.[13]

In 1942, endocrinologist Harry Klinefelter, together with Edward Reifenstein and Fuller Albright, published an article titled "Syndrome Characterized by Gynecomastia [enlarged breasts in a man], Aspermatogenesis without A-Leydigism [one kind of absence of the production of sperm cells], and Increased Excretion of Follicle-Stimulating Hormone." This article described a group of men with imperfect sexual development that could be attributed to a male "gonadal agenesis."[14] Klinefelter became interested in endocrinology during his studies at Johns Hopkins University School of Medicine. In 1941–1942, he became a research fellow in Albright's laboratory at Massachusetts General Hospital in Boston, which at that time was the leading center of endocrinological research in the United States.[15] One of the first patients Klinefelter examined when he arrived at Albright's laboratory was a black boy with "gynecomastia and small testes." Albright was very enthusiastic about this case, and Klinefelter found his enthusiasm to be contagious. Klinefelter soon found two other similar patients, and this strange combination of syndromes became one of his main research topics in Boston.[16] The 1942 article described nine male patients who had enlarged breasts, sparse facial and body hair, small testes (hypogonadism), and an inability to produce sperm. Seven cases were observed at Massachusetts General Hospital, and two in private practice. One of the patients was black, and three were Jewish. Five patients did manual labor (one of them was described as "feeble-minded"), two had nonmanual occupations (a teacher and a merchant), and two were still in school.[17] Klinefelter treated his patients with testosterone to favor the development of secondary sexual traits and to boost their libido. Those with prominent breasts were offered a mastectomy. The treatment was seen as successful; in retrospect, Klinefelter stressed the "normality" of his early patients.[18]

The original name of the syndrome (gynecomastia, aspermatogenesis without a- Leydigism, and increased excretion of follicle-stimulating hormone) was too complex, so it was quickly renamed Klinefelter syndrome (KS).[19] The original name conveyed, however, an important message: this syndrome was a unique combination of several structural anomalies. In Albright's laboratory, KS was firmly integrated into an endocrinological conceptual framework.[20] KS was sometimes aggregated with TS under the heading "gonadal agenesis." However, while TS was from the very beginning linked with manifestations unrelated to sexual development, such as webbing of the neck and generalized edema, and perceptible already in newborns, manifestations of KS were limited to faulty development of sex glands and secondary sex traits.[21] Moreover, frequently the main complaint of people with KS and the reason why they sought medical help was sterility. KS was therefore more readily perceived as a "true" endocrinological manifestation, or, rather, as one among many disorders linked with insufficient development of sex glands.

In the early 1950s, endocrinologists, pediatricians, and general practitioners were not sure what the precise boundaries of TS and KS were, and what the cause of these disorders was, but they were mainly seen as conditions that belonged to the endocrinologists' jurisdiction. The status of these syndromes had, however, dramatically changed in the mid-1950s, as a consequence of Murray Barr's studies of sex chromatin. These studies indicated that TS and KS patients were not what they seemed to be. Turner's conviction that hormonal treatment transformed TS girls into normal (although sterile) women and excellent wives, and Klinefelter's belief that thanks to an appropriate hormonal and occasionally surgical treatment his patients became "normal men" were erroneous.[22] Both TS and KS, Barr and his colleagues claimed, were "nature's freaks": extreme cases of pseudohermaphroditism with a complete sex reversion. TS women, according to Barr and other experts, were, in fact, biological men, and KS men were biological women.

Inversions: Barr Bodies and Origins of the Distinction between Sex and Gender

How doth the telltale chromosome
Make sex distinctions clearer
And sent a doubting Thomas home
A doubting Thomasina?
Rejoice, hermaphroditic folk
In Doc Barr's deed of splendor
A moment glance from him evokes
Your true and proper gender
—*Anonymous (probably circa 1953)*[23]

"Doc Barr's deed of splendor" was the description of the "Barr body": a cellular marker of sex. The anonymous author of this poem speaks about "true and proper gender," but in this context the meaning was in all probability a true and proper biological/chromosomal sex. However, a few years later, psychologists and psychiatrists defined *gender* as a given person's self-perception as being a man or a woman and started to speak about "gender identity" and "gender role." The dissociation between sex and gender was directly linked with "Doc Barr's deed of splendor" and its direct consequence—studies of the presence of Barr bodies in cells of people with TS and KS conducted in the pediatric endocrinology laboratory at Johns Hopkins School of Medicine.[24]

Barr's 1949 observation that a cellular marker, the Barr body (a dark spot visible in the cytoplasm), was present in mammals in female but not in male cells led to the development of a simple method of differentiating between "chromosomal males" and "chromosomal females." Barr and his colleagues assumed that this cellular marker indicated the presence of two X chromosomes.[25] At first, they looked for the presence of "sex chromatin bodies" in skin biopsies, including from humans, which was a tedious and painful procedure. Later, they switched to the study of cells present in a buccal smear. The latter, much simpler test (it was sufficient to take a cotton swab from the interior of the mouth) made it possible to quickly determine whether an individual was a "chromosomal male" or a "chromosomal female."[26] The main clinical importance of tests that determined a chromosomal sex, experts concluded in the 1950s, was to define the "true sex" of individuals with disorders of sexual development who could not be easily defined as typical males or typical females.[27]

In the early 1950s, Barr and his collaborators examined cells from people with TS and KS, and found that those with KS always had chromatin bodies, while those with TS always lacked such bodies. They concluded that TS women were in fact genetic males and KS men were genetic females.[28] The case of TS was readily explained through an analogy with a well-known animal model: the feminization of rabbits castrated at a very young age. The feminization of male rabbits and the presence of a (quasi) feminine body in TS individuals were interpreted as demonstrations of the "Adam principle"—that all living organisms are female by default and acquire masculine traits as a result of the presence of an additional stimulus provided by the development of testes. Individuals with TS suffered from an underdevelopment of sex glands (gonadal agenesis), which explained why their anatomical sex was in contradiction with their chromosomal sex.[29]

The finding that KS patients (i.e., individuals who looked like men) had a female chromosomal pattern was more difficult to explain, because it contradicted the concept that masculinization is not a default condition but can only be achieved as a result of an additional stimulus.[30] Newborn female animals can be masculinized if exposed to high doses of testosterone, but the development of testes—however imperfect—in biological females was in total contradiction to the Adam principle, as was a virilization of these (presumed) biological females in the absence of high levels of male hormones. At first, researchers proposed that KS individuals might be true hermaphrodites (people who have both male and female sex glands or mixed sex glands with ovarian and testicular cells), but this hypothesis was not supported by histological findings. KS individuals had testicular but not ovarian tissue. Researchers had finally decided that KS was probably a consequence of an anomaly at a very early stage of embryonic development, such as an error in the expression of sex-determining genes in a zygote (the first stages of the division of a fertilized egg) that carries two X chromosomes.[31]

The reinterpretation of TS and KS as extreme cases of pseudohermaphroditism favored a radical distinction between biological sex and psychosocial gender. This distinction originated in studies of "intersex" children in the pediatric endocrinology department at Johns Hopkins Hospital. It is usually traced to early attempts of hormonal and chirurgical treatment of children born with ambivalent or sex-inappropriate genital organs. The head of the pediatric endocrinology department at Johns Hopkins Hospital, Dr. Lawson Wilkins, specialized in the treatment of children with congenital adrenal hyperplasia (CAH)—a recessive hereditary condition that leads to excess testosterone secretion in the fetus, and then in the newborn child. Girls with CAH are "biological females"— they have a uterus and ovaries, and are Barr body–positive—but are often born with masculine-looking external genital organs and develop a masculine body build and hair distribution. As a consequence, some were raised as girls, while others were raised as boys.

Wilkins developed a pragmatic approach to the management of CAH girls. Initially, this condition was seen as untreatable because, unlike TS, it did not respond to female sex hormones. Wilkins therefore proposed that a strongly virilized newborn girl with CAH would in all probability be happier if raised in the male sex, since Wilkins believed that it was possible to be a biological female with the psychological sex of a male. By contrast, individuals already socialized as females should be offered corrective surgery that would feminize their external genital organs.[32] Attitudes toward the treatment of CAH girls had changed, however, circa 1950, when physicians discovered that treatment with a newly isolated hormone, cortisol (a steroid hormone secreted by the adrenal gland), attenuated the virilization of CAH girls and helped them develop a more feminine silhouette and menstruate.[33] From that time on, the standard recommendation in the endocrinology department at Johns Hopkins Hospital was to treat all CAH girls with cortisol and, if necessary, to reduce the size of their clitoris through surgery. In 1951, Wilkins hired a young psychologist, John Money, to assess the effects of cortisol treatment on a child's psyche. Money concluded that a child's "gender role," that is, whether a child saw him- or herself as a boy or a girl, was shaped by the sex in which the child was raised. Early education was more important than any single biological variable. The key term was *early*. Gender role, Money and his collaborators Joan and John Hampson proposed, was acquired at a critical age, o to 3 years, when it was imprinted on the child's mind. CAH girls who were socialized from the earliest age as "normal girls," they explained, would develop a female gender role and "gender appropriate" behaviors and aspirations, which in the 1950s included playing with dolls rather than trucks, liking pretty clothes, rejecting a tomboy demeanor, and hoping one day to be a mother.[34]

Money and the Hampsons's research started with observations of CAH girls. This was, however, an imperfect model for the display of a radical dissociation between social and biological sex, because despite their hormonal imbalance and virilized external sex organs, these girls were "true" biological females.[35] People with TS were different because in that case, (presumed) biological men were socialized as women.[36] People with TS, Wilkins and his collaborators stressed in 1955, "should be regarded as the most severe and extreme forms of male pseudohermaphroditism." They added, however, that "the sexual orientation of these patients has been entirely feminine, irrespective of the chromosomal sex pattern," and concluded that "patients and their families should not be informed concerning their chromosomal sex when a male chromatin pattern is found, in view of present-day misconceptions of the importance of chromosomes in determining psychosexual outlook."[37]

Further investigations by Money and the Hampsons consolidated this view.[38] Their study of eleven individuals/women with TS revealed that all these patients "fulfilled completely all the cultural and psychological expectations of femininity." Their behavior and sexual orientation was invariably feminine, an excellent illustration of the principle that "the salient finding to emerge from the study was that a person's conviction of himself as a man or herself as a woman—the gender role and erotic orientation—is a variable quite independent of genes and chromosomes."[39] Then again, Money and the Hampsons believed that TS individuals were able to develop a psychologically sound female gender role because they and their families and friends had no doubts about their sex / gender identity. Were they aware of the discrepancy between their chromosomes and their bodies, the final result might have been less felicitous.[40]

KS individuals were seen by some experts as even more extreme cases of sex reversal. Some TS girls were diagnosed with structural anomalies (edema, webbed neck) as babies or young children. Many others consulted a physician at adolescence because of their short stature, atypical body shape, and, above all, absence of menstruation. By contrast, many KS men, especially those without gynecomastia, looked "normal" and did not view themselves as "different," at least until they attempted to have children. Using buccal smears, researchers found that numerous men treated in infertility clinics had KS.[41] Between 1955 and 1959, researchers who studied KS individuals explained that they investigated the effects of "extreme sex reversal." The adjective "extreme" might have referred to the fact that many among the people with this condition classified as biological females on the basis of the presence of Barr bodies in their cells had unremarkably male bodies. Often the only symptom, which finally led their doctors to the conclusion that they were examining a "biological woman," was their infertility. Since only a fraction of infertile men consulted a specialized clinic, it was probable that the majority of KS men escaped the medical gaze and never learned that they represented the "most severe type of pseudohermaphroditism." KS was technically defined as "male pseudohermaphroditism with gonadal dysgenesis," but, as Barr stressed, "in the practical situation the patients are clearly males, and a terminology that suggests otherwise is best avoided."[42]

Money and the Hampsons's paper on gender role was constructed as a critique of what they called the new dogma that presented chromosomes as the ultimate arbiters of sex.[43] Conversely, the rise of this new dogma was made possible precisely by the diffusion of testing for the presence of sex chromatin in "intersex" individuals. A 1957, a review of the role of human sex chromosomes explained that "the systematic analysis of human intersexes by the cytological diagnosis of the sex chromosomes, in combination with anatomical, endocrinological, and genetic evidence, has made possible a new approach to the study of normal and pathological human sexual development. It can also be seen that this approach has already proved to be of considerable value both from the clinical and the theoretical point of view."[44]

The widespread diffusion of testing for Barr bodies helped resolve earlier controversies about the definition of the syndrome that included claims that TS was found in men, too. A woman who displayed some of the signs of TS, such as gonadal agenesis, short stature, and webbed neck, and who was found to be Barr body–negative (a male chromosomal pattern) was diagnosed with TS. The same symptoms without a male chromosomal pattern were diagnosed as a different endocrinological or physiological condition, as were gonadal agenesis and gynecomastia in "Barr body–negative" men. Studies conducted by Paul Polani and his colleagues at Guy's Hospital in London, which indicated that TS individuals display some predominantly male traits such as the narrowing of the aorta and color blindness, reinforced the claim that TS "women" are, in fact, biological males.[45]

Researchers who studied TS and KS in the 1950s looked for the presence of the Barr body. The presence of this body, they assumed, revealed that an XX chromosomal formula, and its absence, was interpreted as an indication of the presence of an XY chromosomal formula. Some investigators proposed, however, that XX and XY are not the only possible configurations of human sex chromosomes, and that it is highly plausible that some people have other chromosomal patterns, such as Xo, XXY, XYY, and XY and XX with sex reversal and hermaphroditism. It is not excluded that at least some individuals with TS and KS carry one of these atypical configurations.[46] In order to verify this hypothesis, however, scientists had to turn to direct studies of human chromosomes. Such studies became possible in the late 1950s and again radically changed the understanding of TS and KS.

Chromosomes: From Underdeveloped Gonads to Imperfect Gametes

The redefinition of "mongolism" as "trisomy 21" in 1959 was immediately followed by the description of the role of an abnormal number of sex chromosomes in the genesis of TS and KS.[47] In 1959, Charles Ford, Paul Polani, and their collaborators linked TS with an absence of one X chromosome (chromosomal formula 45,oX), and Patricia Jacobs and her colleagues linked KS with the presence of a supplementary X chromosome (chromosomal formula 47,XXY).[48] Jacobs and her colleagues also described girls with an additional X chromosome (47,XXX), a relatively frequent condition later linked with a risk of mild to moderate learning impairment.[49] Other investigators found even rarer multiples of X and Y, conditions usually linked with more serious physical and intellectual disabilities.[50]

The view of TS, KS, and similar syndromes as anomalies of the number of sex chromosomes complicated the understanding of these conditions. Some individuals were found to have a mosaic chromosomal formula—a mixture of cells with a normal and an abnormal number of chromosomes (for TS, 45,Xo/46,XX and for KS, 47,XXY/46,XY). Other individuals developed KS- or TS-like syndromes as a result of a sex chromosome translocation rather than a variation in the number of such chromosomes, a situation similar to trisomy 21 manifestations produced by a translocation.[51] The new definition narrowed the number of cases defined as "true" TS and KS. It also put an end to the perception that these symptoms represented sex reversal and extreme cases of pseudohermaphroditism in humans. For the majority of specialists, TS individuals became women again with some health-related issues, and KS individuals became men again with some health-related issues.

The redefinition of TS and KS as sex chromosome aneuploidies freed physicians from having to hide from their patients that their "biological sex" was at odds with their bodies and their socialization but did not have other practical consequences. Individuals with these conditions, if they were diagnosed at all (this is especially true for KS men, often unaware of their condition), continued to be treated mainly with sex hormones, as they were in the 1940s and 1950s. However, the new understanding of these disorders had an important theoretical consequence: a focus on the role of the Y chromosome. This chromosome replaced the testes as the structure that modulated the (presumed) default female embryonic development and produced male attributes. The Adam principle was maintained in a new, chromosomal version. Another consequence of the shift to a chromosomal definition of TS and KS was a new understanding of the nature of the Barr body. In 1961, British geneticist Mary Lyon proposed that in women, one of the two X chromosomes was always inactivated and that the Barr body represented the inactivated and excluded chromosome. This new view explained why the Barr body was absent in TS women who only had one X chromosome (45,Xo) and was present in KS men who had two X chromosomes (47,XXY).[52] The Barr body was an efficient marker of biological/chromosomal sex, but only in individuals with a "normal" chromosomal formula: it had no diagnostic value in people with an atypical number of sex chromosomes.

The evidence that some birth defects were produced by chromosomal anomalies was presented as a new revolution in medicine. Not all medical practitioners were persuaded that this was the case. Interviewed in 1969 on the history of the discovery of TS, Turner only briefly mentioned the 1959 redefinition of TS as 45,Xo and focused on the hormonal management of this condition.[53] His lack of interest in chromosomes might have reflected the fact that, between 1959 and 1968, sex chromosomes were studied mainly in the framework of fundamental investigations. The central practical value of the search for sex chromosome formulas was differential diagnosis in cases of suspected sex chromosome aneuploidy.[54] Moreover, TS and KS are seen as resulting from an unpredictable accident in the production of sperm and egg cells (de novo mutations). There was no need to study families of affected children in order to provide genetic counseling to these families.[55]

In the early 1960s, chromosomal studies merely confirmed or discarded the diagnosis of TS and KS. In the late 1960s, however, it became possible to diagnose chromosomal anomalies before birth.[56] A gradual extension of amniocenteses for the risk of Down syndrome in women of an "advanced maternal age" led to unexpected diagnoses of sex chromosome aneuploidy, an unintended result of the counting of fetal chromosomes. Women who believed that they knew what they would do if the fetus was diagnosed with trisomy 21 or the nearly uniformly lethal autosomal trisomies 13 or 18 faced an unanticipated dilemma: should they continue a pregnancy with a fetus diagnosed with KS, TS, or another sex chromosome aneuploidy? Their dilemma was amplified by the absence of reliable data on long-term outcomes in children with these anomalies.

In the 1960s and 1970s, the opinion about the severity of impairment induced by a sex chromosome aneuploidy varied greatly. Some researchers were pessimistic about the future of children with these conditions, while others believed that an individual with forty-seven chromosomes (47,XXY, 47,XXX, 47,XYY) would have mild impairment only; a higher number of sex chromosomes was linked with more severe physical and cognitive problems. TS was usually excluded from deliberation on the fate of individuals with sex chromosome aneuploidy, because it was not seen as an "invisible syndrome." TS was often detected immediately after birth, and if that was not the case, it was detected during childhood or at the latest in adolescence. As a consequence, pediatricians and endocrinologists had access to data on the development of girls with this condition. Other sex chromosome aneuploidies, however, were often detected only in adults, or not at all. Moreover, it is reasonable to assume that people diagnosed with sex chromosome aneuploidy had, on average, more severe manifestations of this condition than those who remained "invisible" and were therefore not fully representative of the totality of people with a given condition. The best way to study the effects of sex chromosome aneuploidies on health and intellectual development, experts agreed, was to conduct longitudinal and prospective studies: to follow a cohort of children diagnosed with sex chromosome aneuploidy at birth through childhood, adolescence, and, if possible, into adulthood, and compare them with children with a normal chromosomal formula. One of the most important among such longitudinal studies was the one conducted by Edinburgh geneticist Shirley Ratcliffe.

Ratcliffe started her research in the 1970s. At that time, Edinburgh was an important center of genetics and cytogenetic studies, especially at the Medical Research Council unit led by Michael Court Brown, which employed leading cytogeneticists such as Patricia Jacobs.[57] Ratcliffe, a pediatrician, collaborated closely with a different MRC unit, the Human Genetics Unit of Western General Hospital. In 1967, Ratcliffe initiated a prospective investigation of sex chromosome aneuploidy (mainly Klinefelter and triple X syndromes) focused on the physiological and psychological effects of these conditions. She studied the levels of sex hormones in blood, the acquisition of secondary sexual traits during puberty, and psychological and cognitive development. The study was funded by the MRC and was directly linked to an MRC-sponsored survey of chromosomal anomalies in newborns in Edinburgh. The screening of 34,380 newborns in Edinburgh between 1967 and 1979 identified 53 newborns with sex chromosome aneuploidy (47,XXY, 47,XYY, and 47,XXX); these newborns were enrolled in Ratcliffe's study. The control group for Ratcliffe's longitudinal study was composed of 94 boys and 75 girls with a "normal" chromosomal formula, born at the same time in Edinburgh. The parents of children with XXY and XXX karyotypes were given selective information about sex chromosome aneuploidy. They learned that the purpose of the study was to provide a better understanding of their child's condition. Conversely, infertility in XXY males was not mentioned at the beginning of the study so as not to disturb parents' perception of their child's masculinity. When the popular press started to discuss presumed "criminal tendencies" of XYY males, the MRC decided that information about the presence of this condition in a child should be discussed with the family physician before informing the parents.[58]

Ratcliffe recognized that the children included in her study were not fully representative of the general Scottish population because they were born in hospitals mainly frequented by higher social classes. This was also true, however, for the matched controls. She therefore believed that her research provided important information on the development of XY, XXY, and XYY boys and of XX and XXX girls.[59] Summing up the results of her study in 1999, Ratcliffe pointed to delayed puberty and problems with secondary sex manifestations in XXY boys and the existence of learning difficulties and occasional behavioral problems linked with all the studied sex chromosome aneuploidies: XXY, XXX, and XYY.[60] The IQs of the children with sex chromosome aneuploidy she studied was as a rule ten to twenty points lower than that of their siblings; they needed educational support more often than children in the control group; and their consumption of psychiatric services was higher than that of the controls. Nevertheless, Ratcliffe described these difficulties as "minor." She stressed that if children with sex chromosome aneuploidy receive appropriate parental guidance and professional help, they can live a happy and productive life. Ratcliffe's main conclusion was a strong recommendation for an early diagnosis of sex chromosome aneuploidy. Most people with these conditions remained undiagnosed. Ratcliffe believed that this was regrettable because early intervention could have helped them minimalize their difficulties and maximize their potential.[61]

Sex Chromosome Aneuploidy and "Deviant Behavior"

Probably the most visible expression of dilemmas linked with prenatal diagnosis of sex chromosome aneuploidy was the controversy of the presumed criminal/violent tendencies of XYY men, later extended to the investigation of links between sex chromosome aneuploidy, behavioral problems, and deviance. The XYY controversy started with a 1965 article by Patricia Jacobs (the geneticist who first described 47,XXY and 47,XXX karyotypes) and her collaborators, who claimed that they had found an abnormally high percentage of 47,XYY men among prisoners, especially among those who committed violent crimes. Jacobs and her colleagues affirmed that 3.5% of prisoners in the latter subgroup were XYY males, while the frequency of this condition in the general population was less than 0.2%.[62] Jacobs later explained that since men commit more aggressive crimes than women (or, to put it otherwise, the presence of a single Y chromosome is a marker of a greater probability of aggressive behavior), it was not illogical to think that the presence of two such chromosomes would favor a higher prevalence of aggressive behavior. As she put it in a 2004 interview: "If you stop and think about it, 98% of the prison population are males. So you can't say that Y has got nothing to do with behavior, because why would you find this astonishing figure, which is incontrovertible."[63]

Several other studies, usually performed on a small number of institutionalized men, also pointed to the existence of a link between the XYY karyotype and aggressive behavior or criminality.[64] Inmates of psychiatric hospitals, prisons, and institutions for the mentally impaired were "captive populations" often studied by geneticists. The exact meaning of the studies of these populations was, however, unclear. Some researchers linked the (putative) higher frequency of 47,XYY men among aggressive prisoners with the observation that they tended to be considerably taller than average men. The combination of early puberty, greater height and physical power, and a lower IQ, they argued, might be a recipe for trouble. However, attempts at verifying this hypothesis did not reveal a correlation between height and the suspected greater inclination of XYY men to commit violent crimes (or, to be more accurate, to be jailed in high-security establishments). Moreover, some investigators found that XXY men were also overrepresented in prisons.[65] The latter observation contradicted Jacobs's assumption that an "overdose" of masculinity leads to aggressive behavior. An alternative hypothesis was that other traits found more frequently in men with sex chromosome aneuploidy, such as borderline IQ, tall stature, lower tolerance of stress, and emotional immaturity, could explain the tendency of men with sex chromosome aneuploidy to become involved in illegal activities.[66]

Writing in 1970 on the ethical aspects of prenatal diagnosis, geneticist James Neel used the controversy about XYY syndrome to illustrate the dilemmas linked with the newly developed diagnostic approach. "What should our stance be," Neel asked, "when the condition we detect in utero carries with it only a probability of an untoward outcome, and that this probability is undoubtedly influenced by poorly understood variables?" Neel did not question the evidence that XYY men are unusually prone to criminal aggression; however, he added that until large-scale surveys have been completed, it is impossible to say how frequent deviant behavior is seen in this population, or whether those who are not institutionalized are "normal" or "problematic." "The recognition of XYY syndrome," Neel concluded, "raises in an unusually acute form not only the question of individual responsibility, but the question of responsibility of society for the individual who, for genetic or environmental reasons, has an increased possibility of pathological behavior. And now prenatal diagnosis makes it possible in some case for society to face this problem before the child is even born!"[67]

In the 1970s, the media published many stories about the so-called criminality chromosome, which produced an inborn tendency to develop deviant behavior. Researchers who studied sex chromosome aneuploidy knew that studies on the links between it and criminal behavior were made in mental hospitals and high-security prisons and therefore in all probability greatly exaggerated deviant behavior among XYY men. Studying the behavior of XYY men in the general population was, however, a quasi-impossible task because the great majority of these men were not diagnosed and, one could assume, led ordinary lives. Hence, the key importance of prospective case control studies that compared the development of children diagnosed at birth with the XYY karyotype with normal controls. One such study was, as we have seen, Ratcliffe's investigation in Edinburgh. Another was conducted at Harvard Medical School by psychiatrist Stanley Walzer and geneticist Park Gerald.

Walzer and Gerald's aim was to study XXY and XYY boys. Their study started in 1968. It was funded by the Center for Studies of Crime and Delinquency at the National Institute of Mental Health. In 1974, Walzer and Gerald's investigations met strong opposition from a group of Harvard scientists who argued that parents who learned that their child carried a XYY karyotype, and who already knew from sensational reporting in the media that this karyotype might predispose him to violent behavior, would in all probability treat their child differently, potentially reinforcing his "difference."[68] Researchers who criticized Walzer and Gerald's study, such as geneticist Jon Beckwith, also strongly objected the presentation of the study's goals to parents. Initially, mothers of the studied children received very partial information about the goals of the study. This omission was partly corrected in a new version of consent forms, but parents, as Beckwith and his colleagues argued, were still led to believe that the benefits of taking part in this study outweighed its risks. This was inaccurate. In view of the widespread talk about the "criminal chromosome," such a study could only harm the families involved and propagate the damaging myth of genetic origins of antisocial behavior.[69] Harvard Medical School faculty reviewed Walzer and Gerald's study and renewed the school's support of this investigation, but its main investigator, Stanley Walzer, decided that he was unable to face the unrelenting critique of his work and abandoned the study.[70]

Beckwith and his colleagues were criticized for their supposed antiscientific and doctrinary attitude. The evolution of the rules of experimentation on humans later legitimated many of their objections. Today, it is no longer possible to propose a population-based screening for the presence of an inborn condition without valid proof that such screening is expected to provide individual benefits to the screened persons, and will not harm them. Alternatively, the claim advanced by Beckwith and his colleagues that XYY syndrome was "pure fiction" and an artifact produced by genetic inquiries was later rejected by professionals.[71] Studies of this syndrome indicated that boys with the XYY karyotype are at a higher than average risk of developing learning difficulties and behavioral problems. In 1975, John Hamerton, then-president of the American Society of Human Genetics, insisted in his presidential address at the annual meeting of the American Society of Human Genetics that difficulties faced by children and adults with sex chromosome aneuploidy are well documented.

There was ample confirmation of the overrepresentation of XYY males, and to some extent XXY males, in prisons and similar institutions as well as evidence of an increased frequency of psychiatric treatment in XXX women. These data may be related to lower documented IQs of people with these conditions, possibly coupled with other psychosocial and behavioral difficulties.[72] In the 1970s, some experts continued to defend screening for sex chromosome aneuploidy at birth, arguing that such a screening may single out children in need of special help, and then facilitate the obtention of such help.[73]

A popular book on prenatal diagnosis explained in 1977 that XYY and XXY males end up in mental or penal institutions at a higher frequency than XY males. The reason is not, however, inborn criminal tendency: "The most likely reason for the XYY males ending up in trouble is the low intelligence associated with an anti-social behavior. Boys and men with this configuration tend to be loners, prone to uncontrollable tempers and have problems of attention in school. . . . What about those parents who discover that they have a XYY fetus and have to decide for or against abortion? Many are likely to be swayed by the evidence of low intelligence and anti-social behavior; others may take their chances that their son, like some others, will be a normal, non-violent XYY child."[74]

In a 1979 letter to the *British Medical Journal* titled "What Is to Be Done with the XYY Fetus?," Shirley Ratcliffe affirmed that "we wish to point out that we do not consider the small reduction of IQ to be grounds for selective abortion." She added that because their longitudinal study covered only the first twelve years of any child's life, it might be premature to make any pronouncement on the rate of social deviance.[75] Twenty years later, she confidently attested that the rate of social deviation among XXY boys was moderate and manageable. She did find a fourfold increase in transgressions of XYY boys, but the majority of these transgressions were minor and they were directed against property rather than persons. In the XYY boy, Ratcliffe explained, the combination of lowered intelligence, delayed development of speech, and emotional immaturity with greater body size indeed favored a higher frequency of behavioral problems, but such problems tended to diminish with time and could be controlled by educational help, consistent parental management, and, if needed, psychiatric intervention. She also reiterated her conviction that people with sex chromosome aneuploidy would greatly benefit from an early diagnosis of their condition.[76]

In the 1980s, the accumulation of data from several longitudinal studies, which, besides Ratcliffe's research, included research conducted by Martha Leonard and Sarah Sparrow at Yale, Johannes Nielsen and his collaborators in Copenhagen, and Donald Stewart and his colleagues in Toronto, confirmed that all sex chromosome aneuploidies often produced, but not always, mild to moderate impairment. Some children with sex chromosome aneuploidy developed without any notable problems, but a significant proportion among them faced some psychological, cognitive, and behavioral problems, and, for those with KS, also physiological issues such as changed body image.[77] Walzer, who stopped recruiting new children for his study in the mid-1970s but continued to follow XXY and XYY boys he had begun to observe earlier, also found a higher frequency of learning disabilities and mild cognitive deficiencies in people with both conditions. He therefore stressed the need to provide these individuals with appropriate psychological and educative support.[78]

Turner and Klinefelter Syndromes in the Twenty-First Century

The concept of generalized newborn screening for sex chromosome aneuploidy was abandoned in the 1980s.[79] Instead, specialists proposed to increase awareness of early symptoms of sex chromosome aneuploidy among health professionals and educators in order to favor early diagnosis of these conditions and to promote early intervention.[80] They were persuaded that the benefits of such intervention (hormonal treatment, behavioral therapy, remedial teaching) greatly outweighed the potential disadvantages of early disclosure of a chromosome anomaly and rarely mentioned the possibility that such an early diagnosis may cause negative interactions between parent and child.[81] Sex chromosome aneuploidies are highly variable conditions. Thus, a prenatal diagnosis of TS can predict the existence of some traits (e.g., short stature and sterility in TS women) but not the presence and extent of others (cardiovascular problems, learning difficulties). TS is frequently presented today, especially by its activists, as a nonproblematic condition that at most induces minor health and learning issues easily overcome with appropriate medical treatment and educative intervention. This may be an optimistic evaluation. Many women with TS have ordinary personal lives, hold full-time jobs (including, for some, in highly qualified occupations), and see themselves as "normal" women with some health-related issues, but other women with this condition struggle with difficulties related to their physical and cognitive problems.[82]

With the generalization of diagnostic ultrasound, TS is frequently detected before birth, often following abnormal ultrasound findings such as increased nuchal translucency. Many women who learn that they are carrying a TS fetus decide to terminate their pregnancy. The elevated rates of abortion following a diagnosis of TS (in Europe, from 70% to 90%, according to EUROCAT data) did not change much in the past twenty years.[83] Abortion for this condition is strongly correlated with the presence of "ultrasound markers" of TS. When a diagnosis of karyotype 45,Xo is accompanied by abnormal ultrasound findings such as cystic hygroma or lymphedema (a condition sometimes labeled "severe TS"), nearly all pregnant women elect to terminate the pregnancy.[84] The persistence of high rates of termination for TS was attributed to parents' fears of infertility and "sexual anomaly," and, in some cases, the amplification of these fears by the negative attitude of a genetic counselor.[85] Termination for TS may also reflect the growing popularity of diagnostic ultrasound examination at eleven to twelve weeks of pregnancy. At that stage of pregnancy, it is relatively easy to spot structural anomalies linked with TS, and then to collect fetal cells through chorionic villi sampling and confirm the diagnosis of this sex chromosome aneuploidy. When TS is diagnosed in the first rather than in the second trimester of pregnancy, women may be more inclined to have an abortion, more so because they are often told of the elevated probability of spontaneous miscarriage of a TS fetus.

KS is different. This condition is seldom detected by ultrasound or uncovered during a physical examination of a newborn baby. Until very recently, a prenatal diagnosis of KS was nearly always an accidental consequence of a search for trisomy 21.[86] Rates of termination for prenatally detected KS are, for now, lower than those for prenatally detected TS; they vary greatly among countries and sites.[87] Thus, according to 2011 data of the French Institute de Veille Sanitaire, rates of termination in France were 36% for KS and 75% for TS (and, in this database, 77% for Down syndrome).[88] Postnatal diagnosis of KS is rare before adolescence. Typically, KS is detected following an investigation of puberty troubles or of infertility. Today, too many individuals with KS are never diagnosed.[89] KS is sometimes called "the forgotten syndrome."[90] For many specialists, this is regrettable, because they are persuaded that early hormonal and educational interventions significantly improve outcomes for men with this condition.[91] This view is, however, grounded in studies that compared the fate of children diagnosed with this condition either immediately after birth or during pregnancy with those who were consulted for KS-associated symptoms as adolescents or adults. This view does not take into consideration outcomes in "truly forgotten" people with KS, those who view themselves as "normal" and do not seek medical attention.

Parents of children with "recognized" KS sometimes oscillate between the acceptance of their child's diagnosis, because it opens access to services such as special education, psychological help, and medical treatment, and its rejection, because of its stigmatizing potential. Their child is a "typical Klinefelter" when they discuss the condition with health authorities or an insurance company and an "atypical / minimal Klinefelter" when they speak about their child in a different context. Outside a bureaucratic framework of managing officially recognized disabilities, they focus on the individuality of their diagnosed child, his accomplishments, and other positive aspects that go beyond a genetic diagnosis. The grandmother of a boy with KS explained that "he's really not a full blown Klinefelter, he's just a borderline because I see things that when I look on the website or people have described to me like the facial hair, the hair you know, I'm just amazed at how much hair he has. . . . I go, you know, he's just a little Klinefelter's, he's not a lot Klinefelter's." Parents of children with KS talked about their sons being "sweet" and having a "nurturing personality." They also stressed the diversity of the manifestations of this syndrome: "From what I understand, you know, not one specific case of Klinefelter's is going to be exactly the same as another."[92]

The presence of many undiagnosed KS men is seen both as proof that the presence of an additional X chromosome in men does not produce major impairments and, particularly for specialists who believe that early medical and social intervention improves the outcome for XXY boys, as a problem to be tackled.[93] These specialists argue that many of the difficulties of KS boys are linked with their physical signs of "otherness," such as delayed puberty, effeminate silhouette, and development of male breasts. Preadolescent hormonal therapy attenuates these external signs of otherness. The normalization of the bodies of boys/men with KS reduces, in turn, their psychological and relational difficulties.[94] Occasionally, a "visible" association of KS with deviant behavior, as was seen in the case of the French serial killer Francis Heaulme, has brought to the fore a potential association between an abnormal number of chromosomes and criminality. Articles in the French media described Heaulme as a "freak": very tall, with a feminized body, no body hair, small testes, and a borderline IQ. However, these articles usually added that people with KS were frequently mild-tempered. Heaulme, they explained, was bullied because of his atypical body, but such bullying was but one among many elements that contributed to his chaotic, violent, and deeply unhappy childhood.[95]

Today, 47,XXY children are invariably raised as boys, but researchers have found that some people with KS see themselves as more female than male.[96] The invisibility of intersex/transex XXY people may be related to the fact that many studies of men with KS were conducted with men diagnosed with this sex chromosome aneuploidy during a search for the cause of their infertility. Those men had a male gender identity and were in heterosexual relationships. They were also more inclined see their atypical chromosomal formula as an anomaly and a medical condition that should be treated. However, some individuals, probably influenced by the transex/transgender movement, perceive the possession of the 47,XXY karyotype as a distinct identity and not a pathology. Some scholars therefore proposed to distinguish KS, a condition presented as "incomplete masculinity" and treated with testosterone, from a 47,XXY karyotype, a condition that could lead to an identification with the female gender or an intersex condition and therefore should not be automatically treated with male sex hormone.[97] It is not excluded that certain people with KS will follow the lead of transgender people and reject the perception of their condition as incomplete sexual development that has to be corrected through the administration of "missing" sex hormones. They may replace experts' conviction that KS should be recognized as early as possible because of the putative advantages of early hormonal treatment with a demand that their families accept their "nonhormonally modified" bodies as an expression of the diversity of human sexual development.

Another recent development is the linking of KS with an increase in the risk of psychiatric conditions such as autism spectrum disorders, attention-deficit disorders, schizophrenia, and bipolar disorders, especially their milder variants. The majority of people with KS are free of such conditions or are not bothered enough by them to consult a physician, but some have behavioral problems and others mental health issues. The magnitude of cognitive, psychological, and psychiatric problems in people with KS is difficult to evaluate because the studied samples are usually small and the precise definition of "autistic spectrum disorder" or "attention-deficit disorder" may vary. Nevertheless, specialists seem to agree that children with sex chromosome aneuploidy, especially KS and XYY syndrome, are at a greater risk of such disorders than children with a "normal" chromosomal formula. These studies also confirm that the majority of people with sex chromosome aneuploidy do not suffer from perceptible psychological/psychiatric disturbances.[98]

The diagnosis of sex chromosome aneuploidy (with the exception of very rare cases of more than forty-seven, and especially more than forty-eight, chromosomes) is perceived today as a diagnosis of a risk of "minor" psychiatric and behavioral issues. However, sociologist Linda Blum persuasively argues that "minor" psychiatric and behavioral problems of a child can produce nontrivial difficulties for the child's parents.[99] Some pregnant women facing decisions about the continuation of their pregnancies with KS may assume that potential physiological problems linked with the education of a child with this condition are fully manageable, as is a higher probability of behavior associated with the higher end of the autistic spectrum. Others may feel that even a small risk of a cognitive disorder, especially when coupled with other potential problems such as a lower IQ, impaired executive functions, atypical body shape, and sterility, may be too much and may elect to terminate the pregnancy—if they are allowed to make such a decision.[100]

The history of sex chromosome aneuploidy illustrated the difficulty in defining what masculinity and femininity is, and how these notions are related to anatomy, physiology, and the number of chromosomes. It also displays a dissociation between genetic diagnosis and its concrete meaning. Knowing that the chromosomal formula of a given individual is 45,Xo, 47,XXY, 47 XYY, or 47, XXX does not say much about the consequences of the possession of an "abnormal" number of sex chromosomes for this individual. Lack of precise knowledge on the consequences of being born with sex chromosome aneuploidy, especially an "invisible" condition like KS or XYY syndrome, may sometimes be a blessing.[101] Many people with sex chromosome aneuploidy refuse to "live in diagnosis" and escape scientists' classifications in order to construct their existence elsewhere.[102] Such avoidance of diagnosis may, however, become increasingly difficult, especially with the predicted generalization of new, noninvasive prenatal testing based on the analysis of cell-free DNA (cfDNA) in a pregnant woman's blood. NIPT can detect sex chromosome aneuploidies as early as the ninth and tenth weeks of pregnancy.[103] It is possible that in the near future, a much smaller proportion of children/people with sex chromosome aneuploidy will escape the "tyranny of diagnosis" of their atypical chromosomal formula.

CHAPTER 6

Prenatal Diagnosis and New Genomic Approaches

Chromosomal Anomalies and Microarrays

From 1959 on, cytogeneticists studied the karyotype (stained human chromosomes). This initially heterogeneous domain was gradually made more uniform through international nomenclature workshops. The first two—the Denver workshop of 1960 and the London workshop of 1963—produced a basic agreement on the nomenclature of human chromosomes. Each pair of chromosomes was given a number, and chromosomes were divided into seven groups according to their shape. The next nomenclature conference, held in Chicago in 1966, proposed to divide each chromosome into a long arm (q) and a short arm (p).[1]

The next important step was the development of a new staining technique called banding, which made the identification of specific regions of the chromosomes possible, allowing for a more "anatomical" study of chromosome structure.[2] Banding greatly facilitated the differentiation between chromosomes, especially within the same group. A conference held in Paris in 1972 proposed a nomenclature for the newly observed chromosome bands. The name of each band first presented the number of the chromosome on which it was situated, and then the arm (q or p), the region, and subregion of the chromosome. At first, the banding technique made it possible to identify a small number of large-scale chromosomal anomalies. In the late 1970s and early 1980s, the improvement of the banding technique—more than one thousand bands were identified on human chromosomes—facilitated the identification of smaller changes in the chromosome's structure and greatly expanded the number of detected chromosomal anomalies, such as deletions, duplications, and translocations. This then led to the identification of inborn syndromes linked with these chromosomal changes. New findings about anomalies of the human genome were summarized in the highly complex *Morbid Map of Human Genome*, produced by leading

US geneticist Victor McKusick in 1985. This map was a visual display of the efforts to link new developments in genetics and cytogenetics with traditional clinical practices.[3]

The accomplishment of banding technology opened an era of intensive human cytogenetic studies, and such studies were also extended to fetal cells. The term *mutation*—previously applied to diseases produced by changes in a single gene, such as hemophilia, sickle cell anemia, Tay-Sachs disease, or Gaucher disease—became increasingly associated with "syndromes": a group of anomalies related to changes in a chromosome's structure. Syndromes such as Prader-Willi, Angelman, cri du chat, or Williams often involve changes in numerous genes (associated with missing or duplicated parts of a chromosome) and tend to be associated with a large number of impairments. They are frequently, although not always, linked with developmental delays and the presence of dysmorphic traits.[4]

From the 1980s on, DNA-based technologies, above all, fluorescence in situ hybridization (FISH), have made possible a more refined analysis of chromosomal anomalies. FISH looks for the presence of specific—and known—anomalies in the cell. Segments of DNA ("probes") carrying the genes one is looking for are marked with a fluorescent stain. The probe is then mixed (hybridized) with fixed (in situ), denatured chromosomes (chromosomes with an opened helix structure) of the tested cell and is allowed to attach to its complementary sequence. The presence of a hybridized fluorescent probe—that is, the existence of a complementary sequence on the tested DNA—is then revealed under light that activates the fluorescent dye. Fluorescence is then visible to the naked eye or, alternatively, is measured with specialized instruments.[5] The introduction of FISH and similar technologies such as multiplex ligation-dependent probe amplification (MPLA) facilitated the identification of pathological changes in fetal chromosomes and improved the understanding of some hereditary syndromes and allowed for the expansion of the definition of others.[6] FISH and similar approaches are efficient when physicians have a relatively precise idea of which mutated genes they are looking for, either because they are present in the family or because clinical observations point in the direction of a specific condition (or conditions). When physicians suspect that their patient has a genetic anomaly but they are unable to identify this anomaly, or, alternatively, they previously made a tentative diagnosis but genetic tests disproved their initial suppositions, they frequently apply a different genomic approach: comparative genomic hybridization.

CGH (also called chromosomal microarrays) is an extension of FISH technology used to study the whole genome of a cell. DNA from the tested sample is labeled with red fluorescent dye, while DNA from a reference sample is labeled with green florescent dye. The two samples are then mixed, and the observers measure the ratio of red to green fluorescence at each chromosome. Deviations of the expected 1:1 ratio indicate the presence of an anomaly in the tested DNA. The test was initially employed in the same way as FISH was and was used primarily for the study of isolated cells. It was made more efficient through the use of fragments of DNA printed on a chip (microarrays), an approach that enables a very rapid comparison between DNA sequences. The resolution power of CGH depends on the size of the DNA fragments used: the smaller the size, the greater the resolution, but, additionally, a smaller-size fragment also means a higher probability of observing structural changes that do not have a known clinical meaning and may merely indicate normal variations among individuals. Such deviations from the structure of the reference DNA are called variants of unknown significance. CGH was first introduced in the 1990s and was used to study genetic anomalies of cancer cells. In the early twenty-first century, its use was extended to the investigation of suspected inborn genetic anomalies.[7] FISH and CGH are complementary technologies. FISH answers the question "Is mutation X present in this patient?" CGH answers a different question: "Is the patient's genome normal?" and, if the answer is negative, "Where is the anomaly located?" CGH is especially useful for the search of chromosomal anomalies such as deletions, duplications, and translocations. When, following a display of a structural anomaly by CGH, geneticists suspect the presence of an already-identified mutation, they can use other approaches such as FISH or MPLA to confirm that this indeed is the case.

Genomic approaches were quickly introduced into dysmorphology clinics. Dysmorphologists soon became cutting-edge researchers of clinical genetics, and the study of rare mutations, first in children, and then in fetuses, opened new avenues for genetic research, as well as new opportunities to solve clinical puzzles. Many children seen by dysmorphologists suffered from developmental delays. In the early 2000s, when sociologist Joanna Latimer studied a UK dysmorphology clinic, CGH was mainly viewed as a research tool that was rarely employed in a routine clinical setting. Latimer observed many children who were classified as possibly suffering from a genetic anomaly, but in most of these cases the diagnosis of such an anomaly was not a priority.[8] New genomic technologies, such as CGH and high-throughput DNA sequencing (a high-speed sequencing method that hastened the identification of new mutations), rapidly increased the percentage of inborn syndromes and developmental delays correlated with inborn changes in DNA.[9] The website of Unique, a UK-based charity for parents of children with rare chromosomal syndromes, provides a long (and ever-growing) list of the major anomalies detected on each human chromosome.[10] In the 1970 edition of David Smith's *Recognizable Patterns of Human Malformation*, only a small fraction of the described inborn malformations, mainly major aneuploidies, were attributed to known genetic causes. In the 2013 edition of this book, 80% of the cataloged malformations were linked with identified genetic anomalies.[11]

Recent advances of genetic diagnosis also tend to blur the boundaries between physical health problems and intellectual impairments. For example, inborn heart anomalies, until recently seen only as a potentially treatable health issue, were linked in 2015 with intellectual impairment. Some mutations seem to induce both.[12] Heart anomalies are frequently visible during a diagnostic ultrasound examination. When a woman whose fetus was detected to have such an anomaly is followed in a setting with access to new genetic approaches such as CGH, her doctors may suggest that she undergo amniocentesis and genetic analysis of fetal cells. Such genetic investigation was not systematic: many fetal heart defects were perceived as a surgical problem. Linking heart defects with cognitive problems may favor the extension of genetic testing to all cases of observed fetal heart anomalies. Scientists who describe such a mutation propose that "clinical genotyping may help stratify congenital heart defect patients and identify those at high risk for neurological developmental delays, enabling surveillance and early interventions to improve school performance, employability, and quality of life," carefully avoiding any mention of an additional option—selective abortion.[13]

A pilot study published in 2004 found chromosomal rearrangements in 25% of individuals with severe developmental delays coupled with dysmorphic features.[14] This and other similar observations led to the recommendation, made in 2005 by the American College of Medical Genetics, of a systematic inclusion of genetic and genomic studies in each clinical evaluation of intellectual delays. This recommendation was reinforced in the College's 2012 update.[15] New genetic technologies also favored the "geneticization" of autism. Autism was increasingly being linked with the presence of predisposition genes and with neurological anomalies produced during embryonic and fetal life.[16] It was also increasingly seen as being closely related to the broader category of developmental delays.[17] Some experts even proposed to create a single nosological category called "autism-intellectual disability complex."[18] The link between autism / developmental delays complex and genetic / chromosomal anomalies was reinforced by defining autism as an important trait of several previously described genetic syndromes.

Physicians who treat autistic children today systematically aim to find out whether these children have a genetic condition such as Prader-Willi syndrome, Williams syndrome, Smith-Lemli-Opitz syndrome, Angelman syndrome, Rett syndrome, Smith-Magenis syndrome, or CHARGE syndrome.[19] Moreover, new syndromes linked with changes in chromosomes, such as Phelan-McDermid syndrome, were partly defined through their association with autism.[20] Parents of children with inborn disorders frequently have a positive attitude toward the transformation of a collection of inexplicable physical symptoms and developmental delays into a diagnosis of a well-defined genetic anomaly. They believe that an accurate genetic diagnosis will improve the care of their child. Even if that is not the case, a genetic diagnosis can provide parents with an explanation of the child's condition and a framework for understanding his or her problems.[21]

Fluorescence In Situ Hybridization, Comparative Genomic Hybridization, and the Fetus

FISH and similar genetic approaches were integrated into prenatal diagnosis in the 1980s.[22] At first, these techniques were mainly used for the detection of hereditary diseases that could not be diagnosed through biochemical tests on fetal cells. One such disease was thalassemia. In the 1970s, in order to diagnose thalassemia in the fetus, physicians sampled blood from the umbilical cord: a risky and cumbersome test that can only be performed relatively late in pregnancy. The possibility of using FISH to investigate whether fetal DNA cells carry a mutation for thalassemia greatly facilitated the prenatal diagnosis of this disease and made it possible for women to have abortions much earlier.[23] In the 1990s, with the extension of uses of FISH, this method was employed in the prenatal diagnosis of numerous hereditary monogenic diseases (diseases produced by mutation in a single gene), including those earlier detected through biochemical methods.

When the aim of the study of fetal cells is not to find out whether the fetus has two or three copies of chromosome 21 or two copies of a mutation for thalassemia but to uncover what might have gone wrong, it is reasonable to use chromosomal microarrays, which can uncover a wide range of chromosomal anomalies. The introduction of CGH to prenatal diagnosis is a recent development that was facilitated by the advancement of genomic analysis methods and their growing automatization.[24] The first attempts to use CGH to investigate the anomalies of the fetus were made by obstetrician Arthur Beaudet and his collaborators at Baylor College of Medicine in Houston, Texas. They reported that this approach uncovered many known genetic anomalies but also, in some cases, variants without known meaning, potentially—but not certainly— benign. Other researchers who applied CGH to the study of fetal DNA similarly reported finding sequence variations with unknown meaning. Circa 2010, CGH was nevertheless gradually integrated into a search for fetal anomalies.[25] A pregnant woman may learn about "suspicious" ultrasound findings during the second or third trimester of pregnancy, and her doctor may suggest that she undergo amniocentesis. A pregnant woman who has just learned that something may be seriously wrong with her future child seldom declines such a proposal.[26]

In 2012, US geneticist Ronald Wapner and his colleagues argued that CGH should replace karyotype (the observation and counting of stained chromosomes) as the main method for studying the genetic material of fetal cells because it is more convenient than a karyotype. Karyotypes are read by trained cytotechnicians, while routine CGH produces an automatic reading of results, therefore eliminating subjective evaluations and increasing the reliability of diagnoses. CGH is more informative than a karyotype, because this method indicates where exactly the detected chromosomal anomalies are. Finally, CGH leads to the detection of 10%–15% more DNA anomalies than the classic karyotype and therefore yields more information about potential fetal anomalies: "If the observed 1.7% (1:60) frequency of clinically relevant microdeletions and microduplications in pregnancies sampled for indications other than fetal structural anomalies is confirmed by others, offering invasive testing and microarray analysis to all pregnant women would seem to be appropriate. This is consistent with the recommendations of the American Congress of Obstetricians and Gynecologists, who suggest that all women, regardless of risk, should be offered the option of invasive testing."[27]

In order to undergo a microarray examination of fetal cells, a pregnant woman has to submit to an invasive test. American College of Obstetrics and Gynecology (ACOG) estimated, however, that if a woman wishes accept the associated risks linked with such a test and can afford it (or her insurance is willing to pay for it), the decision should be hers alone and should not be conditioned by the presence of risk factors.[28] In the twenty-first century, debates on amniocentesis in the United States moved from public health considerations that dominated these debates in the 1970s and 1980s to questions of individual choice, the right to know, and the right to take health risks. In Western Europe, gynecologists and obstetricians objected to an unregulated expansion of amniocentesis and CVS during pregnancy, with the double argument of risks to healthy fetuses and costs for the public health system. The introduction of Down syndrome screening aimed to limit, as much as possible, the frequency of these tests and to propose them only to women who had a higher than average risk of having a trisomic fetus: health professionals, not pregnant women, are expected to decide whether an invasive test is justified.[29]

The number of US women who underwent amniocentesis decreased between 2001 and 2007, a trend attributed to the diffusion of Down syndrome screening with serum markers and ultrasound. The number of amniocenteses performed in the United States increased again slightly between 2007 and 2009, and was interpreted to reflect women's lack of confidence in the probabilistic results of Down syndrome screening.[30] An increase in the number of amniocenteses circa 2010 might have been the result of the introduction of the new ACOG guidelines. Then again, only a small fraction of pregnant women in the United States underwent amniocentesis in 2010. Ronald Wapner's 2012 suggestion to transform microarrays into a routine screening technique was probably no more realistic than Stein and Susser's 1973 proposal to offer amniocentesis and testing for Down syndrome to all pregnant women.[31]

In some cases, CGH or other new genetic approaches identify a hereditary condition present in parents or other family members, a situation similar to the detection of a hereditary anomaly in a child in a dysmorphology clinic. In both cases, the child—or the fetus—becomes a "proband" for the display of a hidden condition in a family, sometimes with far-reaching consequences. People who view themselves as perfectly healthy may find out that they carry mutations that may negatively affect not only their children but themselves as well.[32] French researchers studied families in which the diagnosis of a fetal anomaly led to the discovery of the presence of a hereditary disease. Many people were distressed upon learning about the potentially negative consequences of the diagnosis of such a disease for their or their family members' health. Occasionally, such an unanticipated diagnosis destabilized couples and unsettled family relationships.[33]

When genetic studies of fetal cells uncover a hidden hereditary anomaly in the family, the problem may be defined as an excess of knowledge and the imposition of such knowledge on people who might have otherwise elected to remain ignorant. In other cases, the problem is quite the opposite: an insufficient knowledge and persisting diagnostic uncertainty. One of the difficulties of the application of CGH to prenatal diagnosis is the relatively high-frequency detection of variants of unknown significance.[34] CGH of fetal DNA sometimes leads to the diagnosis of a genetic anomaly, much more frequently fails to detect such an anomaly, and in a nonnegligible number of cases uncovers the presence of variants of unknown significance. Uncertain results of CGH may increase maternal stress, especially when women who agree to undergo this test in order to learn more about their future child are not warned that the test may uncover the presence of genetic anomalies with unknown meaning for their child's health.[35] Professionals argue that appropriate genetic counseling for women who undergo CGH will alleviate the stress produced by uncertain results.[36] Conversely, it may be difficult to reassure pregnant women when the professionals may not be sure themselves what a specific CGH result means. Women who learn about the detection of a variant of unknown significance are frequently told that in all probability it is a normal variation of the human genome. Geneticists know, however, that some variants of unknown significance were redefined as new genetic syndromes.[37] They also know that when a mutation detected by CGH has clinical significance, it is not always clear precisely what its presence will mean for a child, especially when a mutation is linked with a rare, arcane condition. The growing resolution of genetic testing, like the growing resolution of obstetrical ultrasound, improves the detection of fetal anomalies but can also increase diagnostic and prognostic uncertainty.

Fetal Cells in Maternal Circulation

In the early days of prenatal diagnosis, this diagnostic approach became synonymous with the study of fetal cells. In order to get access to these cells, however, physicians had to perform an invasive test, either amniocentesis or chorionic villus sampling, both linked with the risk of losing a healthy fetus. From the early days of prenatal diagnosis, researchers attempted to overcome this difficulty and develop a noninvasive—and thus risk-free—way of sampling fetal DNA. For a long time, such efforts were focused on attempts to isolate fetal cells in maternal circulation, but they culminated circa 2012 with the marketing of tests that analyzed cell-free DNA (cfDNA) in a pregnant woman's blood, an approach called noninvasive prenatal testing.[38]

The history of NIPT is an encounter of two parallel stories. One is the story of a scientific-technical endeavor with a long and occasionally bumpy trajectory. The other is a much shorter story of a successful commercial development of new technology, intellectual property wars, and struggles to control markets. The second story may be presented as a continuation of the first: a successful exploitation of scientific results by commercial firms. Such a view is inaccurate. The rapid development and diffusion of NIPT was an industry-driven endeavor. The key role of the industry in developing and marketing a biomedical innovation is far from being unusual, but frequently the development of such an innovation is the result of close cooperation between fundamental researchers, clinicians, and industry. Companies that developed NIPT chose a different approach. All the stages of the expansion and testing of the new diagnostic approach were initiated and fully controlled by NIPT producers. Scientific publications validated industrial achievements, not the other way around.

The story of the commercial development of NIPT and the ongoing struggle (as of this writing) over the ownership of patents and the control of markers is a truly fascinating topic, but it is beyond the scope of this book and the competence of its author. In what follows, I trace the story of scientific developments that paved the way for NIPT and focus on the career of two scientists who played an important role in this story: Diana Bianchi, of Tufts University in Boston, and Denis Lo, of the National University of Hong Kong. Both (but particularly Lo) were important to the development of NIPT, but they were not the sole founders of this approach. Science, especially today, is a collective enterprise with many key players. Nevertheless, the professional trajectories of Bianchi and Lo illuminate the biography of a new technoscientific object.

Bianchi became interested in noninvasive approaches that would allow physicians to examine fetal cells through her collaboration with immunologist Leonard Herzenberg. In the early 1970s, Herzenberg and his collaborators at Stanford University developed (or rather finalized) an instrument called the fluorescence-activated cell sorter (FACS), which made possible an automatic sorting and analysis of cells "marked" with fluorescent antibodies. FACS had numerous applications as a research tool and a clinical diagnostic device.[39] Among other things, this instrument made it possible to isolate and study a small subset of cells, an approach that, according to Herzenberg and his collaborators in 1973, could also be applied to prenatal diagnosis: "the cell separator we have developed can be a very useful tool in a number of biological and clinical areas, ranging from basic research in the immune system, and its role in such problems of transplant rejection, to a routine use as a substitute for amniocentesis in screening for Down syndrome."[40]

In the 1970s, researchers knew that fetal cells are present in maternal circulation. Bianchi, who arrived at the Herzenberg Laboratory a young doctor of medicine in the late 1970s, was given the task of finding a way to use FACS to identify and isolate such cells, with the aim of developing a simple and risk-free diagnosis of fetal anomalies, something that would be accessible to all pregnant women.[41] Herzenberg's interest in the prenatal diagnosis of Down syndrome may have been for personal and professional reasons, as he had a son with this condition, born in 1961, before the development of testing for trisomy 21.[42] For three years, Bianchi attempted to isolate fetal cells from the blood of women known to carry male fetuses. In this cases, the only cells in the pregnant woman's blood, which carried a Y chromosome, were the fetal cells. Bianchi hoped that she could use antibodies against Y chromosome markers to isolate these cells. She and her coworkers were successful—in principle. In 1979, Herzenberg's group attested that they were able to identify fetal cells in maternal circulation as early as the fifteenth week of pregnancy. Such cells, they explained, were potentially usable for prenatal diagnosis. If they could find a way to improve the frequency of the isolation of fetal cells, and then cultivate them and find surface reagents that differentiate fetal and maternal cells,

> FACS sorting . . . could provide a universal noninvasive screening technique for prenatal diagnosis of genetic abnormalities. It could replace (or be used in conjunction with midtrimester amniocentesis techniques currently used to monitor pregnancies with a relatively high empirical risk of chromosomal abnormalities in the fetus). . . . Widespread screening is desirable because the relatively large number of pregnancies in women below 35 years old means that they bear the majority of children with chromosomal abnormalities despite the relatively low risk of such abnormalities in pregnancies in this age group. Thus, if the remaining obstacles can be overcome, FACS sorting of fetal cells from maternal blood could enable early recognition of large numbers of abnormal fetuses that currently go to term before diagnosis.[43]

Herzenberg hoped that the method developed by Bianchi and her colleagues would allow fetal cells in maternal circulation to be used for the routine detection of fetal anomalies. However, in 1981, they recognized that the quantity of fetal cells they isolated from pregnant women's blood was too low for diagnostic purposes. Even more disturbing, they also found that one woman who gave birth to a daughter had cells with Y chromosome markers in her blood. This woman already had a son: the simplest explanation was that fetal cells from an earlier pregnancy do not always disappear after the child's birth. This finding greatly complicated the development of prenatal tests based on the presence of fetal cells in maternal circulation.[44]

In the 1990s, Bianchi turned to the exploitation of her accidental finding that fetal cells can stay in the maternal body for a very long time. The presence of such cells was reported as early as 1969, but this observation was seen as an isolated curiosity and did not lead at that time to further investigations.[45] In the 1990s, Bianchi and other researchers became interested in the reciprocal exchange of cells between a pregnant woman and the fetus, as well as the persistence of these cells, a phenomenon called maternal-fetal microchimerism. They found that microchimerism was a frequent occurrence and that fetal cells, including those originated in a pregnancy that ended with a spontaneous miscarriage or an induced abortion, could sometimes persist in the maternal body for a very long period. Researchers who studied this phenomenon were especially interested in the implications of the observation that many people, and perhaps all people, have chimeric bodies that contain cells with a different genetic makeup.[46] Bianchi and other researchers investigated the links between microchimerism and human disease, especially autoimmune diseases (conditions in which the immune system of an individual turns against the body itself), and published numerous papers on this subject.[47] Microchimerism became very fashionable in the late 1990s and led to much speculation about its beneficial and harmful consequences.[48] Among the researchers interested in this topic was Denis Lo, a Hong Kong biochemist who studied fetal cells in maternal blood at Cambridge University in the 1990s.[49]

Bianchi did not give up hope on isolating sufficient fetal cells from maternal blood to develop a reliable prenatal diagnosis of fetal anomalies. In the 1990s, she and her colleagues attempted to adapt the newly developed FISH technique to improve the isolation of fetal cells. Again, the approach yielded positive results but was not sufficiently sensitive for its use in routine prenatal testing.[50] Nevertheless, these and similar findings persuaded the US National Institute of Child Health and Human Development to conduct a large-scale clinical evaluation of studies that looked for fetal cells in maternal blood: the National Institute of Child Health and Human Development Fetal Cell Isolation Study (NIFTY). The NIFTY multicenter trial, conducted between 1994 and 2002, tested approximately three thousand maternal blood samples.[51] The trial confirmed that it is possible to isolate fetal cells and detect those with an abnormal number of chromosomes.[52] Nevertheless, a workshop held in 2003 at the National Institutes of Health concluded that the method was not sufficiently reliable for routine diagnostic use: more technological advances were needed before it could enter clinics.[53] It was "good, but not good enough."[54]

Circulating Cell-Free DNA

In the 1990s, Bianchi, at that time involved in the NIFTY program, reiterated the hope that the isolation of fetal cells in maternal blood would complete, one day, the existing modalities of screening for Down syndrome: the search for serum markers and the measure of nuchal translucency.[55] In the same year, there was a new development—the description, by Lo, of the presence of an important quantity of cfDNA in the blood of pregnant women unlocked a new possibility of noninvasive prenatal diagnosis (NIPD). Bianchi, a veteran of the efforts to find fetal hereditary material in maternal circulation, was invited to comment on Lo's finding.[56] She quickly grasped the importance of Lo's observations. These observations, she explained, obliged scientists to radically rethink the view that fetal and maternal circulations were tightly separated by the placenta's barrier.[57] Such a view is now replaced by a dynamic one in which fetal DNA continually enters maternal circulation and is rapidly destroyed, only to be replaced by new fetal DNA. Moreover, Bianchi added, Lo's finding could soon lead to the development of diagnostic tests grounded in the analysis of cfDNA.[58]

The passage from observations made in the laboratory to the manufacture of a marketable item is far from simple; however, NIPT had a remarkably fast commercial trajectory. In 2010, summarizing her search for a noninvasive way to detect Down syndrome and other chromosomal anomalies, Bianchi explained that two years earlier Lo and his collaborators in Hong Kong and Steven Quake and his colleagues at Stanford employed a new genomic technology, massive parallel sequencing, to detect extra copies of chromosome 21 in the plasma of pregnant women carrying fetuses with Down syndrome. These two groups produced convincing evidence that a NIPD of Down syndrome was technically feasible. Bianchi added, however, that at that point it remained to be seen whether such a diagnostic test would be cost-effective and could be applied on a large-scale basis.[59] The next year, in 2011, Bianchi joined the staff of Verinata, one of the four companies that commercialized cfDNA-based prenatal testing. Noninvasive testing for aneuploidies received a market permit in 2012, which was unusually quick for the marketing and diffusion of an innovation in prenatal diagnosis, according to Bianchi.[60]

The starting point of Lo's scientific trajectory was similar to Bianchi's: the search for fetal cells in maternal circulation.[61] In 1987, Lo became interested in the diagnostic use of fetal cells in maternal circulation. He applied the newly developed polymerase chain reaction to look for the fetal cells. For ten years, he and his colleagues attempted to isolate and study these cells. They investigated two potentially useful clinical applications of this approach: the detection of fetal sex and the investigation of fetal Rh status. Lo and his collaborators had shown that it was possible to reliably predict fetal sex by studying Y chromosome markers on these cells. Nevertheless, they concluded: "The technique we describe needs further development before any routine clinical application can be envisaged, but our early results indicate that some types of fetal genetic analysis from maternal blood samples may be feasible."[62] Or, to put it another way, their tests, like the earlier ones developed by Bianchi and her collaborators, were not good enough for the use for which they were intended: routine prenatal testing. The attempt to investigate the Rh status of the fetus met a similar fate. The test was successful as a research endeavor but was not reliable enough for routine clinical use.[63]

In the 1980s and 1990s, scientists reported the presence of tumoral DNA in the blood of cancer patients.[64] Inspired by the observation that malignant tumors shed DNA in circulation, in 1997 Lo and his colleagues decided to search for circulating fetal DNA in pregnant women's blood. They were successful beyond their initial hopes and found very high amounts of such DNA in maternal circulation, especially in the late stages of pregnancy.[65] Lo later described their findings as a conceptual revolution, and they started to look for DNA in the plasma, a material they had previously discarded. They discovered that cfDNA does not persist in maternal plasma after birth. This observation solved an additional problem linked with the use of fetal cells in maternal circulation, the possibility that some of these cells might have been originated in a previous pregnancy.[66] The next step for Lo was to repeat his earlier work on fetal Rh markers, this time using cfDNA.[67] The new test was more reliable than those based on the isolation of fetal cells and could be applied in clinics. Conversely, the use of this test was limited to cases in which a marker—such as the Rh antigen on red blood cells—was present in the fetus but not in the pregnant woman's blood. Similar diagnostic use of cfDNA was possible, in principle at least, for a marker of a hereditary condition when such a marker was not present in the pregnant woman's body (e.g., when the father was a carrier of a dominant hereditary condition, while the mother did not carry a mutated gene).

Around 2000, it was not technically possible to produce a test that could measure the presence of three copies of chromosome 21, an entity also present in a pregnant woman's blood. Lo and his group, in collaboration with Bianchi and her colleagues, had shown that women who carried trisomic fetuses had higher levels of cfDNA in their blood, but this finding merely added one more nonspecific serum marker for Down syndrome risk.[68] However, in the 2000s, the increasing power of computers led to the development of a new genomic technology, next-generation sequencing (or high-throughput sequencing). This approach paralleled the sequencing process through a simultaneous analysis of a very high number of sequences (massive parallel sequencing). High-throughput sequencing technologies lowered the cost of DNA sequencing well beyond what was possible with previous approaches.[69] They also reinforced the position of producers of sequencing machines, such as Illumina. Next-generation sequencing made possible the development of routine diagnostic tests grounded in the analysis of cfDNA.[70] In 2008, Lo's group in Hong Kong and Stephen Quake's group at Stanford University demonstrated, separately, the feasibility producing cfDNA-based tests for Down syndrome.[71] Lo and his collaborators, who teamed with the commercial firm Sequenom, and Quake and his colleagues, who teamed with the firm Verinata, immediately took patents for their respective methods. These cfDNA-based tests, renamed NIPT, entered an era of commercial exploitation, patent wars, intense competition on markets, and the promise of radical transformation of prenatal diagnosis.

Industry, Markets, and the State: Noninvasive Prenatal Testing in Context

NIPT was developed, above all, to improve Down syndrome screening. Such screening was described by Cees Oudejans, head of the molecular biology laboratory in the Department of Clinical Chemistry at the Vrije Universiteit Medical Center in Amsterdam, as "truly the holy grail in our field."[72] The initial goal was to replace the existing tests, above all, serum tests for Down syndrome markers with NIPT, and to integrate the new test into the "prenatal diagnosis dispositif" and routine prenatal testing. Accordingly, the diffusion of NIPT followed the highly diversified attitudes toward screening for Down syndrome and the regulation of this activity. NIPT producers, in fierce market competition, then developed tests for additional genetic conditions. These tests further complicated NIPT's uses.[73] The first three years of marketing of NIPT brought to the fore and accentuated elements already present in earlier prenatal diagnosis history: technology- and market-driven developments, important national and local differences in the use of the new tests, and the central role of attitudes toward screening for Down syndrome in the diffusion of NIPT.

The first data from clinical NIPT (at that stage still called NIPD) appeared in 2011.[74] In 2012, researchers also confirmed the validity of this technology to detect trisomy 13 and trisomy 18.[75] In 2012, four tests—Sequenom's MaterniT21 Plus, Verinata's verifi, Ariosa's Harmony, and Natera's Panorama—obtained marketing permits for cfDNA-based prenatal tests in the United States. In 2013, Sequenom's MaterniT21 Plus, Verinata's verifi, and Natera's Panorama proposed testing for trisomy 21, trisomy 18, trisomy 13, sex chromosome aneuploidies, and fetal sex; Ariosa proposed a somewhat cheaper test that only looked for the three autosomal aneuploidies: trisomy 21, 13, and 18.[76] The majority of data on the validity of the new tests were presented on the companies' websites rather than in scientific journals. At that time, the main North American producers of NIPT—Sequenom, Verinata (bought in 2013 by the large producer of new-generation sequencing machines, Illumina), Natera, and Ariosa—became involved in prolonged patent battles.[77] Some of these battles were later resolved through mergers of companies. In 2015, Ariosa Diagnostics was bought by the pharmaceutical firm Roche, while an alliance between Sequenom and Illumina (the owner of Verinata Health) put an end to three years of fighting over patents between these firms (recall that Verinata held Quake's patent, and Sequenom held Lo's patent).[78] The companies continued, however, other disputes on intellectual property, closely connected with their effort to control important parts of the potentially very important market for NIPTs.

All the companies that market NIPT advertise very high specificity and sensitivity of their test (over 99% for Down syndrome; over 98% for other chromosomal anomalies). This may well be accurate, but women (and possibly some health care providers, too) may confuse high specificity and sensitivity—absolute variables—with a high positive predictive value—a variable that depends on the frequency of a given condition in a tested population. A pregnant woman is not interested in abstract data about the accuracy of a commercial test but wants to know what the chances are that she is carrying a fetus with a given genetic anomaly. Let us assume that a NIPT test has 99.9% specificity, something the companies proudly proclaim. If there is a high probability that the tested woman has a given condition (e.g., 1%; this is approximately the risk of a 41-year-old woman giving birth to a child with Down syndrome), a positive predictive value of the test will be high, too, since for every ten thousand women tested there will be one hundred true positive results and ten false positive ones. If there is a very low probability that the tested woman has a given condition (e.g., 0.01%, because this condition is very rare), the positive predictive value of the test will also be low, because for every ten thousand tested women there will be one true positive result and ten false positive ones.[79]

At first, NIPT was proposed only to high-risk women, a subpopulation in which this test has a relatively high predictive value. NIPT producers hoped that it would replace the existing methods of Down syndrome screening. They were therefore very interested in proving that the test was efficient in low-risk women as well. The first studies on the efficacy of NIPT in low-risk women, published in 2014, indicated that NIPT was much more efficient as a "first intention" screening for Down syndrome risk than the existing screening method: serum tests coupled with ultrasound. The positive predictive value of NIPT for Down syndrome in low-risk women was between 40% and 50%, which means that one out of two women who receive a positive NIPT result for this condition and who undergo amniocentesis will learn that the fetus is normal. This was an important improvement on the positive predictive value of the previous method of screening for Down syndrome—serum markers combined with the measure of nuchal translucency, estimated at 4%.[80] Later studies, performed in larger groups of women, have confirmed that NIPT can be used by all pregnant women, regardless of age and risk status.[81] The main advantage of the new method is to drastically reduce the number of amniocenteses, because a negative result of NIPT is seen as quasi-certain.[82] The implicit conclusion may be that NIPT merely provides a better version of an already-existing diagnostic approach. Such a view overlooks, however, two issues linked with the shift from the already-existing combination of serum tests and ultrasound measures to NIPT: the potential enlargement of the scope of prenatal screening and an earlier detection of fetal anomalies.[83]

Discussing in 2011 the future of NIPT, Sequenom's director declared that the company's goal was the development of a test for conditions that are already part of prenatal screening programs: "Our focus is on making existing clinical applications safer. I don't think that we are in the position to say that we should determine what hair color the baby has."[84] This is accurate as far as the baby's hair color goes, but much less accurate when tests propose screening for conditions such as sex chromosomes aneuploidies.[85] It is reasonable to assume that not many prospective parents will consider an abortion because they have discovered that their future child will, for example, have red hair or will lack musical talents: in France, nearly half of all pregnant women elect to terminate a pregnancy following an—often incidental—diagnosis of a sex chromosome aneuploidy.[86] An additional complication are incidental findings. NIPT can lead to the chance discovery of maternal inborn anomalies or diseases. Chinese researchers who investigated 181 cases in which diagnosis of a sex chromosome aneuploidy by NIPT was not confirmed by a direct examination of fetal cells discovered that in 16 of these cases the woman had a sex chromosome aneuploidy, usually Xo mosaicism.[87] NIPT can also lead to a diagnosis of cancer in the pregnant woman. In some cases, discordance between the results of NIPT and those of amniocentesis was produced by an occult maternal cancer. Women were, however, rarely told that looking for fetal anomalies can lead to the discovery of a pathology unrelated to pregnancy.[88]

Another potentially problematic issue is moving prenatal diagnosis forward in time. NIPT results and their confirmation by CVS should be available in the first trimester of pregnancy, when abortion may be perceived by some women as less difficult.[89] A first trimester pregnancy is often perceived as "tentative," not only because of the possibility of the detection of a fetal anomaly but also because women know that many pregnancies end with an early miscarriage.[90] For this reason, women frequently make their pregnancy public only in the beginning of the second trimester, when their body starts to undergo visible changes, they feel fetal movements, and they are more confident that the pregnancy will lead to the birth of a child. The loss of a well-formed fetus in the second trimester of pregnancy may be perceived as qualitatively different and more distressing than an early miscarriage.[91]

In countries such as Denmark or France, where nearly all pregnant women already undergo first trimester screening for Down syndrome, the predicted replacement of serum tests with NIPT will probably not produce an important change in existing screening practices. Such change may be more meaningful if NIPT will also encompass the detection of additional fetal anomalies, such as sex chromosome aneuploidies or chromosomal deletions. In countries in which a much smaller proportion of pregnant women are screened for Down syndrome risk in the first trimester, such as the United States, the rapid diffusion of NIPT from 2014 on led to an increase in the number of women who undergo such a screening.[92] Some women aware of the need to confirm NIPT's results by an invasive test elected to have an early termination of pregnancy without such a test in order to avoid the stress of an invasive test and a later abortion, especially if, in their case (e.g., testing for Down syndrome in an older pregnant woman), NIPT has a high positive predictive value.[93] One study found that 6% of US women at high risk of a chromosomal anomaly terminated their pregnancy without a confirmation of the result by amniocentesis.[94] The possibility that a woman will decide to have an abortion, even on the basis of an imperfect indication of the risk of a fetal anomaly, may be particularly elevated in countries in which abortion is illegal. In these countries, access to a secure late-term abortion is very difficult, and such abortions are available to affluent women only. It is much easier for a pregnant woman, especially in Latin America, to have access to the abortive drug misoprostol (Cytotec), which is reasonably safe when used in the first trimester of pregnancy.

In the spring of 2014, when several producers of NIPT included screening for certain chromosomal deletions in this test, they presented this development as a nonproblematic extension of NIPT's scope.[95] The new tests were frequently proposed to users as an "opt out" rather than an "opt in" possibility (as were tests for sex chromosomes aneuploidies): the users were offered a "complete" test, with the option to receive only selected results (e.g., the presence of trisomies

21, 13, and 18).[96] The enlargement of the scope of NIPT may reflect companies' aspirations to extend their markets and their wish to present a more advanced product than their main competitors. It may be compared to manufacturers' efforts to put on the market a new model of their product, with additional features. There is, however, an important difference between shopping for a new smartphone and testing for fetal anomalies. Tests offered by NIPT producers can have a deep impact on people's lives.[97]

National differences in the use of Down syndrome screening shape the NIPT market. According to Bianchi, in the United States, the increase in recommendations to test for Down syndrome allow for large-scale diffusion of NIPT:

> The reason that NIPT is important is that it is currently standard of care for all obstetricians to offer pregnant women screening for Down syndrome (DS). That was a decision made by the American College of Obstetrics and Gynecology (ACOG) in 2007. OB/GYN is one of these specialties in which there are "edicts" from their professional organization. You pretty much have to follow their recommendations, otherwise you're liable to be sued for malpractice. So, all obstetricians offer their patients the current version of screening for aneuploidy, which includes the measurement of certain proteins in the blood and an ultrasound examination of a fluid-filled space at the back of the fetal neck.[98]

Despite the initial absence of proof of the efficacy of NIPT in low-risk women, from 2013 on US gynecologists and fetal medicine experts prescribed this test frequently, including to their low-risk patients.[99] NIPT became popular in the United States among women who can afford it or have health insurance that covers it. This test reassures many women because a negative result of NIPT provides a quasi-certitude of the absence of the tested anomalies. In addition, NIPT frees many women from the stress of amniocentesis.[100] An industry-sponsored survey of NIPT in a large number of "low-risk" US women confirmed the validity of this technology as a first screen test.[101] It also indirectly confirmed that doctors were prescribing NIPT to low-risk women well before the official validation of its efficacy. NIPT quickly became an important commercial success in the United States. Surveys conducted in 2015 estimated that the three main US firms that produced this test sold 800,000 tests per year (3,932,181 babies were born in the United States in 2013).[102]

European specialists were more reluctant to rapidly adopt NIPT, especially its variants that go beyond the detection of autosomal trisomies.[103] The existence of generalized screening for Down syndrome in many European countries molded the marketing strategies of NIPT manufacturers. Commercial firms interested in persuading European health providers to replace routine serum tests with their product are developing simplified, less expensive tests. Such tests, especially when coupled with the predicted sharp decrease in the use of amniocentesis, can make NIPT cost-efficient. Sequenom developed a cheaper version of its MaterniT21 Plus test, called VisibiliT, targeted toward women at average risk. VisibiliT reports only Down syndrome and Edwards syndrome (trisomy 18); Patau syndrome (trisomy 13) was probably not included because of a reported lower predictive value of this test but also because malformations induced by trisomy 13 can nearly always be detected during an ultrasound examination early on in pregnancy. Several other NIPT producers also announced that they planned to move to cheaper tests; some also planned to develop inexpensive diagnostic kits.[104] In 2015 and 2016, additional players appeared in the NIPT marketplace: European firms such as LifeCodexx and Premaitha Health and Chinese firms such as Berry Genomics and BGI. BGI's NIFTY test, which tests only for trisomies 21, 13, and 18, is competitively priced and explicitly targets the market of screening for Down syndrome through agreements with numerous European and North American service providers.[105]

European guidelines for the use of NIPT, published in 2014, stress the need for appropriate pre- and posttest counseling and, if applicable, bereavement support for couples that elect to have an abortion. These guidelines also highlight the importance of culturally sensitive counseling, especially for women of non-European origins.[106] A shared position document on the uses of NIPT, issued in 2015 by the European Society of Human Genetics and the American Society of Human Genetics, points to some of the potential pitfalls of NIPT. It explains that when the testing reveals the presence of conditions that are mild, highly variable, or uncertain, couples may face very difficult decisions, incidental genetic findings may affect the parents and other family members, and a prenatal detection of an impairment that might otherwise have remained undetected may violate the child's right to an open future. The document adds that it is difficult to adequately explain the goals and limitations of an "enlarged NIPT test" during a routine clinical encounter between a health provider and a pregnant woman. The growing complexity of interpretations of the test, and the increasing costs of such interpretations, may mean that even if NIPT will be accessible to all, the possibility of receiving an appropriate follow-up of the results will vary among individuals and societies. Because of such difficulties, the 2015 position document proposed to limit the use of NIPT to the detection of major autosomal trisomies: "Expanding NIPT-based prenatal screening to also report on sex chromosomal abnormalities and microdeletions not only raises ethical concerns related to information and counseling challenges but also risks reversing the important reduction in invasive testing achieved with implementation of NIPT for aneuploidy, and is therefore currently not recommended."[107]

It is not very likely that NIPT producers will radically change their marketing strategies and stop selling a "complete" test that includes testing for deletions, or that all physicians will follow the recommendation to propose to their patients only NIPT for trisomies 21, 13, and 18, because they may fear that if they fail to mention the possibility of testing for rare fetal anomalies, a woman who gives birth to a severely impaired child may turn against them. In countries in which screening for Down syndrome as part of routine pregnancy supervision is funded by the National Health Service, governmental agencies can influence the implementation of diagnostic tests through decisions about the diffusion of and reimbursement for such tests.[108] The first four years of the rapid increase in the volume of NIPT were, however, dominated by a swift diffusion of this technology on free, unregulated markets. Brazil is an example of such a market.

Fetal DNA on the Free Market: Noninvasive Prenatal Testing in Brazil

The diffusion of NIPT in the United States was mostly guided by commercial logic. Such logic was partly tempered by major health insurance companies' decisions about whether, and under which conditions, they will cover NIPT's costs. In Brazil, the introduction of this technology was primarily outside the sphere of control not only of the state but also of major Brazilian health insurance companies that are unwilling (as of the time of this writing) to pay for noninvasive prenatal screening. NIPT became one of the signs of "quality care of pregnancy" in Brazil, offered exclusively to affluent women. The marketing of NIPT in a middle-income country as an upscale product for the rich was not an obvious development. According to the authors of a 2015 article, NIPT can improve the detection of autosomal aneuploidies, especially in rural areas, in middle- and low-income countries because it can greatly reduce the need for physicians who perform ultrasound screening for Down syndrome and amniocenteses. With the advent of NIPT, it may become possible for community health workers in prenatal care clinics to take blood samples of pregnant women and send them to central laboratories. Only the few who will test positive will be invited to undergo amniocentesis and/or diagnostic ultrasound.[109] Such a scenario assumes, however, a willingness to induce a screening for fetal anomalies and, implicitly, the possibility for a woman who carries a fetus diagnosed with such an anomaly to elect to have an abortion. Neither element exists in Brazil.

As of this writing, abortion for a fetal indication is illegal in Brazil, with the sole exception of anencephaly.[110] As a consequence, there are no official rules regarding prenatal screening for fetal anomalies in the public health system (Sistema Único de Saúde) employed by the majority of Brazilians.[111] This system is interested in cfDNA-based tests that can lead to efficient treatment of a fetal anomaly. In 2012, selected public hospitals began to offer tests for fetal sex to pregnant women known to be carriers of the mutation for congenital adrenal hyperplasia. If a woman carries a female fetus, she may be a candidate for treatment with dexamethasone, designed to prevent the "virilization" of external genital organs of the female fetus.[112] In the same year, a small number of pilot institutions introduced cfDNA-based testing for fetal Rh markers in the blood of a Rh-negative mother (in that case, like in the case of a search for markers on chromosome Y, the cfDNA-based test looks for a marker absent from the maternal DNA, and thus relatively easy to detect). If such markers are found, the woman's physicians supervise the fetus for signs of destruction of the red blood cells.[113] By contrast, public hospitals and clinics did not show interest in the use of NIPT for the detection of incurable fetal conditions, such as Down syndrome.

The situation in the private health sector in Brazil is very different. The private sector provides services to 25%–30% of the Brazilian population. In many domains, among them gynecology and obstetrics, the quasi-totality of middle- and upper-class women use exclusively private health services. Women treated in the private sector usually undergo some variant of screening for Down syndrome risk, often a combination of a serum test and an ultrasound examination. If these tests uncover a high risk of Down syndrome or other inborn anomaly, the woman often undergoes amniocentesis, and if the fetus has a chromosomal anomaly she can chose to have an illegal but safe abortion. The low number of children with congenital anomalies born in private hospitals and clinics indirectly attests to the popularity of abortions for fetal anomalies in the private health sector.[114] As Brazilian physician and author Drauzio Varella explained when speaking about fetal malformations induced by the Zika virus, abortion for a fetal indication is freely accessible in Brazil—for those who have money.[115]

Circa 2006, several private Brazilian laboratories started to offer noninvasive tests of fetal sex: such tests can be performed as early as the fifth or sixth week of gestation.[116] The fact that Brazilian laboratories were able to perform this text is unremarkable. Brazil has highly skilled molecular biologists often trained in the best North American and European centers. It also has well-equipped clinical biology laboratories. The unusual element was the widespread diffusion of a test for fetal sex. This test, developed circa 1999, became available in numerous industrialized countries in the first years of the twenty-first century.[117] In many Western European countries, diagnosis of fetal sex early in pregnancy is, however, strictly regulated and is limited to cases in which the woman is at risk of carrying a fetus with an X-linked hereditary condition, such as hemophilia and fragile X syndrome, and those in which an early diagnosis of the fetus' sex helps to decide whether the pregnant woman will receive treatment aiming to prevent a fetal anomaly.[118] Diagnosis of fetal sex is less stringently controlled in the United States. It is, however, relatively expensive, and since future parents can learn what the fetus' sex is from an ultrasound scan a few weeks later, the market for very early determination of fetal sex is not very large. An additional argument against such an early identification of fetal sex is the existence of a significant risk of a spontaneous early miscarriage. Pregnancy loss, even a very early one, is frequently a distressing event. Knowing the sex of a miscarried fetus can endow that fetus with a firmer identity as a future son or daughter, therefore making coping with pregnancy loss more difficult.[119]

In Brazil, a test that detects fetal sex early in pregnancy had a different fate: it became a popular consumption item. It is proposed to women in private maternity clinics, together with other blood tests such as a serum test for Down syndrome risk as a part of routine supervision of pregnancy. The test is relatively inexpensive—in 2015, its price was around 300–400 real, that is, approximately $80–$100. Its popularity may be linked with its competitive pricing. Many women take this test because knowing the future child's sex is seen in Brazil as a key step in the integration of this child into the family. The fetus, redefined as a male or a female, acquires a name and an identity.[120] Health professionals affirmed that Brazilians do not have a strong preference for boys, and that it is highly unlikely that a woman would abort a fetus because it was the "wrong" sex. Alternatively, it is difficult to exclude the possibility that a woman who, for personal reasons, strongly desires to have a child of a given sex will not abort a fetus of a different sex. It is even more difficult to exclude the possibility that a woman who knows that she is a carrier of an X-linked condition, such as hemophilia or fragile X, will elect not to give birth to a boy.

US producers of NIPT became very interested in the Brazilian market.[121] In 2013, two US firms, Ariosa and Natera, signed agreements with Brazilian laboratories, and private clinics started to introduce NIPT.[122] In early 2013, the Brazilian press presented the new test to their readers with headlines such as "Looking for the Perfect DNA?" or "Blood Test That Detects Down Syndrome

Arrives in Brazil." The latter article explained that the test will help families be better prepared for the arrival of a child with Down syndrome and was illustrated with a photograph of a smiling young middle-class couple with a very cute little girl with Down syndrome.[123] Private laboratories such as Centro Paulista de Diagnóstico, Pesquisa e Treinamento, and Laboratório Gene de Belo Horizonte began to include information about NIPT for Down syndrome in their publicity leaflets. The uptake of NIPT was not regulated. Every woman who wanted to have this test and was able to pay for it could ask her doctor to take a blood sample and send it for testing. Conversely, initially only few gynecologists were familiar with NIPT. In the fall of 2013, specialists from the private sector were not sure whether NIPT would became popular in Brazil. One possible obstacle for the diffusion of this test was its price—between 2,000 and 3,000 real for a test for trisomies 21, 18, and 13, and fetal sex—and the test was not reimbursed by health insurance. The price of a serum test for Down syndrome risk (usually PAPP-A) was at that time 200–300 real, 300–400 real for a test for fetal sex, and 1,000–1,200 real for amniocentesis (if needed). Women could therefore obtain comparable information at a much lower cost.

One year later, NIPT became part of the prenatal testing landscape in Brazil, and this trend was amplified in 2015 and 2016. Ariosa and Natera were very active, and successful, in dispersing information about their respective tests through targeted activities such as information meetings and dinners for doctors. Some professionals said they were surprised how fast the new technology was accepted among pregnant women treated in private clinics. The test's price did not seem to discourage affluent women who wanted to be sure that their child would be "all right." Interviewed professionals (not a representative sample) also thought that the acceptance of this test was not limited to women older than 35 who wished to avoid amniocentesis. It also became popular among young women with a very low risk of giving birth to a child with Down syndrome. Not infrequently, women arrived at their first diagnostic ultrasound examination, conducted at eleven to twelve weeks of pregnancy, with NIPT results in hand. The test is usually prescribed by their gynecologist.

Brazilian physicians, especially those who work in upper-class private clinics, tend to prescribe numerous advanced diagnostic tests. Such tests are partly seen as a status symbol and markers of cutting-edge medicine. Private Brazilian hospitals often purchase expensive diagnostic equipment, such as sophisticated ultrasound and MRI machines. NIPT in Brazil became one of numerous "status-related" diagnostic tests, intended to reassure affluent users. The prescription of NIPT was dissociated from a calculus of individual risk and became a test that aims to reassure the pregnant woman that her baby is all right. NIPT producers took into account this specificity of the Brazilian market. An advertisement for Natera's Panorama test, produced by the laboratory that distributes this test in Brazil, Laboratório Gene, and titled "Healthy Baby, Serene Pregnancy," stated that there are two versions of the Panorama test: a "standard" test, which detects trisomies 21, 13, and 18, and sex chromosomes anomalies, and an "amplified" test, which also includes testing for five major chromosomal deletions.[124] The advertisement then explained that while Down syndrome is more frequent in older women, the risk of microdeletions is not determined by a woman's age: women younger than 30 therefore have a higher risk of having a child with a microdeletion than one with Down syndrome.[125] The implicit message is that a savvy pregnant woman of any age should invest in NIPT if she wants to avoid a reproductive disaster.

For upper-middle-class women, NIPT can indeed be seen as a good investment. Services provided by high-end maternity clinics are usually not reimbursed by private health insurance companies. Women who choose such clinics because of their excellent reputations are already prepared to pay significant sums of money out of pocket for quality prenatal care. In 2016, the price of NIPT was not very high when compared to other health-related expenses such as an ultrasound examination. In a subculture that strongly stresses the consumer aspect of pregnancy, the purchase of a NIPT may be seen as similar to, but less frivolous than, the purchase of a luxury baby stroller. NIPT was smoothly integrated into the high-tech supervision of pregnancy accessible to upper-class Brazilian women, which includes testing for fetal anomalies and (illegal) abortions for such anomalies.

Noninvasive Prenatal Testing and DiGeorge Syndrome

In the spring of 2014, biotechnology companies started to market tests for chromosomal deletions.[126] Natera's Panorama test, the first to offer the detection of chromosomal anomalies, included testing for 22q11 deletion syndrome (DiGeorge syndrome, frequency of 1 in 2,000 live births), 1p36 deletion syndrome (frequency 1 in 5,000 live births), Angelman syndrome (maternal 15q11-q13 deletion, frequency 1 in 12,000), and Prader-Willi syndrome (paternal 15q11-q13 deletion, frequency 1 in 20,000). These syndromes are rare; nevertheless, Natera's leaflet that presents these new developments explains that in aggregate they produce inborn anomalies in 1 in 1,000 children. Their frequency may be compared with the estimated 1 in 830 frequency of Down syndrome in the general population.[127] Ariosa's Harmony test offers testing of the same five mutations as

Panorama, Illumina's verifi test added on Wolf-Hirschhorn syndrome (4p, frequency 1 in 50,000), and Sequenom's MaterniT21 Plus test offered the largest spectrum of anomalies, including the five conditions included in the Panorama test plus Wolf-Hirschhorn syndrome, Langer-Giedion syndrome (8q, rare but its precise frequency is unknown), and Jacobsen syndrome (11q, frequency 1 in 100,000)—it also added testing for two rare autosomal trisomies: trisomy 16 and trisomy 22. Full trisomy 16 or 22 is incompatible with life, but children with mosaic forms of these trisomies (a mixture of normal and trisomic cells) can survive. The severity of their clinical manifestations depends on the proportion of trisomic cells.[128]

Publicity leaflets for Panorama, MaterniT21 Plus, Harmony, and verifi tests provide accurate descriptions of the tested chromosomal anomalies; however, they tend to accentuate the negative consequences of these mutations and do not explain that because of the great rarity of the majority of the described conditions, a "positive" NIPT result has a low positive predictive value—it is at most an indication of advisability of further investigation. Conversely, the majority of these rare syndromes produce severe health problems and developmental delays. Therefore, one may assume that a great majority of woman who test positive for one of these syndromes will undergo an invasive test (usually CVS) that confirms or informs NIPT's results; a 5% probability that the fetus carries a deletion that produces a severe impairment is much higher than a 0.01% chance of a child being born with such a deletion in the general population.

Many of the chromosomal anomalies detected by NIPT are new mutations, but some may be inherited from a parent. People who carry a chromosomal anomaly usually have a 50% probability of transmitting it to their offspring. If a given chromosomal anomaly produces a very serious impairment, the chances are low that people who carry this anomaly will have children. However, if it has a variable expression, there is a much higher chance that some of its carriers will have children. DiGeorge syndrome stands out among the chromosomal anomalies included in expanded NIPT tests of 2014 because of its relatively high frequency, the great variability of its expression, and the important number of "hidden" cases of DiGeorge syndrome in the general population.

DiGeorge syndrome is the most frequently employed name for a deletion—the absence of a segment of the long arm of one of the pair of chromosomes 22, on region 1, band 1, and subband 2—usually abbreviated as 22q11.2del.[129] The length of such a deletion may vary, but as of the time of this writing scientists have not uncovered a clear-cut correlation between the size of the deletion and its location, as well as the severity of the impairments it produces. Until recently, few people other than clinical geneticists, patients, and their families have heard about this condition: DiGeorge syndrome was seen as one among many rare and obscure genetic anomalies. Thanks to the development of new genomic approaches, it has become somewhat less obscure, decidedly less rare, and, with the possibility of detecting it in the fetus, more problematic. DiGeorge syndrome is linked with numerous physical defects and mild to moderate cognitive impairments (the mean IQ of people with DiGeorge syndrome is in the low 70s, but approximately one-third are in the normal range of 80 to 100) as well as psychiatric disorders, above all, schizophrenia.[130]

DiGeorge syndrome was first described in 1968 by Italian pediatrician Angelo DiGeorge.[131] It was defined as a distinct genetic condition in the 1990s, following the finding that several inborn anomalies given different names—ovelocardiofacial syndrome, Shprintzen syndrome, conotruncal anomaly face syndrome, Strong syndrome, third and fourth pharyngeal pouch syndrome, congenital thymic aplasia, and thymic hypoplasia—were manifestations of a single chromosomal anomaly, the 22q11.2 deletion.[132] A deletion on the long end of chromosome 22, according to scientists, influences the development of the embryo during weeks six to eight of gestation, affecting cells in sites (e.g., bronchial arch, pharyngeal pouch, and neural crest) that are important for the development of numerous regions of the body.[133] DiGeorge syndrome was initially associated with a long list of physical impairments such as heart defects (especially tetralogy of Fallot, four interconnected heart anomalies that can be treated with surgery), dysmorphic features, cleft palate, anomalies of calcium metabolism, insufficient activity of the thyroid and of the thymus, autoimmune disorders, hearing loss, laryngo-tracheo-esophageal anomalies, growth hormone deficiency, seizures, and skeletal anomalies and chronic dental problems.[134] Later, it was also linked with intellectual disability and a high risk of mental illness in young adults. In the twenty-first century, the latter conditions became the defining traits of this syndrome in adults.[135]

New developments in medicine and biomedical sciences often produce new classifications. When syphilis was defined as a disease produced by the bacillus *Spirochaeta pallida*, it was separated from other venereal diseases such as gonorrhea and aggregated with neurological and cardiac pathologies that were shown to be late manifestations of the infection with *Spirochaeta*.[136] A new classification of a pathological condition may primarily affect the concerned person (e.g., when the new classification of the normal range of blood pressure redefined an individual previously seen as healthy as somebody who has to be treated), it may be of importance for the community (this is especially true for infectious diseases), and, when dealing with genetic conditions, it may affect not only the diagnosed individuals but also their families. The rapid increase in the number of individuals diagnosed with DiGeorge syndrome, a direct consequence of a wider diffusion of genomic diagnosis techniques, also increased the number of people concerned about the transmission of this condition. Scientists estimate that about 30% of DiGeorge syndrome cases are transmitted in families (mainly by people with a mild variant of this condition), while 70% are new mutations.

Experts stress the importance of multidisciplinary management of this complex condition. Children with DiGeorge syndrome suffer from feeding difficulties and infections, and many need surgeries for congenital heart and pharynx anomalies. In later life, people with this syndrome have difficulties with long-term communication and have learning, behavioral, and mental problems: many correspond to the definition of autistic spectrum disorders.[137] Nearly all affected adolescents and adults need some kind of educational and psychiatric support, as do their caretakers, nearly always their parents. Many adults with DiGeorge syndrome are in psychiatric care.[138] Another challenging problem is reproductive guidance of people with DiGeorge syndrome. As a rule, people diagnosed with this syndrome following its diagnosis in a child or a fetus have a milder form of this condition. Conversely, since a 22q11.2 deletion has variable expression, it is impossible to predict the severity of pathological manifestations of this mutation in an affected person's children. Genetic counseling for people with DiGeorge syndrome may be complicated by the presence of learning difficulties and neuropsychiatric disorders, not infrequently coupled with a denial of their existence. Such a denial, some experts argue, may be facilitated by the fact that people with this condition usually do not have marked dysmorphic traits (they look "normal") and have good language skills, which may mask the severity of underlying cognitive difficulties and psychiatric problems.[139]

The majority of parents of children with DiGeorge syndrome were favorable to a prompt postnatal diagnosis of this condition. Genetic diagnosis, they explained, saved them from a long and often stressful diagnostic journey and helped them get appropriate help and support for their child. At the same time, genetic counselors were often reluctant to tell parents of a young child that their child has a high probability of developing a psychiatric illness later in life. Instead, they preferred to concentrate on solutions to the child's immediate physical health problems.[140] Parents of people with a 22q11.2 deletion thus attested that they were rarely informed by health professionals about the high risk of schizophrenia, severe anxiety disorder, and other psychiatric manifestations of this condition, and often received this information from nonmedical sources such as the internet. They found psychiatric conditions especially difficult to manage and complained about the scarceness of support for people with Di George syndrome and their families.[141]

Before the generalization of genomic diagnostic approaches, the prenatal diagnosis of DiGeorge syndrome was grounded in the observation of morphological anomalies associated with this condition, above all, heart and palate defects.[142] As late as 2010, fetal medicine specialists recommended the search for a 22q11.2 deletion in a fetus only when there were several concurring ultrasound signs that strongly pointed to the possibility of DiGeorge syndrome. If there was only one ultrasound sign that pointed to this possibility, they did not propose a costly and complicated genetic inquiry.[143] Four years later, with the generalization of new genomic approaches, searching for a 22q11.2 deletion was no longer seen as expensive or complicated. Searching for this mutation became a standard procedure, recommended in each case when ultrasound examination revealed morphological anomalies that might be linked with DiGeorge syndrome.

A French study indicated that 69% of couples who received a diagnosis of DiGeorge syndrome in a fetus decided to terminate the pregnancy, 3% of fetuses were lost through miscarriages and death in utero, and 28% of pregnancies ended with the birth of a live child. The main elements that favored the decision to abort an affected fetus were the presence of more severe morphological anomalies and an earlier diagnosis of fetal DiGeorge syndrome. The presence of the mutation in one of the parents did not seem to affect decisions about termination, possibly because the presence of a mild variant of this condition in a parent does not predict the severity of the impairment in a child.[144] Conversely, an article published in 2016 by a Canadian group that specializes in following up with people with a 22q11.2 deletion stressed the importance of prenatal diagnosis of this condition, because it favors early psychological and psychiatric care of affected children. Such early psychiatric intervention can attenuate their risk of schizophrenia (estimated at 25%), anxiety disorders (40%), and intellectual impairment (30%). The article does not mention the possibility that some parents may elect to abort a fetus with a 22q11.2 deletion.[145]

Prenatal diagnosis of DiGeorge syndrome is one of the first cases of a prenatal detection of a serious risk of mental disease. In 2016, mutations linked with DiGeorge syndrome were found in less than 1% of people diagnosed with schizophrenia and similar conditions; as of the time of this writing, their prenatal diagnosis is not expected to diminish the frequency of psychiatric diseases in the general population.[146] Nevertheless, NIPT for DiGeorge syndrome paves the way for prenatal screening for the risk of severe mental disease in children in the future.[147] Another complex issue linked with the prenatal diagnosis of this condition is an incidental finding of a 22q11.2 deletion in one of the parents. The diagnosis of DiGeorge syndrome in a fetus is nearly always followed by testing the parents for the presence of this mutation. Uncovering the presence of a 22q11.2 deletion in a parent can lead to a reinterpretation of his or her behavioral or psychiatric difficulties, previously seen as temporary and curable, as symptoms of an underlying severe structural defect that will not go away. Such reinterpretation may have distressing consequences for the diagnosed person and his or her family.[148]

The story of a 22q11.2 deletion started as the description of a typical syndrome, an inborn association of several structural impairments. It shifted to the detection of morphological anomalies of the fetus by obstetrical ultrasound, and then was transformed into a story about the detection of mutation, 22q11.2 del. The latter development led to an increase in the number of people—and fetuses—diagnosed with this condition. The new focus on genetics did not abolish the key role of the clinic (and also psychiatric clinics) in the management of DiGeorge syndrome. New genomic technologies lead, however, to a redefinition of the normal and the pathological, as well as a reclassification of complaints, syndromes, and risks. They can also reshape disease-specific activism.

The diagnosis of some well-known genetic conditions, such as Down syndrome, achondroplasia ("dwarfism"), or hereditary deafness, relies mainly on clinical signs. Its confirmation by genetic tests may be important for procedural and administrative reasons and may affect the reproductive decisions of mutation carriers, but it does not play an important role in the care of affected individuals. Activists of disease-specific associations for these "older" genetic conditions usually do not develop close collaborations with geneticists, and some energetically oppose prenatal diagnosis. In Europe, Down syndrome associations, composed mainly of parents of children with this condition, strongly resisted the introduction of NIPT.[149] In June 2012, two months before the company Life-Codexx, based in Konstanz, Germany, commercialized its PrenaTest for Down syndrome, thirty Down syndrome organizations from sixteen European countries formally objected in the European Court of Human Rights the sale of the test.[150] The French National Consultative Ethics Committee ended its opinion that recommended the introduction of NIPT for Down syndrome screening with a passionate argument in favor of the extension of the rights of disabled people, perhaps as an attempt to deflect accusations advanced by French associations of parents of children with Down syndrome that this technology would lead to a "eugenic" elimination of impaired people.[151]

Activism developed around "new" genetic diseases is often different. The new ethos of linking advanced genetic technologies with clinics favored an alliance between researchers interested in genetic puzzles and speedy progress of their domain of expertise and patients/parents interested in a better understanding of the causes of their / their children's problems.[152] Activists—very often parents of children with severe genetic anomalies—hope that the progress of genetic knowledge will promote a search for cures. They also hope that the uncovering of mutations responsible for a given genetic condition will facilitate their children's access to medical and extramedical resources.[153] Parental input may be one of the driving forces behind the double movement of a growing "geneticization" of inborn conditions and a predicted extension of testing for the presence of genetic anomalies in children with developmental delays.[154]

An alliance between geneticists and parents/activists can favor new genetic diagnoses. It can also lead to tensions between groups of activists who advocate different models of disease-centered "biosociality."[155] In the 1960s and 1970s, women aware of the presence of an "old" hereditary disease in the family, such as hemophilia or thalassemia, frequently supported prenatal diagnosis and selective abortion of affected fetuses, because these approaches allowed them to free themselves from a "family's malediction" and give birth to healthy children. Later, associations of parents of children with inborn genetic conditions, such as Down syndrome, strongly rejected prenatal diagnosis followed by an abortion of trisomic fetuses and presented such abortion as a "eugenic" elimination of people with disabilities as well as a statement about the lesser worth of disabled individuals. NIPT favors the detection of rare genetic anomalies. It remains to be seen whether associations of parents of children with "new" genetic impairments will support prenatal detection of such impairments coupled with a possibility to elect to abort an affected fetus, oppose prenatal diagnosis and selective abortion, or be divided on this question.

Imperfect Pregnancies in the Genomic Era

In 1971, geneticist James Neel praised the advent of prenatal diagnosis. Before the development of this technology, genetic counselors could at best provide rough estimates of the risk of having a child with a hereditary condition.[156] With the development of prenatal diagnosis, it became possible to provide a positive alternative to genetic counseling, remove what some experts called "the Russian roulette atmosphere" that previously shaped reproductive decisions in families affected by hereditary disorders, and replace previously shaky risk evaluations with certainty.[157] In retrospect, this was a very optimistic evaluation. Prenatal diagnosis and prenatal screening did eliminate some reproductive dilemmas but in other cases exchanged one set of difficult choices with another.

Dilemmas produced by the prenatal diagnosis of DiGeorge syndrome resonate with those linked with the detection of Klinefelter syndrome during pregnancy.[158] Specialists have divergent opinions concerning the level of impairment induced by the presence of an additional X chromosome and hold discordant views on abortion for this anomaly. Some highly qualified experts perceive KS as a source of minor dysfunctions only. They point to the fact that the great majority of people with this condition live fully independent lives, and that many are unaware that they have an abnormal chromosomal formula. Accordingly, these experts view the termination of pregnancy for this indication as an irresponsible quest for a "flawless" child. Other, equally qualified experts view KS as a condition that besides sterility is linked with a nonnegligible risk of health and behavioral problems and cognitive difficulties. Accordingly, these experts believe that only a pregnant woman can decide whether such a risk justifies terminating a pregnancy. In 2016, the great majority of US women who underwent NIPT opted for a test that included sex chromosome aneuploidies. If this trend continues, it will probably lead to an important augmentation in the number of people with KS whose parents have been aware of their condition from the day they were born. These children/people may benefit from early educational and psychological interventions. Alternatively, they may lose the right to have a childhood unburdened by parental knowledge of their genetic anomaly and may suffer from the consequences of parental overprotection, problematic relations with other family members, diminished self-esteem, and stigmatization.[159]

The expansion of genomic approaches in the late twentieth and early twenty-first centuries led to an increase in the number of people diagnosed with inborn genetic disorders and a parallel increase in the number of fetuses diagnosed with such disorders. Conversely, when a given mutation is diagnosed during pregnancy, it is often impossible to predict what its effects will be. It is possible that in the near future, a woman will not only learn that she carries a fetus with a 22q11.2 deletion but will also learn what the probable consequences of this deletion will be. However, the example of Down syndrome illustrates the difficulty of making such predictions. Close to half a century of prenatal diagnosis of this condition has not improved physicians' ability to predict the degree of impairment of a trisomic fetus. At the same time, public images of Down syndrome have become strongly polarized. People with this condition are depicted either as severely impaired or able to function well in daily life; as disturbed and difficult or happy and easygoing; or as a source of excessive misery or great joy for their families. Such a polarization of images, which may be contrasted with more nuanced views of impairment that arise after birth, probably reflects attempts to put pressure on pregnant women faced with a "positive" prenatal diagnosis to make specific choices. The extension of NIPT and other technologies that will allow the scrutiny of fetal DNA may deepen women's quandaries and intensify attempts to influence them to make the "right" decision.

Foreseeing the future of a newly developed biomedical technology is a perilous task. Reading predictions of the future of specific medical innovations, one can readily grasp how inaccurate the majority of such predictions were. This is not, however, the way people usually see them. The ability to cherry-pick successful predictions and conveniently overlook the others is not very different from vividly recollecting a premonitory dream two days before an accident and forgetting all the dreams about disasters that never happened. The flood of forecasts about a swift end to infectious diseases that followed Pasteur's and Koch's findings about the role of pathogenic bacteria in the late nineteenth century can be retroactively seen as an accurate foreseeing of the future. Such a view is not false. Asepsis, vaccination, and antibiotics dramatically diminished mortality and morbidity from infectious diseases. It is also grossly inaccurate. Antibiotics, the first truly antibacterial agents, were developed more than fifty years after the description of pathogenic bacteria; improvement of sanitation, nutrition, and life conditions played a key role in reducing mortality from infectious diseases; the Spanish influenza pandemic of 1918–1919, the worst since Black Death, was not affected by the rise of bacteriology; and in the twenty-first century, the persistence of high mortality from AIDS, tuberculosis, malaria, and many other transmissible diseases continues to interrogate the nineteenth-century optimistic vision of a rapid elimination of such diseases.

The story of NIPT deals with a new, rapidly changing domain, an especially tricky subject. This chapter is, at best, a series of blurred snapshots of a fast-moving target. Many statements about the potential uses of NIPT made between 2008 and 2010 quickly became outdated because they failed to foresee the central role of commercial firms in the production of knowledge and practices in this area, and underestimated the speediness of the development of marketable—and aggressively promoted—tests. It is possible that cfDNA-grounded tests developed between 2010 and 2017 will become obsolete in the next few years, as a result of, for example, the successful development of accurate and inexpensive prenatal tests based on the study of fetal cells in maternal circulation, a sharp decrease in costs of the sequencing of complete fetal DNA, or totally unpredicted developments that could radically change the domain of NIPT. Conversely, it is probably not too risky to propose that new genomic techniques will continue to favor the extension of the scrutiny of the unborn. It also may not be too hazardous to argue that these technologies will continue to be shaped by commercial considerations sometimes at odds with users' interests. Geneticists Mark Evans and Joris Vermeesch argued in 2016 that the rush to extend cfDNA-based tests to low-risk populations is an especially clear example of the potentially negative effects of commercial strategies. In these populations, the incidence of microarray-detectable anomalies is actually ten times that of Down syndrome. The replacement of previous diagnostic procedures (microarrays performed on fetal cells collected through CVS or amniocentesis) with cfDNA-based tests, according to Evans and Vermeesch, will cost more and find less.[160]

NIPT, a technology developed during a period of intensive scrutiny of the ethic dimension of prenatal diagnosis, was discussed by scientific and medical journals, professional bodies, and the media.[161] These debates were centered on two points: Down syndrome activists' opposition to an increase in screening for this condition and the perils of the use of cfDNA to sequence the whole fetal genome.[162] The flood of information about the future child produced by such a sequencing, some geneticists, bioethicists, and jurists argued, may be confusing and unsettling for future parents.[163] It may also, especially if available early in pregnancy, allow for a "eugenic" selection of desirable traits of children.[164] In a typical statement, French molecular biologist Bertrand Jordan explained that with the recent advances of possibilities to predict the health and behavior of people from analyzing their genome and the expected drastic decrease in the cost of sequencing fetal genomes, we are nearing the vision—outlined in Andrew Niccol's 1997 film *Gattaca* and Lee Silver's 1997 book *Remaking Eden*—of a society with a swiftly growing gap between genetic haves and have-nots.[165]

However, the use of NIPT for producing "flawless" offspring seems, for the time being, remote from the already-existing applications of this diagnostic technology. Dealing with present-day developments rather than with hypothetical futures, debates on NIPT often focus on the dangers of an insufficient understanding of this approach by users.[166] A 2015 editorial of the *British Medical Journal* argued that while NIPT provides important advantages, its generalization raises serious concerns about informed consent of cfDNA-based tests. Women easily confuse probabilistic testing with diagnosis and fail to understand that a positive NIPT test denotes probability and not certainty of changes in fetal DNA.[167] Luckily, as the editorial added, these concerns may be overcome by careful pretest and posttest counseling, accurate information provided to users, and adequate training of health providers.[168]

Researchers sometimes keep silence on a selected topic that may hinder the progress of their studies. Sidelined contentious issues become unmentionable "public secrets." Debates on new technologies often mention the "known knowns" (what we know), the "known unknowns" (what we know that we do not know), and the "unknown unknowns" (what we do not know that we do not know). Researchers may systematically eschew a fourth important category, the "unknown knowns," that is, the things we do know but elect to evacuate from ongoing discussions in order to favor further advancement of a given domain and avoid complications.[169] In 2016, debates on NIPT tended to neglect "unknown knowns" that could hamper the diffusion of this diagnostic approach, such as an increase in pregnant women's anxiety and stress, the impact of prenatal diagnosis of inborn anomalies on parents' relationships with their "genetically marked" children, the effect of such early knowledge on the child's self-image, or the consequences of an incidental finding of hereditary anomalies for families. If mentioned at all, these and similar contentious issues tend to be quickly dismissed with the argument that NIPT's present-day difficulties will disappear thanks to pregnant women's access to high-quality counseling and the education of health professionals.[170] Uneasy knowledge about NIPT has become a "known unknown" because of a widely shared conviction that problems produced by the intensification of scrutiny of the fetus will be solved through further enlargement of networks of experts in prenatal diagnosis and the expansion of their jurisdiction.

Prenatal Diagnosis' Slippery Slopes, Imagined and Real

Screening for Risks and Screening as a Risk

In a general medical discourse, screening is usually defined as the use of a test that does not provide a final diagnosis. In the health policy discourse, the main distinctive trait of screening is that a given test is systematically offered, at the initiative of medical or public health professionals, to yet unburdened populations. Prenatal diagnosis, or, rather, prenatal screening, is offered today in many countries to pregnant women without any indication of a fetal anomaly or risk of an anomaly. It thus corresponds to the second definition, which may include large-scale programs offered to whole populations but also routine tests offered by practitioners to users of their services.[1] Screening is seen as acceptable when there is clear evidence that its benefits outweigh its harms, and, for some experts, also where there is evidence of its clinical utility. Screening pregnant women for treatable conditions that may lead to an unfavorable pregnancy outcome, such as infectious diseases, abnormal blood pressure, or Rhesus factor incompatibility, corresponds to criteria of clinical utility. Screening for the majority of fetal abnormalities does not lead to a better fetal outcome. It has two goals: preparing the future mother for the arrival of a "special needs" child and giving her the option to terminate the pregnancy. In addition, such screening reassures the great majority of pregnant women. Luckily, imperfect pregnancies are relatively rare.[2]

Women who have accepted prenatal screening—and by extension prenatal diagnosis—often explain that they did it to "ease their mind." Women who refused prenatal diagnosis believed that scrutiny of the fetus would have the opposite effect. It could put an end to their enjoyment of pregnancy and produce undue stress and worry, and such stress might in turn harm their unborn child. Some pregnant women refused a serum screening test for Down syndrome risk because they did not wish to embark on a medical journey that may force them to decide whether they wanted to undergo amniocentesis and put their future child at risk or continue a pregnancy knowing that something may be amiss.[3] However, with the generalization of high-resolution obstetrical ultrasound, fewer women were free to make such a choice. Diagnostic ultrasound is not formally labeled "screening," but in many countries the generalization of its use coupled with improved resolution of ultrasound machines and developed skills of ultrasound experts has transformed it into a de facto screening tool. Ultrasound examinations were initially introduced mainly to search for pregnancy-related problems. The increasing frequency of the detection of fetal anomalies during such examinations has blurred the boundaries between "maternal- and child-health related" and "autonomy-related" goals, but also between prenatal diagnosis and prenatal screening.[4] Nearly all pregnant women in industrialized countries, and many in "intermediary" countries, have at least one, and often several, ultrasound tests during their pregnancy. Each additional test increases the chance of revealing a potential fetal problem. Fetal medicine experts who observe suspicious changes in the fetus often suggest that pregnant woman undergo an invasive test to investigate the genetic material of fetal cells. Few women who learn that something may be wrong with their future child reject further tests, because at that point the risk of an inborn anomaly is not an abstract number but something their doctors can see.[5]

Modern medicine is increasingly oriented toward the management of risks rather than the treatment of already-existing functional impairments. Blockbuster drugs that lower cholesterol and blood pressure manage future disease risks, while cancer treatment often transforms a healthy person into a very sick individual in the hopes of preventing future harm.[6] The screening of "asymptomatic individuals," who before the screening era were called healthy people, is inscribed in this logic. It aims at identifying potentially diseased individuals in a large population and aspires to separate those at high risk of a screened condition from all the others, not infrequently with significant margins of error.[7] Despite its limitations, on the population level screening is perceived as an efficient collective management of health problems, and on the individual level it is perceived as an efficient way of helping people take control of their lives.

Enthusiasm for screening, according to bioethicists Darren Schicle and Ruth Chadwick, is grounded in a widely accepted principle that prevention is always better than a cure. Screening is presented as a neutral technique. However, screening incorporates preexisting concepts and values. It often promotes a specific view of the natural history of a given disease. Thus, screening for cancer implicitly assumes that malignant tumors have a linear trajectory that starts with a localized premalignant lesion and ends with generalized cancer, a perception that leads to a logical conclusion that all premalignant lesions need to be treated aggressively. The enthusiasm for screening frequently fails to take into account its material and emotional costs. A screening test cannot guarantee the absence of false negatives and false positives. It can generate false reassurance for some people and initiate an unnecessary, costly, and distressing diagnostic odyssey for others. It can also produce screening-related stress.[8] Sociologists and anthropologists who study screening are interested in surveillance medicine, citizenship, and responsibility; embodiment; decision-making and informed choice; and risk and uncertainty.[9]

There is abundant scholarly literature on the problematic aspects of screening, such as overdiagnosis, diagnostic uncertainty, incidental findings, costs of complex medical trajectories, and the blurring of boundaries between an already-existing pathology and its risk.[10] However, this literature seldom discusses prenatal diagnosis. Sociologists, anthropologists, and policy experts who study prenatal diagnosis rarely present this approach as an example of the screening of unburdened individuals. The absence of an analysis of a population-based search for fetal anomalies as a screening technology may mirror the ambiguous status of such a screening, rooted in the uncertain status of a pregnant woman as "not an in/dividual." It is not certain who the screened patient/subject is for two distinct reasons. First, the status of the fetus is fluid and indeterminate, perceived in some circumstances as being a part of the maternal body and in others as a distinct, autonomous subject of medical intervention—and sometimes as both.[11] Second, screening for fetal anomalies can reveal maternal problems or, as bioethicist Wybo Dondorp and his colleagues put it, "the reality of irreducible double purpose screening."[12] Such a reality is especially frequent in obstetrical ultrasound examinations, which can display fetal anomalies but also pregnancy-related problems and potential obstacles to childbirth. Prenatal diagnosis combines "maternal- and child-oriented goals" and "autonomy-oriented goals."[13] The inseparability of these two elements maintains an ambivalence about who the target of such a screening is: the pregnant woman or her future child. This ambivalence was aptly captured in the title of Rayna Rapp's pioneering study of prenatal diagnosis, *Testing Women, Testing the Fetus*.[14] Finally, the typical goal of screening is to prevent and/or cure a pathology. This is not the case of screening for fetal anomalies.

Screening for the presence of a hidden disease was initially a public health measure developed to protect populations from transmissible diseases such as tuberculosis or syphilis. Screening allows people previously unaware of their infection to get access to treatment. Still, such personal benefit, however important, is not a precondition for a population-based screening for transmissible pathologies, especially in emergency situations. Screening for noninfectious pathologies is very different. It is seen as legitimate only when the diagnosis of a given condition provides a direct advantage for the diagnosed individual and when the advantages of the screening are greater than its drawbacks.[15] These criteria are difficult to apply to screening for fetal malformations. Despite official discourse that focuses on prenatal diagnosis' role in favoring treatments and preparing parents for the birth of a special needs child, in 2017 the most frequent consequence of a diagnosis of a severe fetal malformation is an abortion. It is problematic to describe this consequence as an unqualified "positive outcome" of screening, especially in light of the uncertainty about who the screened "patient" is. Selective abortion for fetal indications is an uncomfortable and contested topic. It continues to be viewed by many public health experts as a privately managed solution for a public health problem, but this view, openly discussed in the 1970s and 1980s, is rarely made explicit in the twenty-first century. Uneasiness about the consequences of screening for fetal anomalies may explain, at least partly, the scarcity of debates on prenatal diagnosis as a population-based screening approach and specific problems produced by screening fetuses—and the women who carry them.

"Collateral Damage" of Prognostic Uncertainty

Women who receive a diagnosis of a fetal anomaly or a serious risk of such an anomaly have to quickly make a difficult decision about the future of the pregnancy.[16] It is not surprising that researchers have found high levels of distress in women diagnosed with severe fetal impairments as well as in their partners.[17] Such distress may be enhanced by diagnostic and prognostic uncertainty. The improvement of the resolution power of prenatal diagnosis techniques also increases the probability that pregnant women may receive indeterminate results and may face a diagnostic journey that may or may not decrease the initial qualms about the child's future. If the problem is defined as hereditary, diagnostic uncertainty may be extended to the parental couple and other members of the family.[18] Often, women and their partners struggle to understand the precise significance and potential implications of the results of prenatal testing. A typical response of people who received an ambivalent result of analysis of fetal DNA was: "I understood what they told me, but I wish we could have found out more about what it meant. . . . I wanted to know more."[19]

Women may consent to a specific prenatal test without being fully aware of its consequences. This was especially true for women who underwent comparative genomic hybridization, a test that may reveal unsuspected chromosomal anomalies, some without clear meaning. Many women had heard about Down syndrome, but only a few knew what the consequences of chromosomal deletions or translocations were. Women who agreed to undergo amniocentesis and were offered CGH in addition to karyotype readily agreed to an "offer too good to pass [up]": learning more about their future child. Some were reassured by the results, including by a diagnosis of a severe genetic anomaly, which occasionally facilitated the decision to terminate a pregnancy, since "at this point it was written on the wall." Other women felt that when they received a "positive" diagnosis, professionals pressured them to terminate the pregnancy even though they did not want to. Others still became severely stressed. As one woman explained, "I started getting really panicky that the child that I was carrying was going to be severely autistic with seizures and schizophrenia. . . . I would look online and I met with a geneticist and talked to an autism specialist. And frankly, nobody could really tell me."[20]

An uncertain diagnosis made some women apprehensive about the future of their child. Even after delivering what appeared to be a "normal" baby, eight of the sixteen women who continued their pregnancies admitted to lingering worries about their child's development: "Since I had this uncertain microarray result . . . if anything happens to him in the future . . . that will always pop up in my mind. . . . You just have to have a 'wait and see' attitude. . . . I'm a lot more vigilant."[21] Lingering stress after an uncertain result of a genetic test is not just an overreaction of anxious pregnant women. It may also mirror the professional's awareness of the limits of genetic knowledge, especially when dealing with rare disorders. Moreover, many genetic syndromes produce effects expressed only later in life. A healthy-looking newborn does not necessarily mean that the child will live without serious health problems: this child may be just a "patient in waiting."[22]

Uncertain results of ultrasound examinations are another source of anxiety for women. Detection of "soft markers" of a fetal anomaly—indirect signs that the fetus may have a genetic defect—during an obstetrical ultrasound examination can also induce long-term stress, especially in women unprepared for such findings.[23] A French study compared levels of maternal anxiety and maternal involvement with a child's care in women who learned about the presence of soft markers of possible fetal impairment and were reassured later and in matched controls without such episode. This study found that the stress linked to an abnormal ultrasound finding can persist long after the pregnant woman has learned that the result was reclassified as a false positive. Women who at some point in pregnancy learned about potential health problems of their future child had much higher depression scores and anxiety scores than the controls. They also had more difficulty relating to their newborn baby. The authors of this study concluded that "there may be a gap between the way the fetal ultrasound scan is generally represented as 'harmless' and its potential impact on both the psychological state of the pregnant mother and mother-infant interaction. [The authors] found that the impact of a false positive ultrasound screening persists after birth until two months postpartum. Given the frequency with which fetal scans are used to detect at-risk pregnancies, preventative measures should be recommended in case of soft markers detection, in particular when pregnant women express high emotional distress after soft markers diagnosis."[24] In other words, routine prenatal diagnosis can be an iatrogenic intervention that produces long-lasting effects.

With the advancement of technology and research, British activist Jane Fisher, who directs the charity Antenatal Results and Choices, explained that screening is becoming increasingly complex and stress-generating: "The poignancy of ultrasound images for many parents means that it can be especially difficult to manage the anxiety when an ultrasound marker is highlighted as potential cause for concern. They can then face a journey of anxiety-laden uncertainty, which can extend through much of the pregnancy, and even beyond. Professionals involved in screening need to recognize and acknowledge such adverse side-effects."[25]

The generalization of noninvasive prenatal testing and the precision of genetic tests on fetal cells collected through invasive testing may further increase women's anxiety. Fisher's 2011 article is titled "First Trimester Screening: Dealing with the Fallout." Advertisements for noninvasive prenatal testing in Brazil affirm that this test allows a pregnant woman to be reassured that she will have a serene pregnancy and that her baby will be healthy, a double omission of the original goal of prenatal testing, the detection of chromosomal anomalies and thus of impairment of the future child, and the vexing question of what will happen if the test produces a "positive result."[26] With the advent of new genomic technologies, the question of who is going to deal with the fallout of prenatal screening may become even more urgent. A focus on the moral dimensions of prenatal diagnosis has diverted attention from other problematic aspects of this diagnostic technology and transformed them into "known unknowns," hidden in plain sight.

Dreams and Nightmares about Future Children

Debates on innovation in the domain of human reproduction tend to disproportionally focus on relatively rare developments such as preimplantation diagnosis or futuristic risks such as human cloning but tend to overlook the already-existing—and frequent—problematic developments and difficult choices produced by the diffusion of prenatal diagnosis. As sociologist Anne Kerr explained, speaking about assisted reproduction technologies: "There is no need to reign in dark imagining or potentially frivolous thought experiments about choices that may become possible in the future. We need to concentrate upon the messiness and complexity of the present in a time of uncertainty, or else we risk losing from sight what really matters to people in the business of reproduction."[27]

The same argument can be made about present-day development in the similarly untidy and complex business of scrutinizing the living fetus. The prenatal diagnosis dispositif, like other biomedical technologies, is shaped by the context in which it is embedded and in turn shapes this context. The history of prenatal diagnosis is characterized by a rapid diffusion of a specific set of biomedical techniques: amniocentesis, culture of fetal cells, chromosome studies, biochemical studies, obstetrical ultrasound, DNA analysis, and sequencing. It is also characterized by a great diversity of local uses of these techniques. The amplification of the resolution power of diagnostic techniques, which has greatly increased doctors' ability to predict "bad outcomes" of pregnancy, coupled with changing parental expectations about the information they should have about their future child and the acceptability of abortion for a fetal indication favored a speedy diffusion of scrutinizing the fetus and its transformation into a routine and often quasi-invisible diagnostic approach.

In many industrialized countries, prenatal diagnosis became in the late twentieth century a technological imperative and a new standard of care.[28] At the same time, prenatal diagnosis remained a contested area of medical intervention. These two statements are not contradictory: they refer to different meanings of the term *prenatal diagnosis*. The transformation of prenatal diagnosis into a widely diffused diagnostic and screening technology was viewed as a simple extension of the physician's gaze, a view that greatly facilitates a smooth integration of prenatal diagnosis into the medical supervision of pregnancy. Physicians always wanted to be able to assess whether a woman would give birth to a healthy child, but until the 1970s they could only use indirect means of achieving this goal: the study of a woman's family history and close supervision of her behavior during pregnancy. The development of diagnostic approaches that made possible a direct scrutiny of the unborn child was portrayed as a technical solution for a long-sought medical problem, while its extension was presented as a highly desirable improvement of already-existing diagnostic methods. Criticism of prenatal diagnosis focused on its links with selective abortion, an element usually radically divorced from an analysis of situated applications of prenatal diagnosis.

Public debates on the present and future of prenatal diagnosis are frequently centered on the risks of a gradual and imperceptible sliding into increasingly selective reproduction. The parental "dream of a perfect child" opens a "backdoor to eugenics."[29] Some of the goals of the historical eugenic movement, or, rather, the loose associations of diverse entities gathered in the first half of the twentieth century under the heading "eugenics," indeed resonate with certain present-day uses of clinical genetics.[30] Such resonances, historian of science Susan Lindee argued, fails, however, to explain what is most important for the understanding of present-day developments: the complex nexus of the relationship between academic science and private industry that made possible the incorporation of ideals of individual choice, risk management, and responsible parenthood into circulating, marketable items.[31] The use of the term *eugenic* in contemporary debates, according to scholars who studied the history of eugenics, muddles rather than clarifies these debates. The term *eugenics*, Danish sociologist Lene Koch explained, "is open to pejorative use because it is rarely, or only superficially, defined. . . . It seems that the reference to eugenics, perhaps precisely because it is poorly defined, serves the purpose of rendering the activity in question ethically unacceptable."[32] According to historian of eugenics Diane Paul, to assert that a policy with undesirable effects is also "eugenic does not add anything substantive to the accusation. What it does add is emotional charge."[33]

A critique of "backdoor eugenics," omnipresent in debates on prenatal diagnosis, produced an objective, although unintentional, alliance between radical opponents of abortion and disability rights activists.[34] The emotional charge of the claim—or sometimes a battle cry—that the ultimate logic of prenatal diagnosis is an inexorable descent into a Nazi style of eugenics favored an exclusive focusing of these discussions on the risk of a slippery slope that started with a diagnosis of major fetal anomalies and will end with excessive parental demands and a full-blown eugenic agenda. Parents who use prenatal diagnosis to achieve the birth of a "flawless child," according to feminist scholar Joan Rothschild, have the entirely illusory impression that they can control the future child's fate.[35] Prenatal diagnosis, bioethicist Arthur Caplan proposed, produces a conflict between an individual's right to make decisions regarding his or her reproductive and procreative behavior, which entitles him or her to the right to have as much information as possible, and the morally contentious option of terminating the pregnancy, which may be the result of obtaining such information.[36] The availability of such information, Caplan explained, may lead to an increasingly narrow definition of the desirable fetus:

> Prenatal diagnosis will identify conditions, traits and behaviors which parents, for various reasons, might find simply undesirable. It is not at all clear what the dividing line is between normality and disorder. Nor is it clear whether medicine should take as part of its mandate fulfilling all the dreams and desires of parents about their children. . . . Just as the line between health and disease is often blurry, so is the line dividing self-determination from the indulgence of preferences, whims, fancies or biases. . . . To the extent to which the line between choice and whim remains vague, the potential exists for prenatal testing to be enmeshed in the pursuit of the frivolous or to be put in the service of ignorance, prejudice and bigotry.[37]

Caplan's concerns, shared by other bioethicists, focus on what might happen, or perhaps what is already happening, in a small number of cases. Such concerns are remote from dilemmas of the majority of pregnant women who undergo prenatal diagnosis. The brave new world of babies produced to conform to a specific parental design remains (at least for now) exactly where it was in the 1930s: in science fiction books.[38] Not many parents are worried about religious inclinations or musical abilities of their future child, but many pregnant women are confronted with a diagnosis of a fetal condition with an uncertain prognosis and/or a small, but not insignificant, risk of a truly disastrous outcome. Some bioethicists expressed concern that pregnant women will gradually switch from termination of pregnancy for a severe fetal malformation to its termination for less severe malformations, then for minor impairments, and finally to the elimination of all fetuses that do not correspond to their vision of the ideal child.[39] Bioethicist Evelyne Shuster thus explained that there is a serious risk that the list of conditions that will disqualify a fetus from being born will finally make it impossible for a parent to have a child at all: a "normal" child, that is, one devoid of detectable flaws, is a nonexistent child.[40]

The supposition that prenatal diagnosis will inexorably lead to an escalation in parental demands for a "flawless product," and a transition from the search for major fetal impairments to an aspiration to eliminate all possible fetal imperfections, is not grounded in empirical data. Indications of abortion for fetal indications in the twenty-first century are not much different than such indications in the 1970s and 1980s. French professionals estimated in 2010 that 93.6% of the decisions to terminate a pregnancy were made by women and professionals as a result of anomalies that were lethal or would lead to substantial physical and/or mental disabilities.[41] Only in slightly more than 6% of cases was an interruption of pregnancy motivated by fetal anomalies classified by the authors of this study as "borderline," such as a late-onset disease, the absence of a limb, sex chromosome aneuploidy, or cleft palate. All other terminations of pregnancy for nonlethal conditions were for anomalies in which there was a certainty or high probability that the child would have a serious impairment and would need lifelong care.[42] Disability activists' critique of aborting "defective" fetuses is rooted in a distressing reality. Despite official discourse about disability rights, many people with disabilities receive only scant societal support and continue to face disdain and discrimination. An exclusive focus on their point of view may, however, deflect attention from the practical, material, and emotional difficulties of care for severely impaired children and adults, delegated mainly to their family members, above all, mothers.

There is a powerful argument in favor of rejecting selective abortion of impaired fetuses in the name of human diversity and the right of all human beings to live a full life, independently of their inborn capabilities. Nevertheless, in societies that fail to take full responsibility for the well-being of all their disabled members, there is also a powerful argument against forcing a pregnant woman to unconditionally accept any fetus that develops in her womb, regardless of the risk that the birth of an impaired child may negatively affect her own and other family members' lives.[43] Such risk is extremely variable—it depends on the family's socioeconomic status; the availability and quality of external support; the psychological makeup of the family's members, their values, and intrafamily dynamics; and the nature of the child's impairment. Many families who happily raise children with disabilities strongly protest the very notion of "disability risk." Conversely, if one accepts the principle that a woman has the right to decide whether, in a given moment of her life, she is ready for the lifelong duties and obligations of motherhood, it is difficult to argue that she is not entitled to decide which motherhood-related risks she is willing/able to accept.[44] As Anna Quindlen explained, many people are persuaded that they know what "good mothers" and "good people" should do, and then leave women to live with the consequences of their convictions.[45]

In the half-century of its existence, prenatal diagnosis has undergone important transformation: from testing women who were at high risk of giving birth to an impaired child to the screening of all pregnant women; from detection of confirmed fetal impairments to uncovering conditions with highly variable expressions and anomalies with unknown clinical meaning; and from the search for relatively frequent conditions, such as Down syndrome (estimated prevalence: 1:800 live births), to the search for very rare ones, such as "cri du chat" (estimated prevalence: 1:50,000 live births). Critique of the supposed parental aspiration to produce "perfect" children deflects attention from the very real parental aspiration to detect all severe fetal impairments, however rare. The "medical utopia" that favored the rapid extension of prenatal diagnosis is not an effort to produce flawless children but an effort to achieve perfect control over health risks of the future child. It is reasonable to assume that the main motivation of parents who adopted new diagnostic technologies was not an aspiration to ascertain the "superior quality" of their offspring but fear of giving birth to a severely impaired child.[46]

Fear of catastrophic results of a pregnancy may be linked to the ancient fear of "monstrous births" and the modern fear of hidden genetic flaws. Such fear is not limited to affluent, industrialized societies. Anthropologist Tine Gammeltoft movingly showed how Vietnamese women's very frequent use of diagnostic ultrasound despite the fact that it is perceived as potentially dangerous for the fetus is fueled by apprehension of the birth of an impaired child. Such an apprehension persists during the whole pregnancy. Vietnamese women undergo frequent ultrasound scans, despite their worry about the consequences of such scans for the fetus, in order to attenuate their much greater fear of a calamitous outcome of pregnancy.[47] Vietnamese women's reactions are perhaps extreme, but the phenomenon described by Gammeltoft is not limited to Vietnam. The advent of prenatal diagnosis heightened the perception of risks for the fetus and increased the demand for prenatal tests for fetal anomalies, including rare ones and those with variable expression. Large-scale diffusion of prenatal diagnosis, and the possibility of detecting a growing number of fetal anomalies, increases the probability of uncovering new anomalies and new suspicious conditions. It leads to an amplification of diagnostic and prognostic uncertainty, and magnifies prenatal diagnosis–related anxiety, an accurate description of an already-existing slippery slope.

A Path-Dependent, Situated Diagnostic Technology

The aim of prenatal diagnosis, explicit in the 1970s and 1980s, and less explicit, but nevertheless omnipresent, in 2017, is to promote the birth of healthy children. Positive and negative "selective breading" that aims to optimize reproductive outcomes is a millenary practice seen in animal husbandry and human mating. The radical innovation of prenatal diagnosis was to shift the focus of a negative selection from progenitors to fetuses. Debates on prenatal diagnosis became dominated—or perhaps phagocyted—by discussions on the latter topic, often presented as a eugenic threat. Such a framing of discussion about prenatal diagnosis did not leave much space to reflect on the unique history of this diagnostic technology, on developments that shaped this history, and on specific elements that affect its present-day uses. It also does not favor investigations of path-dependent trajectories that lead to the highly divergent situated uses of prenatal diagnosis. The paucity of debates on the technical and material aspects of scrutiny of the living fetus, as this book argues, hampers the understanding of the consequences of the widespread diffusion of this biomedical technology. It also hinders the investigation of its sociocultural and ethical aspects, and the incorporation of norms and values into material practices. According to Bruno Latour, technologies are active agents, forms of mediation, and translation devices. They make possible "being as another" and produce multiple, often unforeseen functions between the intended use of a new technology and its unavoidable transformations: "If we fail to recognize how much the use of a technique, however simple, has displaced, translated, modified, or inflected the initial intention, it is simply because we have changed the end in changing the means, and because, through a slipping of the will, we have begun to wish something quite else from what we at first desired."[48]

The history of prenatal diagnosis displays such displacement, translation, modification, and inflection of its original intentions. The exclusive interest in its role in the selective abortion of "flawed" fetuses deflected attention from its role as a highly productive technology that produced new heterogeneous assemblages of material and social techniques, images, and institutions that, taken together, made possible the definition of some pregnancies as "imperfect."

Biomedical knowledge and practices are situated, as is their study. When Ludwik Fleck warned in the 1930s about the dangers of disconnection of the study of science from the observation of concrete practices of scientists, he did it from his situated standpoint as a physician and public health expert. Fleck's best-known work, the book *Genesis and Development of a Scientific Fact* of 1935, investigated the origins and development of a new diagnostic approach: the Wassermann test for the detection of syphilis. Fleck's pioneering investigations displayed the importance of studying how precisely a unique combination of material and social techniques, professional and institutional factors, and political considerations produced the first laboratory-based screening for the presence of a pathological condition.[49]

Fleck's injunction to pay close attention to the details of the genesis and development of a scientific fact is no less important today than it was in the 1930s. New, powerful biomedical technologies increase the ability of health professionals to help and to harm.[50] The predicted radical transformation of the prenatal diagnosis dispositif by the advent of new genomic technologies makes it even more urgent to carefully examine the material, institutional, organizational, sociocultural, and political variables that shape this dispositif, as well as important differences among its situated applications. It also highlights the importance of the study of the history of prenatal diagnosi and of material cultures of medicine that, to use anthropologist Sarah Franklin's felicitous expression, are a "feeder layer" that favors the consolidation and dissemination of this biomedical innovation.[51] Scrutiny of the living fetus produces many stratums of meaning, but all these meanings came into being through the development, stabilization, modulation, and wide-scale diffusion of a cluster of medical technologies. Debates on prenatal diagnosis centered on the (presumed) dangers of the homogenization of bodies, the rejection of human imperfection, and a slippery slope that will inexorably lead to a new eugenics overlook a crucial element: prenatal diagnosis is a diagnosis.

Preface · A Biomedical Innovation

1. Faye Ginsburg and Rayna Rapp discuss "stratified reproduction": local uses of new reproductive technologies. Faye Ginsburg and Rayna Rapp, eds., *Conceiving the New World Order: The Global Politics of Reproduction* (Berkeley: University of California Press, 1995).

2. A high level of pregnancy-associated plasma protein A (PAPP-A) in a pregnant woman's blood indicates a higher-than-average probability that the fetus has Down syndrome (trisomy 21). A woman diagnosed with an elevated risk of Down syndrome is invited to undergo an invasive test, either amniocentesis or chorionic villus sampling (CVS), to sample fetal cells. A study of these cells can tell whether the fetus has an abnormal number of chromosomes.

3. Magdalena Radkowska-Walkowicz, "Potyczki z technologią: Badania prenatalne w ujęciu antropologicznym" [Grappling with technology: Prenatal tests—an anthropological approach], in *Etnografie Biomedycyny* [Ethnographies of biomedicine], ed. Magdalena Radkowska-Walkowicz and Hubert Wierciński (Warsaw: Zakład Antropologii Kulturowej, 2014), 175–90.

4. All the women interviewed by Radkowska-Walkowicz learned that the fetus was not trisomic.

5. Posted on the *DNA Exchange* blog: http://thednaexchange.com/2014/11/02/guest -post-nips-microdeletions-macro-questions/#comment-53822 (accessed March 20, 2016). All the syndromes mentioned in the posts—cri du chat, DiGeorge, and Prader-Willi, Angelman—are produced by the absence of part of a chromosome (deletion). Angelman and cri du chat syndromes are always linked with severe developmental delays, while Prader-Willi and DiGeorge syndromes have a more variable expression. Maternity and Panorama are commercial NIPT tests. CVS can be performed earlier in pregnancy than amniocentesis and is the more frequently used method employed to sample fetal cells.

6. UK National Screening Committee (NSC) of the National Health Service, *Screening Tests for You and Your Baby*, leaflet, 2012. On the other hand, the leaflet was described as too complicated for many of its users. Clare Williams, Priscilla Alderson, and Bobbie Farsides, "What Constitutes 'Balanced' Information in the Practitioners' Portrayals of Down's Syndrome?," *Midwifery* 19, no. 1 (2003): 230–37.

7. See, for example, Carine Vassy, "From a Genetic Innovation to Mass Health Programmes: The Diffusion of Down's Syndrome Prenatal Screening and Diagnostic

Techniques in France," *Social Science and Medicine* 63, no. 8 (2006): 2041–51; Nete Schwennesen, Mette Nordahl Svendsen, and Lene Koch, "Beyond Informed Choice: Prenatal Risk Assessment, Decision-Making and Trust," *Clinical Ethics* 5, no. 4 (2010): 207–16.

Introduction · *Scrutinized Fetuses*

1. Ilana Löwy, "How Genetics Came to the Unborn: 1960–2000," *Studies in History and Philosophy of Biological and Biomedical Sciences* 47, part A (2014): 154–62; Ilana Löwy, "Prenatal Diagnosis: The Irresistible Rise of the 'Visible Fetus,'" *Studies in History and Philosophy of Biological and Biomedical Sciences*, part B (2014): 290–99.

2. Jacques Gelis, *L'arbre et le fruit: La naissance dans l'occident moderne* (Paris: Fayard, 1984); Judith Leavitt, *Brought to Bed: Childbearing in America, 1750–1950* (Oxford: Oxford University Press, 1988).

3. Irvine Loudon, *Death in Childbirth: An International Study of Maternal Care and Maternal Mortality, 1800–1950* (Oxford: Oxford University Press, 1992).

4. This is a privilege of the affluent. Maternal mortality rates in countries such as Afghanistan (1,575 per 100,000 live births) or the Central African Republic (1,570 per 100,000 live births) remind us of the situation in Europe and North America not so long ago. Margaret C. Hogan, Kyle J. Foreman, Mohsen Naghavi, et al., "Maternal Mortality for 181 Countries, 1980–2008: A Systematic Analysis of Progress towards Millennium Development Goal 5," *The Lancet* 375, no. 9726 (2010): 1609–23.

5. Irvine Loudon, "On Maternal and Infant Mortality, 1900–1960," *Social History of Medicine* 4, no. 1 (1991): 29–73.

6. Centers for Disease Control and Prevention, Birth Defects Homepage, http://www.cdc.gov/ncbddd/birthdefects/data.html (accessed January 18, 2017).

7. Salim Al-Gailani, "The Making of Antenatal Life: Monsters, Obstetrics and Maternity Care in Edinburgh, c. 1900" (PhD diss., University of Cambridge, 2010).

8. After all, a book that in the mid-1980s criticized the overmedicalization of pregnancy was titled *The Captured Womb*, not *The Captured Fruit of the Womb*: Ann Oakley, *The Captive Womb: A History of the Medical Care of Pregnant Women* (Oxford: Blackwell, 1984).

9. Laury Oaks, "Smoke-Filled Wombs and Fragile Fetuses: The Social Politics of Fetal Representation," *Signs: Journal of Women in Culture and Society* 26, no. 1 (2000): 63–108.

10. Michel Foucault, "Le jeu de Michel Foucault" (1977), in *Dits et Ecrits (1954–1988)*, ed. Daniel Defert and François Ewald, vol. 3 (Paris: Gallimard, 1994), 298–329, see esp. 299. English translation: Michel Foucault, "The Confession of the Flesh" (1977), in *Power/Knowledge: Selected Interviews and Other Writings, 1972–1977*, ed. Colin Gordon (New York: Pantheon, 1980), 194–228. I'm indebted to Christiane Sinding, who pointed out that prenatal diagnosis can be seen as a dispositif.

11. See, for example, Barbara Duden, *Disembodying Women: Perspectives on Pregnancy and the Unborn* (Cambridge, MA: Harvard University Press, 1993); Karen Newman, *Fetal Positions: Individualism, Science, Visuality* (Stanford, CA: Stanford University Press, 1996).

12. Nick Hopwood, "Visual Standards and Disciplinary Change: Normal Plates, Tables and Stages in Embryology," *History of Science* 43, no. 3 (2005): 239–302; Lynn Morgan, *Icons of Life: A Cultural History of Human Embryos* (Berkeley: University of California Press, 2009); Sara Dubow, *Ourselves Unborn: A History of the Fetus in Modern*

America (Oxford: Oxford University Press, 2011), 10–66; Emily Wilson, "Ex Utero: Live Human Fetal Research and the Films of Davenport Hooker," *Bulletin of the History of Medicine* 88, no. 1 (2014): 132–60.

13. For examples of illustrations in these books in the 1950s, see Solveig Jülich, "The Making of a Best-Selling Book on Reproduction: Lennart Nilsson's *A Child Is Born*," *Bulletin of the History of Medicine* 89, no. 3 (2015): 491–525, see esp. 500–503.

14. These photographs were first published in Nilsson's 1965 *Life Magazine* photo essay "Drama of Life before Birth" and a few months later in Nilsson's book *A Child Is Born*, mainly intended for expecting mothers. Jülich, "The Making of a Best-Selling Book on Reproduction." Few among the millions of readers who admired Nilsson's aesthetically compelling photographs knew that, despite his essay's title, Nilsson photographed miscarried and aborted fetuses: his true subject was death before birth.

15. X-rays were also employed to display major fetal malformations. The first diagnosis of such malformations using X-rays was made in 1917. This approach, however, was confined mostly to the third trimester of pregnancy and had limited practical use. Robert Resta, "The First Prenatal Diagnosis of a Fetal Abnormality," *Journal of Genetic Counseling* 6, no. 1 (1997): 81–84; Ann Oakley, "The History of Ultrasonography in Obstetrics," *Birth* 13, no. 1 (1986): 8–13.

16. Stuart Blume, *Insight and Industry: The Dynamics of Technological Change in Medicine* (Cambridge, MA: MIT Press, 1992); Bettyann Kevles, *Naked to the Bone: Medical Imaging in the Twentieth Century* (Reading, MA: Addison-Wesley, 1998); Angela Creager, *Life Atomic: A History of Radioisotopes in Science and Medicine* (Chicago: University of Chicago Press, 2014).

17. Sharon Kaufman, Janet Shim, and Ann Russ, "Revisiting the Biomedicalization of Aging: Clinical Trends and Ethical Challenges," *Gerontologist* 44, no. 6 (2004): 731–38; Sharon Kaufman, *Ordinary Medicine: Extraordinary Treatments, Longer Lives, and Where to Draw the Line* (Durham, NC: Duke University Press, 2015).

18. Sarah Franklin makes a similar argument about in vitro fertilization. Sarah Franklin, *Biological Relatives: IVF, Stem Cells and the Future of Kinship* (Durham, NC: Duke University Press, 2013), 5.

19. According to UN data, in 2011, 38% of "developing" countries and 86% of "developed" countries legalized abortion for fetal malformation. United Nations, Department of Economic and Social Affairs, Population Division, *World Abortion Policies, 2013*. http://www.un.org/en/development/desa/population/publications/policy/world-abortion-policies-2013.shtml (accessed January 18, 2017).

20. On risk-driven medicine and the circular effects of a search for risks that uncovers more risks and leads to increased stress and more medicalization, see Jeremy Greene, *Prescribing by Numbers: Drugs and the Definition of Disease* (Baltimore: Johns Hopkins University Press, 2007); H. Gilbert Welch, Lisa Schwartz, and Steven Woloshin, *Overdiagnosed: Making People Sick in the Pursuit of Health* (Boston: Beacon Press, 2011); Robert Aronowitz, *Risky Medicine: Our Quest to Cure Risk and Uncertainty* (Chicago: University of Chicago Press, 2015).

21. Bruno Latour, "Morality and Technology: The End of the Means," *Theory, Culture and Society* 19, no. 5/6 (2002): 247–60 (first published in French as "La fin des moyens," *Reseaux* 18 [2000]: 39–58).

22. I borrow the term *technoscientific entity* from Annemarie Mol's description of blood as being not a stable, preexisting entity but something that comes into existence as a "separated, distinct thing" entirely in relation to its specific sociotechnical milieu. Annemarie Mol, *The Body Multiple* (Durham, NC: Duke University Press, 2002).

23. Sarah Franklin, "Fetal Fascinations: New Dimensions of Medical-Scientific Constructing of Fetal Personhood," in *Off Centre: Feminism and Cultural Studies*, ed. Sarah Franklin, Celia Lury, and Jackie Stacey (London: HarperCollins, 1991), 190–205.

24. Dubow, *Ourselves Unborn*.

25. In the twenty-first century, the viability limit is usually fixed at twenty-two or twenty-four weeks of pregnancy.

26. J. M. Jørgensen, P. L. Hedley, M. Gjerris, and M. Christiansen, "Including Ethical Considerations in Models for First-Trimester Screening for Pre-eclampsia," *Reproductive Biomedicine Online* 28, no. 5 (2014): 638–43; Wybo Dondorp, Guido de Wert, Yvonne Bombard, et al., "Non-invasive Prenatal Testing for Aneuploidy and Beyond: Challenges of Responsible Innovation in Prenatal Screening," *European Journal of Human Genetics* 23, no. 11 (2015): 1438–50; Wybo Dondorp, G. C. Page-Christiaens, and G. M. de Wert, "Genomic Futures of Prenatal Screening: Ethical Reflection," *Clinical Genetics* 89, no. 5 (2015): doi:10.1111/cge.12640.

27. Dondorp, de Wert, Bombard, et al., "Non-invasive Prenatal Testing for Aneuploidy and Beyond," 1145–46.

28. Ann Rudinow Saetnan, "To Screen or Not to Screen? Science Discourse in Two Health Policy Controversies, as Seen through Three Approaches to the Citation Evidence," *Scientiometrics* 48, no. 3 (2000): 307–44.

29. Peter Gøtzsche and Karsten Juhl Jørgensen, "Screening for Breast Cancer with Mammography," *Cochrane Database of Systematic Reviews*, no. 6 (2013): doi:10.1002/14651858 .CD001877.pub5; Nikola Biller-Andorno and Peter Jüni, "Abolishing Mammography Screening Programs? A View from the Swiss Medical Board," *New England Journal of Medicine* 370, no. 21 (2014): 1965–67.

30. On the widespread diffusion of ultrasound technology in Vietnam (where abortion for fetal indication is encouraged), see Tine Gammeltoft, *Haunting Images: A Cultural Account of Selective Reproduction in Vietnam* (Berkeley: University of California Press, 2014), and in Brazil (where abortion for fetal indication is illegal), see Lilian Krakowski Chazan, "'É . . . tá grávida mesmo! E ele é lindo!' A construção de 'verdades' na ultra-sonografia obstétrica," *História, Ciências, Saúde—Manguinhos* 15 (2008): 99–116.

31. This is a very schematic division. One of the goals of this study is to display the great variability of patterns of implementation and diffusion of different approaches to prenatal diagnosis and the important differences between countries, institutions, and sites.

32. This expression was attributed to Dr. Everett Kopp, who later became US surgeon general. Charles Bosk, *All God's Mistakes: Genetic Counseling in a Pediatric Hospital* (Chicago: University of Chicago Press, 1992), 26.

33. Kristin Luker, *Abortion and the Politics of Motherhood* (Berkeley: University of California Press, 1984), 236. Luker hints that the "genocide against disabled" language migrated from pro-life activists to disability activists, not the other way around.

34. Gena Corea, *The Mother Machine: Reproductive Technologies from Artificial Insemination to Artificial Wombs* (New York: Harper and Row, 1985).

35. Barbara Katz Rothman, *The Tentative Pregnancy: Prenatal Diagnosis and the Future of Motherhood* (New York: Viking, 1986).

36. Bonnie Steinbock, "Disability, Prenatal Testing and Selective Abortion," in *Prenatal Testing and Disability Rights*, ed. Eric Parens and Adrienne Asch (Washington, DC: Georgetown University Press, 2000), 108–23.

37. Judith McCoyd, "'I'm Not a Saint': Burden Assessment as an Unrecognized Factor in Prenatal Decision Making," *Qualitative Health Research* 18, no. 11 (2008): 1489–1500. Women who decided to terminate pregnancy for nonlethal fetal malformation often saw their decision as the only one possible under the circumstances but at the same time felt guilty for not being the kind of person who could withstand the rigors of parenting a child with special challenges. Ibid., 1495.

38. Veronique Mirlesse, "Diagnostic prénatal et médecine fœtale: Du cadre des pratiques à l'anticipation du handicap: Comparaison France–Brésil" (PhD diss., Université Paris Sud–Paris XI, 2014), 57.

39. Annemarie Mol, *The Logic of Care: Health and the Problem of Patient Choice* (London: Routledge, 2008), xi. The Netherlands has a low level of uptake of screening for Down syndrome and a low level of full-time employment of mothers of young children, perhaps the reason for Mol's insistence that she is fascinated by her work and is reluctant to give it up to became a full-time caretaker for a special needs child.

40. Rayna Rapp and Faye Ginsburg, "Enabling Disability, Rewriting Kinship, Reimagining Citizenship," *Public Culture* 13, no. 3 (2001): 533–56, see esp. 542.

41. Dorothy Wertz and Joseph Fletcher, "A Critique of Some Feminist Challenges to Prenatal Diagnosis," *Journal of Women's Health* 2, no. 2 (1993): 173–88.

42. Helen Statham, "Prenatal Diagnosis of Fetal Abnormality: The Decision to Terminate the Pregnancy and the Psychological Consequences," *Fetal and Maternal Medicine Review* 13, no. 4 (2002): 213–47.

43. Abby Lippman, "Prenatal Genetic Testing and Screening: Constructing Needs and Reinforcing Inequities," *American Journal of Law and Medicine* 17, nos. 1–2 (1991): 15–50; Margarete Sandelowski and Julie Barroso, "The Travesty of Choosing after a Positive Prenatal Diagnosis," *Journal of Obstetric, Gynecologic, and Neonatal Nursing* 34, no. 3 (2005): 307–18.

44. See, for example, Carine Vassy, Sophia Rosman, and Bénédicte Rousseau, "From Policy Making to Service Use: Down's Syndrome Antenatal Screening in England, France and the Netherlands," *Social Science and Medicine* 106 (2014): 67–74.

45. Tom Shakespeare, *Disability Rights and Wrongs Revisited* (New York: Routledge, 2014); Isabelle Ville, "Politiques du handicap et périnatalité: La difficile conciliation de deux champs d'intervention sur le handicap," *ALTER: European Journal of Disability Research / Revue Européenne de Recherche sur le Handicap* 5 (2011): 16–25.

46. Anne Kerr and Sarah Cunningham-Burley, "On Ambivalence and Risk: Reflexive Modernity and the New Human Genetics," *Sociology* 34 (2000): 283–304.

47. Tsipy Ivry, "The Ultrasonic Picture Show and the Politics of Threatened Life," *Medical Anthropology Quarterly* 23, no. 3 (2009): 189–211.

48. Silja Samerski, "Genetic Counseling and the Fiction of Choice: Taught Self-Determination as a New Technique of Social Engineering," *Signs: Journal of Women in Culture and Society* 34, no. 4 (2009): 735–61.

49. Nete Schwennesen and Lene Koch, "Representing and Intervening: 'Doing' Good Care in First Trimester Prenatal Knowledge Production and Decision-Making," *Sociology of Health and Illness* 34, no. 2 (2012): 283–98.

50. Dymphie van Berkel and Cor van der Weele, "Norms and Prenorms on Prenatal Diagnosis: New Ways to Deal with Morality in Counseling," *Patient Education and Counseling* 37, no. 2 (1999): 153–63.

51. Susan Markens, "'It Just Becomes Much More Complicated': Genetic Counselors' Views on Genetics and Prenatal Testing," *New Genetics and Society* 32, no. 3 (2013): 302–21.

52. José Van Dijck, *The Transparent Body: A Cultural Analysis of Medical Imaging* (Seattle: University of Washington Press, 2005), 116.

53. Marilyn Strathern, *After Nature: English Kinship in the Late Twentieth Century* (Cambridge: Cambridge University Press, 1992).

54. Tsipy Ivry, Elie Teman, and Ayala Frumkin, "God-Sent Ordeals and Their Discontents: Ultra-Orthodox Jewish Women Negotiate Prenatal Testing," *Social Science and Medicine* 72, no. 9 (2011): 1527–33.

55. Numerous scholars studied the history of obstetrical ultrasound, genetic diagnosis, and genetic counseling, but few examined the intersections between all the approaches that led to the development of the prenatal diagnosis dispositif. Ruth Cowan studied the beginnings of prenatal diagnosis, but then focused exclusively on genetic testing for hereditary pathologies. Ruth Cowan, *Heredity and Hope: The Case for Genetic Screening* (Cambridge, MA: Harvard University Press, 2008), 71–116.

56. There are numerous excellent sociological and anthropological studies of scrutiny of fetuses and prenatal diagnosis. See, for example, Rayna Rapp, *Testing Women, Testing the Fetus: The Social Impact of Amniocentesis in America* (New York: Routledge, 1999); Clare Williams, "Framing the Fetus in Clinical Work: Rituals and Practices," *Social Science and Medicine* 60, no. 9 (2005): 2085–95; Lynn Morgan, *Icons of Life: A Cultural History of Human Embryos* (Berkeley: University of California Press, 2009); Tine Gammeltoft, *Haunting Images: A Cultural Account of Selective Reproduction in Vietnam* (Berkeley: University of California Press, 2014). I'm especially indebted to Kristin Luker's argument that debates on abortion rights are above all discussions about women's role in society. Kristin Luker, *Abortion and Politics of Motherhood* (Berkeley: University of California Press, 1984). I also benefited greatly from numerous other studies on the history of women's reproductive decisions, fertility and pregnancy, genetic and medical imagery technologies, diagnostic tools, management of risk, and uncertainty in medicine. My research stands on the shoulders of an impressive crowd.

57. In the early twenty-first century, both chromosomal anomalies—above all, Down syndrome—and structural malformations of the fetus accounted for the great majority of pregnancy termination for a fetal indication, with an approximately equal contribution from each group. For example, in 2010 in France 38.5% of abortions were decided based on chromosomal anomalies (trisomies 21, 13, and 18, as well as sex chromosome aneuploidies), and 44% were decided based on structural anomalies. *Rapport Annuel de l'Agence de la Biomedicine*, 2011, p. 72, http://www.agence-biomedecine.fr/IMG/pdf/rapport_reinvdef.pdf (accessed March 20, 2006).

58. Stefan Timmermans and Mara Buchbinder studied the complex effects of a similar extension of the number of detected inborn anomalies in newborn children. Stefan

Timmermans and Mara Buchbinder, *Saving Babies? The Consequences of Newborn Genetic Screening* (Chicago: University of Chicago Press, 2013).

59. This argument was persuasively developed by Sharon Kaufman in *Ordinary Medicine: Extraordinary Treatments, Longer Lives, and Where to Draw the Line* (Durham, NC: Duke University Press, 2015).

60. Diane Paul discussed the unavoidably political nature of debates on scientific subjects such as the one on eugenics. Diane Paul, "Culpability and Compassion: Lessons from the History of Eugenics," *Politics and the Life Sciences* 15, no. 1 (1996): 99–100.

61. Didier Fassin, "A Case for Critical Ethnography: Rethinking the Early Years of the AIDS Epidemic in South Africa," *Social Science and Medicine* 99 (2013): 119–26.

62. Ludwik Fleck, "Zagadnienie teorii poznania," *Przeglad Filozoficzny* 39 (1936): 3–37. English translation: "The Problem of Epistemology," in *Cognition and Fact: Materials on Ludwik Fleck*, ed. Robert Cohen and Thomas Schnelle (Dordrecht: Reidel, 1986), 79–112.

63. Paul Veyne, "Foucault Revolutionizes History," in *Foucault and His Interlocutors*, ed. Arnold Ira Davidson (Chicago: University of Chicago Press, 1997), 146–82. On "estrangement," see Carlo Ginzburg, *Wooden Eyes: Nine Reflections on Distance*, trans. Martin Ryle and Kate Soper (New York: Columbia University Press, 2001).

Chapter 1 · Born Imperfect

1. Irvine Loudon, "On Maternal and Infant Mortality, 1900–1960," *Social History of Medicine* 4, no. 1 (1991): 29–73.

2. Carlos Lopez-Beltran, "The Medical Origins of Heredity," in *Heredity Produced: At the Crossroads of Biology, Politics, and Culture, 1500–1870*, ed. Staffan Müller-Wille and Hans Joerg Rheinberger (Cambridge, MA: MIT Press, 2007), 105–32.

3. Katharine Park and Lorraine Daston, "Unnatural Conceptions: The Study of Monsters in Sixteenth- and Seventeenth-Century France and England," *Past and Present* 92 (August 1981): 20–54; Lorraine Daston and Katharine Park, *Wonders and the Order of Nature, 1150–1750* (New York: Zone Books, 1998).

4. Daston and Park, *Wonders and the Order of Nature*, 57, 65, 180.

5. Ibid., 177.

6. Ambroise Paré, "Le vingt cinquiesme Livre, traitant des Monstres and Prodiges," in *Oeuvres*, fourth ed. (Paris: G. Buon, 1585), MXX, quoted by Sandrine Lely, "Corps défigurés, corps figurés: Le regard des artistes avant l'invention du "handicap," XVIe–XVIIIe s.," in *L'approche de genre dans la déconstruction sociale du handicap*, ed. Marie-Claude Saint-Pé et Sandrine Lely (Paris: 2IRA, 2009), 21–34, see esp. 23. In the twentieth century, the absence of a hand was more often attributed to an accident of fetal development, such as the presence of amniotic bands (protein "ropes" in amniotic fluid), while an abnormal number of fingers or short limbs was more often linked with genetic anomalies.

7. Daston and Park, *Wonders and the Order of Nature*. On the history of embryology in the nineteenth century, see, for example, Nick Hopwood, "Producing Development: The Anatomy of Human Embryos and the Norms of Wilhelm His," *Bulletin of the History of Medicine* 74, no. 1 (2000): 29–79.

8. Camille Dareste, "Préface," in *Précis de tératologie: Anomalies et monstruosités chez l'Homme et chez les animaux*, ed. L. Guinard (Paris: J. B. Balière et fils, 1893), vii.

9. See, for example, Charles Feré, *La Famille névropathique: Théorie tératologique de l'hérédité et de la prédisposition morbides et de la dégénérescence* (Paris: F. Alcan, 1894); Charles Féré, "Essai expérimental sur les rapports étiologiques, de l'infécondité, des monstruosités, de l'avortement, de la morti-natalité, du retard de développement et de la débilité congénitale," *Teratologia: A Quarterly Journal of Antenatal Pathology* 2, no. 4 (1895): 245–55.

10. Antje Kampf, "Times of Danger: Embryos, Sperm and Precarious Reproduction, ca. 1870s–1910s," *History and Philosophy of the Life Sciences* 37, no. 1 (2015): 68–86. On the history of heredity, see Staffan Müller-Wille and Hans-Jörg Rheinberger, "Heredity—the Formation of an Epistemic Space," in *Heredity Produced: At the Crossroads of Biology, Politics, and Culture, 1500–1870*, ed. Staffan Müller-Wille and Hans Joerg Rheiberger (Cambridge, MA: MIT Press, 2007), 3–33.

11. Thomas Cunnane, "The Mentally Defective Child," *California and Western Medicine* 43, no. 1 (1935): 32–36; John Waller, "Parents and Children: Ideas of Heredity in the 19th Century," *Endeavour* 27, no. 2 (2003): 51–56; Lopez-Beltran, "The Medical Origins of Heredity."

12. See, for example, Hopwood, "Producing Development"; Nick Hopwood, "Visual Standards and Disciplinary Change: Normal Plates, Tables and Stages in Embryology," *History of Science* 43 (2005): 239–303; Caroline Arni, "Traversing Birth: Continuity and Contingency in Research on Development in Nineteenth-Century Life and Human Sciences," *History and Philosophy of Life Sciences* 37, no. 1 (2015): 50–67.

13. On the evolution of Ballantyne's ideas, see Salim Al-Gailani, "Teratology and the Clinic: Monsters, Obstetrics and the Making of Antenatal Life in Edinburgh, c. 1900" (PhD diss., University of Cambridge, 2010). Ballantyne continues to be seen as the "founding father" of teratology. J. Bruce Beckwith and Ronald J. Lemire, "John William Ballantyne—a Biographical Sketch (1861–1923)," *Teratology* 1 (1968): 1–3.

14. John Ballantyne, *The Diseases and Deformities of the Foetus: An Attempt towards a System of Antenatal Pathology*, 2 vols. (Edinburgh: Oliver and Boyd, 1892–1895). John William Ballantyne, *Manual of Antenatal Pathology and Hygiene: The Foetus* (Edinburgh: William Green, 1902); John William Ballantyne, *Manual of Antenatal Pathology and Hygiene: The Embryo* (Edinburgh: William Green, 1904).

15. There were exceptions to this rule. For example, the French doctor Charles Féré (1852–1907) was interested both in teratology and experimental embryology and in pathological births. Arni, "Traversing Birth."

16. Ballantyne, *The Diseases and the Deformities of the Foetus*, 1:19–23.

17. Ballantyne, *Manual of Antenatal Pathology and Hygiene of the Foetus*, 1:292–97.

18. Ibid., 1:486.

19. Al-Gailani, "Teratology and the Clinic," 170–71.

20. Ibid., 196.

21. Ibid., 206–7.

22. On Pinard's activity as a eugenist, see Anne Carol, *Histoire de l'eugénisme en France: Les médecins et la procréation, XIXe–XXe* (Paris: Seuil, 1995).

23. Adolphe Pinard, *A la jeunesse, pour l'avenir de la race française* (Paris: La Ligue nationale française contre le péril vénérien, 1925), leaflet.

24. On Pinard's contribution to the care of newborns and young babies, see Anne Cova, *Maternité et droits des femmes en France: XIX–XX siècles* (Paris: Anthropos, 1997).

25. Specialists assume that the majority of premature babies develop normally until their birth. They can suffer from severe physical, neurological, and cognitive impairments, but the cause of these impairments is usually their untimely birth. Conversely, a genetic or developmental anomaly can be at the origin of prematurity.

26. Jane Lewis, "Gender and the Development of Welfare Regimes," *Journal of European Social Policy* 2, no. 3 (1992): 159–73; Anne-Marie Daune-Richard, "Les femmes et la société salariale: France, Royaume-Uni, Suède," *Travail et Emploi* 100 (2004): 69–84; Anne Cova, "Où en est l'histoire de la maternité?," *Clio: Femmes Genre, Histoire* 21 (2005): 189–211.

27. Adolphe Pinard, *De la puériculture* (Lyon: Imprimeries Réunies, 1908).

28. See, for example, Edward John Chance, *On the Nature, Causes, Variety and Treatment of Bodily Deformities* (London: Smith, Elder and Company, 1905); R. Birnbaum, *A Clinical Manual of the Malformations and Congenital Diseases of the Foetus* (London: J. & A. Churchill, 1912; first published in German in 1909, translated by G. Blacker).

29. There are numerous social histories of mental handicap, for example: Philip M. Ferguson, *Abandoned to Their Fate: Social Policy and Practice toward Severely Retarded People in America, 1820–1920* (Philadelphia: Temple University Press, 1994); James W. Trent, *Inventing the Feeble Mind: A History of Mental Retardation in the United States* (Berkeley: University of California Press, 1994); Steven Noll, *Feeble-Minded in Our Midst: Institutions for the Mentally Retarded in the South, 1900–1940* (Chapel Hill: University of North Carolina Press, 1995); David Wright and Anne Digby, eds., *From Idiocy to Mental Deficiency: Historical Perspectives on People with Learning Disabilities* (London: Routledge, 1996); Mathew Thomson, *The Problem of Mental Deficiency: Eugenics, Democracy, and Social Policy in Britain, c. 1870–1959* (Oxford: Clarendon Press, 1998); Steven Noll and James W. Trent Jr., eds., *Mental Retardation in America: A Historical Reader* (New York: New York University Press, 2004); Mical Raz, *What's Wrong with the Poor? Psychiatry, Race, and the War on Poverty* (Chapel Hill: University of North Carolina Press, 2013).

30. Cunnane, "The Mentally Defective Child," 35–36.

31. Samuel Gridley Howe, Horatio Byington, and Gilman Kimball, *The Causes of Idiocy* (Edinburgh: MacLachlan and Stewart, 1858), 27–28.

32. Ibid., ix. Howe and his collaborators blamed the parents of "idiots" but at the same time strongly supported decent treatment of the mentally impaired. Helping these people, they argued, is a moral imperative, not only because they are on public charge but because many are so badly treated and cruelly wronged through ignorance that though born with a spark of intellect, this spark is gradually extinguished. Ibid., xiii.

33. Ibid., 46–52.

34. Peter Martin Duncan and William Millard, *A Manual for the Classification, Training, and Education of the Feeble-Minded, Imbecile, and Idiotic* (London: Longmans, Green, 1866), 6.

35. From the 1970s on, experts refer to this diagnosis as "dysmorphic features."

36. Édouard Séguin (1812–1880), a student of Jean Marc Gaspard Itard (famous for his study of the "wild child of Aveyron"), first worked with impaired children in Paris, where he established a school for children with cognitive deficiencies. His innovative pedagogy combined physical and mental training and aimed at increasing the pupil's autonomy and self-reliance. Séguin emigrated to the United States in 1848 for political reasons. In the United States, he established several schools for mentally impaired

children; he also collaborated with US experts such as Samuel Gridley Howe. G. E. Shuttleworth, *In Memory: Édouard Séguin* (London: H. H. Wolf, 1881), leaflet.

37. B. A. Lond, "Obituary: George Edward Shuttleworth," *The Lancet* i (1928): 1203.

38. George Edward Shuttleworth, *Mentally-Deficient Children: Their Treatment and Training* (London: H. K. Lewis, 1895).

39. George Edward Shuttleworth, *Mentally-Deficient Children: Their Treatment and Training*, second edition (London: H. K. Lewis, 1900), 56–69.

40. George Edward Shuttleworth and William Alexander Potts, *Mentally Deficient Children: Their Treatment and Training*, third edition (London: H. K. Lewis, 1910), 51–119.

41. George Edward Shuttleworth and William Alexander Potts, *Mentally Deficient Children: Their Treatment and Training*, fifth edition (London: H. K. Lewis, 1922), 86–89.

42. Ibid., 265.

43. M. D. Durch, "Obituary: Alfred Frank Tredgold," *The Lancet* ii (1952): 642–43; Bond, "Obituary: George Edward Shuttleworth."

44. Alfred Frank Tredgold, *Mental Deficiency (Amentia)* (London: Baillière, Tindall and Cox, 1908), 79–80. After the Second World War, geneticists who rejected Tredgold's eugenic views, such as Lionel Penrose, nevertheless investigated links between characteristic physical manifestations of hereditary syndromes and mental deficiency. Lionel Penrose, *The Biology of Mental Defect* (London: Sidgwick and Jackson, 1949), 128–39.

45. Tredgold, *Mental Deficiency (Amentia)* (1908), 357–62.

46. Ibid., 36–38.

47. Alfred Frank Tredgold, *Mental Deficiency (Amentia)*, second edition (London: Baillière, Tindall and Cox, 1914), 432–62.

48. Alfred Frank Tredgold, *Mental Deficiency (Amentia)*, third edition (London: Baillière, Tindall and Cox, 1920); Alfred Frank Tredgold, *Mental Deficiency (Amentia)*, fourth edition (London: Baillière, Tindall and Cox, 1922).

49. Alfred Frank Tredgold, *Mental Deficiency (Amentia)*, fifth edition (London: Baillière, Tindall and Cox, 1929), 500–504.

50. Tredgold's views, especially his negative attitude toward mentally impaired people, were strongly criticized in the 1930s by Penrose. Lionel Penrose, *Mental Defect* (London: Sidgwick and Jackson, 1933), 3.

51. Alfred Frank Tredgold, *Mental Deficiency (Amentia)*, sixth edition (London: Baillière, Tindall and Cox, 1937), 520.

52. Ibid., 522.

53. Ibid., 518. The hardening of Tredgold's stance may be related, perhaps, to the 1930s economic crisis. Penrose stated in 1933 that thanks to good institutional care, some mentally defective people greatly improved and could, in principle, return to society and find employment, but "in the present period of economic depression, unemployment and lack of commercial enterprise, it is not to be expected that persons who have been ejected from the community for inefficiency will be favourably received back again even if they have been taught wisdom in the meantime." Penrose, *The Biology of Mental Defect*, 160.

54. Alfred Frank Tredgold, *A Textbook of Mental Deficiency (Amentia)*, seventh edition (London: Baillière, Tindall and Cox, 1947), 491. The same recommendation appears in the last edition of *A Textbook of Mental Deficiency*, edited by Tredgold (with the assis-

tance of his son, Roger Francis Tredgold) in 1952. Alfred Frank Tredgold, assisted by Roger Francis Tredgold, *A Textbook of Mental Deficiency (Amentia)*, eighth edition (London: Baillière, Tindall and Cox, 1952), 503. Tredgold's continuation of support of a physical elimination of "helpless" and "repulsive" idiots and imbeciles after the Second World War may be unsettling. However, in the 1940s and early 1950s, Nazi genocide and the role of the Nazi program of euthanasia of the "unfit" in preparation of the extermination of Jews and Roma were not as widely known as they are today, and not many people immediately recognized the name Auschwitz. Only later did extermination camps become a central element in the Second World War's history. Tredgold and his son explain that they regretted the fact that eugenic considerations are not very popular today, because "doctors' training and inclination alike make them more concerned with the welfare of the individual patient than with the effect he has on the community." They do not mention recent history as a possible factor in the decline of eugenics' popularity. A. F. Tredgold and R. F. Tredgold, *A Textbook of Mental Deficiency* (1952), 474.

55. Roger Francis Tredgold and Kenneth Soddy, *Tredgold's Mental Deficiency (Subnormality)*, tenth edition (London: Baillière, Tindall and Cox, 1963), 470. The same argument is repeated in the eleventh edition of this book. Roger Francis Tredgold and Kenneth Soddy, *Tredgold's Mental Retardation*, eleventh edition (London: Baillière, Tindall and Cassell, 1970), 27.

56. On the use of photography in psychiatry, see Sander Gilman, *Health and Illness: Images of Difference* (London: Reaktion Books, 1995); Sander Gilman, *Seeing the Insane: A Cultural History of Madness and Art in the Western World* (Nebraska: University of Nebraska Press, 1996).

57. Mark Jackson, "Images of Deviance: Visual Representations of Mental Defectives in Early Twentieth-Century Medical Texts," *British Journal for the History of Science* 28, no. 3 (1995): 319–37, see esp. 320.

58. Jackson, "Images of Deviance."

59. Renata Laxova, "Lionel Sharples Penrose, 1898–1972: A Personal Memoir in Celebration of the Centenary of his Birth," *Genetics* 150, no. 4 (1998): 1333–40.

60. On the production of such photographs, see, for example, Alice Domurat Dreger, "Jarred Bodies: Thought on the Display of Unusual Anatomies," *Perspectives in Biology and Medicine* 43, no. 2 (2000): 161–72.

61. Lionel S. Penrose Papers, University College Archives, London, File 74C. The file contains notebooks from 1964; the photographs are probably from the same time period.

62. Positive Exposure, "About the Program," http://positiveexposure.org/about-the-program-2/ (accessed January 25, 2017).

63. Unique, http://www.rarechromo.org/html/home.asp (accessed January 25, 2017). Most of the photographs on the Unique site were taken by parents, not by professionals, and therefore are often less stylized than the ones seen on the Positive Exposure site.

64. David Wright, *Downs: The History of a Disability* (New York: Oxford University Press, 2011).

65. On problems with presenting Down syndrome children as invariably "cute," see, for example, David M. Perry, "Down Syndrome Isn't Just Cute: How the Down Community Sugarcoats Difficult Realities about the Condition," *Aljazeera America*, October 15, 2014, http://america.aljazeera.com/opinions/2014/10/down-s-behind-thesmiles.html.

Perry, the father of a child with Down syndrome, criticized the "inspiration porn" literature, which masks difficulties faced by parents of disabled children. In a debate that followed this article, parents expressed opinions such as "Yes, my son is cute, [but] he also has health issues, autism, is nonverbal, and will always be dependent on myself, and one day his brothers, for his care"; or "Disabilities certainly are painful, the experience is complex, and those who do not have that experience should be informed that individuals with it need empowerment, not supporters armed with cute images." Parents also expressed their love for and attachment to their disabled children, and talked about the multiple ways these children enrich their lives.

66. Jackson, "Images of Deviance," 319.

67. On the history of Down syndrome, see Peter Volpe, "Is Down Syndrome a Modern Disease?," *Perspectives in Biology and Medicine* 29, no. 3 (1986): 423–36; Wright, *Downs*.

68. Francis Graham Crookshank, *The Mongol in Our Midst: A Study of Man and His Three Faces* (London: Kegan Paul, 1924); the second, enlarged edition was published in 1935. For more on Crookshank's view, see Lilian Serife Zihni, "The History of the Relationship between the Concept and Treatment of People with Down's Syndrome in Britain and America, from 1866 to 1967" (PhD diss., University of London, 1989).

69. For example, E. B. Sherlock explained that one of the prominent varieties of the feeble-minded is the mongolian, kalmuc, or tartar type but immediately added that the resemblance to any of the Chinese types of physiognomy is largely fanciful. E. B. Sherlock, *The Feeble-Minded: A Guide to Study and Practice* (London: Macmillan, 1911), 208–11. Kate Brousseau stressed that "mongolism" is present among the Chinese and the Japanese, and people with this condition look very different from their parents and siblings. Kate Brousseau, *Mongolism: A Study of the Physical and Mental Characteristics of Mongolian Imbeciles* (London: Baillière, Tindal and Cox, 1928), 14. In 1930, geneticist Lionel Penrose disproved the "mongolian" hypothesis through the study of blood types. He showed that people with this condition have the same distribution of blood types as the general population from which they are issued. Lionel Sharples Penrose, "The Blood Grouping of Mongolian Imbeciles," *The Lancet* 219, no. 5660 (1932): 394–95. Crookshank acknowledged that specialists rejected his explanation. Crookshank, *The Mongol in Our Midst*, 31.

70. Sherlock, *The Feeble-Minded*, 208–11.

71. Tredgold, *Mental Deficiency (Amentia)* (1908), 189. The term *idiots* described individuals with severe mental impairment.

72. Henry Herd, *The Diagnosis of Mental Deficiency* (London: Hodder and Stoughton, 1930). After the introduction of the Stanford-Binet Intelligence Scales, *idiots* were usually defined as having a mental age of 3 years or less, *imbeciles* as having a mental age of between 3 and 7 years, and *morons* as having a mental age of between 7 and 11 years. Canadian National Committee for Mental Hygiene poster depicting "Types of Mental Deficiency, including Mongolism," ca. 1920, reproduced in Wright, *Downs*, 102.

73. Cunnane, "The Mentally Defective Child," 34. In the 1930s, colleges did not have programs to support students with intellectual impairments; it is possible that the diagnosis of Down syndrome in these cases was inaccurate, or that these pupils had "mosaic Down syndrome" and minor intellectual impairment.

74. Brousseau, *Mongolism*, 43–44.

75. G. A. Sutherland, "The Differential Diagnosis of Mongolism and Cretinism," *The Lancet* 155, no. 3984 (1900): 23–24.

76. J. M. Berg, "Lionel Sharples Penrose (1898–1972): Aspects of the Man and His Works, with Particular Reference to His Undertakings in the Fields of Intellectual Disability and Mental Disorder," *Journal of Intellectual Disability Research* 42, no. 2 (1998): 104–11. On the history of medical genetics in the interwar era and the role of the Colchester Survey, see Jean-Paul Gaudillière and Ilana Löwy, "The Hereditary Transmission of Human Pathologies between 1900 and 1940: The Good Reasons Not to Become 'Mendelian,'" in *Heredity Explored: Between Public Domain and Experimental Science, 1850–1930*, ed. Staffan Müller-Wille and Christina Brandt (Cambridge, MA: MIT Press, 2016), 331–36.

77. Penrose, *The Biology of Mental Defect.*

78. Lionel Penrose, *A Clinical and Genetic Study of 1,280 Cases of Mental Defects* (London: Special Report Series, Medical Research Council, no. 229, 1938). Materials on the Colchester Survey can be found in Penrose's papers, UCL archives, File 59-2.

79. Siegried Centerwall and Willard Centerwall, "The Discovery of Phenylketonuria: The Story of a Young Couple, Two Retarded Children, and a Scientist," *Pediatrics* 105, no. 1 (2000): 89–103.

80. This was the first formal proof that PKU is a recessive disorder that runs in families. Lionel Penrose, "Two Cases of Phenylpyruvic Amentia," *The Lancet* 225, no. 5810 (1935): 23–25; Lionel Penrose, "Inheritance of Phenylpyruvic Amentia (Phenylketonuria)," *The Lancet* 226, no. 5839 (1935): 192–94.

81. Lionel S. Penrose, "Phenylketonuria: A Problem in Eugenics," *The Lancet* 247, no. 6409 (1946): 949–53; Diane Paul and Jeffrey Brosco, *The PKU Paradox: A Short History of a Genetic Disease* (Baltimore: Johns Hopkins University Press, 2013), 17–20.

82. Peter Coventry, "The Dynamics of Medical Genetics: The Development and Articulation of Clinical and Technical Services under the NHS, Especially at Manchester, c. 1945–1979" (PhD diss., University of Manchester, 2000), chapter 5.2.2. In the 1950s, even strong supporters of eugenics, such as London geneticist Cedric Carter, believed that common mental deficiency syndromes such as "mongolism" reflect complex interactions between genes and environment. The definition of this condition as stemming from a single error of cell division came as a surprise to many specialists. K. Codell Carter, "Early Conjectures That Down Syndrome is Caused by Chromosomal Nondisjunction," *Bulletin of the History of Medicine* 76, no. 3 (2002): 528–63.

83. Today, the rare familiar cases of Down syndrome are explained as inherited translocation on the chromosome 21; this phenomenon was described by Penrose and his colleagues in early 1960. L. S. Penrose, J. R. Ellis, and Joy D. A. Delhanty, "Chromosomal Translocation in Mongolism and in Normal Relatives," *The Lancet* 276, no. 7147 (1960): 409–10; E. Hanhart, Joy D. A. Delhanty, and L. S. Penrose, "Trisomy in Mother and Child, *The Lancet* 277, no. 7173 (1961): 403. The great majority of cases of Down syndrome originate in an error of distribution of chromosomes during the formation of an egg or sperm cell ("nondisjunction") that leads to the presence of two chromosomes 21 in such a cell.

84. Lionel Penrose, "The Relative Effects of Paternal and Maternal Ages in Mongolism," *The Journal of Genetics* 27, no. 2 (1933): 219–24.

85. Lionel Penrose, "Observations on the Etiology of Mongolism," *The Lancet* 267, no. 6836 (1954): 505–509. The hypothesis that "mongolism" is linked with an abnormal number of chromosomes was proposed in the 1930s following the observation that this condition links a great number of traits. It was, however, rejected by most experts, among other things, philosopher of science K. Codell Carter argued, because experts were not aware that experiments with the fruit fly (*Drosophila*) supported this hypothesis. Moreover, before 1956 human chromosomes could not be studied in the laboratory. K. Codell Carter, "Early Conjectures That Down Syndrome Is Caused by Chromosomal Nondisjunction."

86. Clemens Benda, manuscript of a talk on "Medical Aspects of Mental Deficiency: A Clinico-pathological Study Based on 200 Autopsies," presented at a meeting of the North Carolina Neuropsychiatric Society, October 25, 1946. Clemens E. Benda papers, 1895–1975. B MS c97. Boston Medical Library, Francis A. Countway Library of Medicine, Boston (henceforth Benda's Papers), box 4, folder 154.

87. Clemens Benda, "Studies in the Endocrine Pathology of Mongoloid Deficiency," *Proceeding of the American Association on Mental Deficiency* 43, no. 8 (1938): 151–55; Clemens Benda, *Mongolism and Cretinism: A Study of the Clinical Manifestations and the General Pathology of Pituitary and Thyroid Deficiency* (London: William Heinemann, 1947); Clemens Benda, *Mongolism and Cretinism*, second edition, revised (New York: Grune and Stratton, 1949).

88. Benda, *Mongolism and Cretinism* (1949), 288–89. In 1959, when "mongolism" was redefined as "trisomy 21," Penrose immediately and enthusiastically adopted the new view of this condition. Benda acknowledged that a chromosomal anomaly may play a role in the origins of "mongolism," but in the 1960s, he continued to believe that the clinical manifestations of this condition were related to hormonal disequilibrium, and that hormonal treatment improved the physical health of children with this condition. See, for example, a letter from Benda to H. D. Frederiks from the research division of the Oregon State system of higher education, October 18, 1967, on the efficacy of pituitary-thyroid mixture in the treatment of mongoloid children. Benda's Papers, Box 2, folder 65, correspondence 1966–75.

89. Clemens Benda, manuscript of a talk titled "Medical Progress in the Understanding and Treatment of Retarded Children," presented in 1952 at the Convention of National Association for Retarded Children. Benda's Papers, box 4, folder 169.

90. Mendel Schachter, "À propos de la psychologie des parents d'enfants mongoliens," *Proceedings of the London Conference on the Scientific Study of Mental Deficiency*, 2 vols. (Danghem, UK: May and Baker, 1960, 1962), 1:502–507, see esp. 503.

91. Schachter, "À propos de la psychologie des parents d'enfants mongoliens," 2:506. Many French doctors adopted in the 1960s and 1970s a bleak view of "mongolism," which contrasts with earlier views of British and US specialists who brought to the fore the great variability of mental impairment in "mongols" and the progress many can make with appropriate education. For French specialists' views on this condition in the 1960s and 1970s, see Lynda Lotte and Isabelle Ville, "Histoire de la prénatalité et de la prévention des handicaps de la naissance en France," report of the contract ANR 09-SSOC-026, French National Research Agency, 2014.

92. The observation that the number of newborns with fatal inborn malformations did not change much over the past one hundred years despite impressive pro-

gress in the overall reduction of perinatal mortality was employed to support a "gene-tic"/"hereditary" hypothesis of origins of a majority of such malformations. J. W. Pryce, M. A. Weber, M. T. Ashworth, S. E. A. Roberts, M. Malone, and N. J. Sebire, "Changing Patterns of Infant Death over the Last 100 Years: Autopsy Experience from a Specialist Children's Hospital," *Journal of the Royal Society of Medicine* 105, no. 3 (2012): 123–30.

93. Douglas Power Murphy, *Congenital Malformations: A Study of Parental Character-istics with Special Reference to the Reproductive Process* (Philadelphia: University of Penn-sylvania Press, 1940), 83.

94. Douglas Power Murphy, *Congenital Malformations: A Study of Parental Charac-teristics with a Special Reference to the Reproductive Process*, second edition (Philadelphia: J. B. Lippincott, 1947), 106. Murphy argued that women who were accidentally irradiated or infected with the rubella virus early in pregnancy should have the right to legally ter-minate the pregnancy.

95. Ibid., 113.

96. Ibid., 81–83. Murphy makes this rather surprising claim on the basis of personal observations. He does not provide details on conditions included in his definition of "congenital malformation."

97. D. Boyd, ed., *First International Conference on Congenital Malformations, London, 18-22.7.1960* (Philadelphia: J. B. Lippincott, 1961).

98. Josef Warkany, "Environmental Teratogenic Factors," in *First International Con-ference on Congenital Malformation*, 99–105.

99. Lionel Penrose, "Genetic Causes of Malformations and the Search for Their Origins," in *First International Conference on Congenital Malformation*, 294–99.

100. Robert Debré, "Medical Problems, Psychological and Social," in *First Interna-tional Conference on Congenital Malformation*, 300–301.

101. Ibid., 301.

102. Douglas Gairdner, "The Rhesus Story," *British Medical Journal* 2, no. 6192 (1979): 709–11; Doris Zallen, Daphne Christie, and Elisabeth Tansey, eds., *The Rhesus Factor and Disease Prevention*, Wellcome Witnesses to Twentieth Century Medicine (London: The Wellcome Trust, 2004), 3–24; Coventry, "The Dynamics of Medical Genetics," chapter 2.1.

103. Zallen, Christie, and Tansey, eds., *The Rhesus Factor and Disease Prevention*, 15.

104. Margaret Muriel Pickles, *Haemolytic Disease of the Newborn* (Springfield, IL: Thomas, 1949).

105. In the 1980s, the development of drugs that favor the maturation of premature babies' lungs greatly improved the survival of such babies.

106. David Goodner, "Prenatal Genetic Diagnosis: An Historical Perspective," *Clini-cal Obstetrics and Gynecology* 19, no. 4 (1976): 837–40.

107. D. C. Bevis, "Composition of Liquor Amnii in Haemolytic Disease of Newborn," *The Lancet* 2, no. 6631 (1950): 443; D. C. Bevis, "The Antenatal Prediction of Haemolytic Disease of the Newborn," *The Lancet* 1, no. 6704 (1952): 395–98. Bevis, according to Lisle Gadd, his collaborator in Manchester, was a somewhat controversial figure: he did not respect authority and sometimes performed amniocenteses without asking permission either from the woman or from his superiors. Coventry, "The Dynamics of Medical Genetics," chap. 2.

108. Albert William Liley, "The Use of Amniocentesis and Fetal Transfusion in Erythroblastosis Fetalis," *Pediatrics* 35 (1965): 836–47. In 1963, Liley performed the first successful transfusion in the womb of a fetus affected with severe hemolytic disease.

109. A. H. C. Walker, "Liquor Amnii Studies in the Prediction of Haemolytic Disease of the Newborn," *British Medical Journal* 2, no. 5041 (1957): 376–78; A. E. Walker and R. F. Jennison, "Antenatal Prediction of Haemolytic Disease of Newborn: Comparison of Liquor Amnii and Serological Studies," *British Medical Journal* 2, no. 5313 (1962): 1152–56.

110. In the 1970s, hematologists developed a new approach: the treatment of a Rh-negative mother with anti-Rh antibodies immediately after the birth of her first Rh-positive child (and today also during pregnancy). Women were immunized against fetal Rh-positive cells, especially during childbirth. Treatment with anti-Rh antibodies eliminated these cells and prevented anti-Rh immunization, and therefore prevented hemolytic disease of the newborn. Zallen, Christie, and Tansey, eds., *The Rhesus Factor and Disease Prevention*, see esp. table on page 23.

111. A. E. Claireaux, P. G. Cole, and G. H. Lathe, "Icterus of the Brain in the Newborn," *The Lancet* 265, no. 6798 (1953): 1226–30; W. W. Zuelzer, "Neonatal Jaundice and Mental Retardation," *Archives of Neurology* 3, no. 2 (1960): 127–35; W. F. Windle, "Neuropathology of Certain Forms of Mental Retardation," *Science* 140, no. 3572 (1963): 1186–89.

112. In the early 1960s, obstetricians were aware of the risks of amniocentesis and strongly recommended its use only when absolutely necessary. Walker and Jennison, "Antenatal Prediction of Haemolytic Disease of Newborn."

Chapter 2 · Karyotypes

1. The first PubMed article with "prenatal diagnosis" in its title is from 1948. It discusses the use of X-rays to diagnose the absence of a brain in a fetus: "Prenatal Diagnosis of Anencephaly and Report of a Case." In the 1950s, several articles with "prenatal diagnosis" in their titles describe diagnosis of hemolytic disease of the Rh-incompatible fetus.

2. Bettyann Holtzmann Kevles, *Naked to the Bone: Medical Imaging in the Twentieth Century* (New York: Basic Books, 1998), 230.

3. Robert Resta, "The First Prenatal Diagnosis of a Fetal Abnormality," *Journal of Genetic Counseling* 6, no. 1 (1997): 81–84. Resta speaks about *prenatal diagnosis*, while James Thomas Case employed the term *diagnosis before birth*.

4. Ann Oakley, *The Captured Womb: A History of the Medical Care of Pregnant Women* (Oxford: Blackwell, 1984), 95–107.

5. Alice Stewart, Josephine Webb, Dawn Giles, and David Hewitt, "Preliminary Communication: Malignant Disease in Childhood and Diagnostic Irradiation In-Utero," *The Lancet* 268 (1956): 44–46.

6. Murray L. Barr and Ewart G. Bertram, "A Morphological Distinction between Neurons of the Male and the Female, and the Behaviour of the Nuclear Satellite during Accelerated Nucleoprotein Synthesis," *Nature* 163 (1949): 676–77. For more on Barr's studies, see Fiona A. Miller, "A Blueprint for Defining Health: Making Medical Genetics in Canada" (PhD diss., York University, Toronto, 2000); Fiona Alice Miller, " 'Your True and Proper Gender': The Barr Body as a Good Enough Science of Sex," *Studies in History and Philosophy of Biological and Biomedical Sciences* 37, no. 3 (2006): 459–83.

7. Fritz Fuchs and Povl Riis, "Antenatal Sex Determination," *Nature* 177, no. 4503 (1956): 330; Leo Sachs, David Serr, and Mathilde Danon, "Analysis of Amniotic Fluid for Diagnosis of Fetal Sex," *British Medical Journal* 2, no. 4996 (1956): 795–98; David Serr, Leo Sachs, and Mathilda Danon, "The Diagnosis of Fetal Sex during Pregnancy," *Surgery, Gynecology and Obstetrics* 104, no. 2 (1957): 157–62.

8. If a mother is a carrier of an X-linked disease, half the girls born to the couple will be carriers and half the boys will have the disease. If the father has an X-linked disease, all the girls will be carriers and all the boys will be healthy. In the rare cases in which the father has an X-linked condition and the mother is a carrier of the same condition, half the boys and half the girls will have the disease, and the other half of the girls will be carriers.

9. In 1960, scientists knew how to stain and count human chromosomes but did not have a reliable method to cultivate fetal cells in a test tube, an indispensable step in the visualization of human chromosomes in these cells. Barr bodies are visible following a simple staining of fetal cells on a slide.

10. It is not excluded that the Israeli group that demonstrated the feasibility of prenatal diagnosis of fetal sex at the same time as Riis and Fuchs also used this technique to diagnose the sex of fetuses of women carriers of an X-linked condition. Danon and Sachs explained in 1957 that "applied to fetal cells in amniotic fluid from pregnant women heterozygous for a sex-linked hereditary disease, the test indicates the sex of the fetus and thus whether the child will be free from the hereditary abnormality or has a one-in-two chance of manifesting it." Mathilde Danon and Leo Sachs, "Sex Chromosomes and Human Sexual Development," *The Lancet* 273, no. 6984 (1957): 20–25, see esp. 20. In the 1950s, abortion was illegal in Israel but was tolerated in practice, especially when doctors deemed it necessary for medical reasons. Israeli doctors might have aborted male fetuses of carriers of an X-linked disease, but, unlike their Danish colleagues, they could not openly admit that they did it.

11. Ruth Schwartz Cowan, *Heredity and Hope: The Case for Genetic Screening* (Cambridge, MA: Harvard University Press, 2008), 91–95.

12. Povl Riis and Fritz Fuchs, "Antenatal Determination of Fetal Sex: In Prevention of Hereditary Diseases," *The Lancet* 276, no. 7143 (1960): 180–82.

13. Fritz Fuchs, "Comment," in *Early Diagnosis of Human Genetic Defects: Scientific and Ethical Considerations*, ed. Maureen Harris (Bethesda, MD: National Institutes of Health, 1971), 143.

14. Ibid., 141–45.

15. Riis and Fuchs, "Antenatal Determination of Fetal Sex."

16. Diane B. Paul, *Controlling Human Heredity, 1885 to the Present* (Amherst, NY: Humanity Books, 1995), 114–35.

17. Joe Hin Tjio and Albert Levan, "The Chromosome Number of Man," *Hereditas* 42, no. 1–2 (1956): 1–6.

18. On the history of early studies of human chromosomes, see Peter S. Harper, "The Discovery of the Human Chromosome Number in Lund, 1955–1956," *Human Genetics* 119, no. 1 (2006): 226-32; María Jesús Santesmases, "Samples, Cultures and Plates: Early Human Chromosomes," in *Microscope Slides: Reassessing a Neglected Historical Resource*, ed. Ilana Löwy (Berlin: Max Planck Institute for the History of Science, 2011), 25–34; Soraya de Chadarevian, "Chromosome Photography and the Human Karyotype," *Historical Studies in the Natural Sciences* 45, no. 1 (2014): 115–46.

19. Aryn Martin, "Can't Any Body Count? Counting as an Epistemic Theme in the History of Human Chromosomes," *Social Studies of Science* 34, no. 6 (2004): 923–48.

20. Soraya de Chadarevian, "Putting Human Genetics on a Solid Basis: Chromosome Research, 1950s–1970s," in *Human Heredity in the Twentieth Century*, ed. Bernd Gausemeier, Staffan Müller-Wille, and Edmund Ramsden (London: Pickering and Chatto, 2014), 141–52.

21. Simone Gigenkrantz and E. M. Rivera, "The History of Cytogenetics: Portraits of Some Pioneers," *Annales de Génétique* 46, no. 4 (2003): 433–42; Marthe Gautier and Peter S. Harper, "Fiftieth Anniversary of Trisomy 21: Returning to a Discovery," *Human Genetics* 126 (2009): 317–24; Peter S. Harper, *First Years of Human Chromosomes: The Beginnings of Human Cytogenetics* (Bloxham: Scion, 2006).

22. Harper, *First Years of Human Chromosomes*.

23. J. H. Edwards, D. G. Harnden, A. H. Cameron, V. M. Crosse, and O. H. Wolff, "A New Trisomic Syndrome," *The Lancet* 1, no. 7128 (1960): 787–90; K. Patau, D. Smith, E. Therman, S. Inhorn, and H. P. Wagner, "Multiple Congenital Anomaly Caused by an Extra Autosome," *The Lancet* 1, no. 7128 (1960): 790–93. The two articles were published together.

24. Daphne Christie and Doris Zallen, eds., *Genetic Testing*, Witness Seminar in Twentieth-Century Medicine (London: Wellcome Trust, 2002); Harper, *First Year of Human Chromosomes*; Susan Lindee, *Moments of Truth in Genetic Medicine* (Baltimore: Johns Hopkins University Press, 2005); Nathaniel Comfort, *The Science of Human Perfection: How Genes Became the Heart of American Medicine* (New Haven, CT: Yale University Press, 2012).

25. F. Clarke Fraser, "Of Mice and Children: Reminiscences of a Teratogeneticist," *American Journal of Medical Genetics* 146A (2008): 2179–202, see esp. 2188 (emphasis original). Fraser added: "In fact, there was something of an overreaction; genetics was regarded by some as synonymous with cytogenetics, genetic diseases with chromosomal diseases." Ibid.

26. Quoted in Christie and Zallen, eds., *Genetic Testing*, 7.

27. Howard W. Jones and William Wallace Scott, *Hermaphroditism, Genital Anomalies and Related Endocrine Disorders*, second edition (Baltimore: Williams and Wilkins Company, 1971), vii.

28. Jérôme Lejeune, "Le mongolisme, maladie chromosomique," *La Nature* 3296 (1959): 521–23.

29. M. Susan Lindee, "Genetic Disease in the 1960s: A Structural Revolution," *American Journal of Medical Genetics* 115, no. 2 (2002): 75–82.

30. See, for example, P. A. Jacobs, D. G. Harnden, W. M. Court Brown, et al., "Abnormalities Involving the X Chromosome in Women," *The Lancet* 1, no. 7136 (1960): 1213–16; Eeva Therman, Klaus Patau, David W. Smith, and Robert I. DeMars, "The D Trisomy Syndrome and XO Gonadal Dysgenesis in Two Sisters," *American Journal of Human Genetics* 13, no. 2 (1961): 193–204.

31. L. S. Penrose, J. R. Ellis, and J. D. Delhanty, "Chromosomal Translocations in Mongolism and in Normal Relatives," *The Lancet* 2, no. 7147 (1960): 409–10; P. E. Polani, J. H. Briggs, C. E. Ford, C. M. Clarke, and J. M. Berg, "A Mongol Girl with 46 Chromosomes," *The Lancet* 1, no. 7127 (1960): 721–24. For an early description of translocation, see María Jesús Santesmases, "Size and the Centromere: Translocations and Visual Cul-

tures in Early Human Genetics," in *Making Mutations: Objects, Practices, Contexts*, ed. Luis Campos and Alexander von Schwerin (Berlin: Max Plank Institute for the History of Science, 2010), 189–208.

32. Equilibrated (Robertsonian) translocation is a reciprocal exchange of genetic material between two chromosomes. Its frequency in humans is estimated at 1:1,000. In "hereditary Down syndrome," the Robertsonian translocation is frequently a fusion of a long arm of chromosome 21 with a long arm of chromosome 14 or 15. Geneticists estimate that a couple with a balanced translocation who already has one Down syndrome child has a 15% chance of having another child with this condition.

33. David Smith, Klaus Patau, Eeva Therman, and Stanley L. Inhorn, "A New Autosomal Trisomy: Two Cases of Multiple Congenital Anomaly Caused by an Extra Chromosome," *Journal of Pediatrics* 57, no. 3 (1960): 338–345; David Smith, Klaus Patau, Eeva Therman, Stanley L. Inhorn, and Robert I. DeMars, "The D1 Trisomy Syndrome," *Journal of Pediatrics* 62, no. 3 (1963): 326–41.

34. Denver Study Group, "A Proposed Standard System of Nomenclature of Human Mitotic Chromosomes," *The Lancet* 275, no. 7133 (1960): 1063–65.

35. Andrew Hogan, "The 'Morbid Anatomy' of the Human Genome: Tracing the Observational and Representational Approaches of Postwar Genetics and Biomedicine," *Medical History* 58, no. 3 (2014): 315–36, see esp. 321. Andrew J. Hogan, *Life Histories of Genetic Disease: Patterns and Prevention in Postwar Medical Genetics* (Baltimore: Johns Hopkins University Press, 2016). In the late 1960s, an important technical innovation, the introduction of new staining methods of chromosomes, fluorescent Quinacrine (Q) banding in 1968, and later Giemsa (G) banding and reverse (R) banding, produced unique banding effects on each chromosome. It then became possible to differentiate similarly shaped chromosomes and better identify chromosomal anomalies, such as deletion or duplication of specific segments. Ibid., 322–23.

36. Triplication of other autosomal chromosomes is lethal, as is triploidy—the triplication of all chromosomes.

37. Patau, Smith, Therman, Inhorn, and Wagner, "Multiple Congenital Anomaly Caused by an Extra Autosome"; David Smith, Klaus Patau, Eeva Therman, and Stanley Inhorn, "A New Autosomal Trisomy Syndrome: Multiple Congenital Anomalies Caused by an Extra Chromosome," *Journal of Pediatrics* 57, no. 3 (1960): 338–45. In 1961, Klaus and his colleagues consolidated their findings through the description of two additional cases. Klaus Patau, Eeva Therman, David Smith, and Stanley Inhorn, "Two New Cases of D1 Trisomy in Man," *Hereditas* 47, no. 2 (1961): 239–42.

38. When no genetic material is lost, people with an equilibrated Robertsonian translocation do not suffer ill effects, but they do have an increased risk of producing offspring with genetic anomalies, because some gametes may receive an abnormal set of chromosomes during the production of sperm and egg cells.

39. Klaus Patau to Irène Uchida, July 5, 1960, Patau's papers, University of Wisconsin, Madison (henceforth, Patau's papers). I'm grateful to Diane Paul for her invaluable help in obtaining copies of Patau's correspondence. Uchida worked at the Children's Hospital of Winnipeg in Canada. In 1965, Patau mentioned the collection of data for a "trisomy index" he was constructing. Patau to Uchida, April 5, 1965, Patau's papers.

40. Uchida to Patau, August 5, 1960; Patau to Uchida, August 10, 1960, Patau's papers.

41. Patau to Uchida, November 22, 1960, Patau's papers.

42. Patau to Uchida, December 14, 1960, Patau's papers. Before the development of banding, even highly experimented cytogeneticists were not always sure what chromosome they were observing because many chromosomes look alike. It was especially difficult to differentiate chromosomes within each group. Group D included chromosomes 13 to 15, group E included chromosomes 16 to 18, and group G included chromosomes 21, 22, and Y. In the 1960s, the standard method of studying chromosomes was to prepare a microscope to view all the chromosomes, photograph the chromosomes, cut the photograph, rearrange the chromosomes in couples, and count them. The classification of chromosomes relied on the training of the observer's eye. De Chadarevian, "Chromosome Photography and the Human Karyotype." On the role of training the scientist's eye, see Lorraine J. Daston and Peter Galison, *Objectivity* (New York: Zone Books, 2007).

43. Uchida to Patau, undated (probably winter 1960), Patau's papers.

44. Uchida to Jim Miller, December 6, 1961, Patau's papers. Later geneticists agreed that trisomy 13 always produces severe anomalies and is usually incompatible with survival.

45. Patau to Uchida, February 6, 1961, Patau's papers.

46. Patau to Uchida, April 5, 1965, Patau's papers.

47. Patau to Uchida, April 20, 1960, Patau's papers.

48. Patau to Penrose, November 20, 1961; Penrose to Patau, November 29, 1961, Patau's papers.

49. Penrose to Patau, December 6, 1961, Patau's papers.

50. Lionel Penrose's papers, UCL Archives, file 62/5.

51. C. E. Ford, K. W. Jones, O. J. Miller, U. Mittwoch, L. S. Penrose, M. Ridler, and A. Shapiro, "The Chromosomes in a Patient Showing Both Mongolism and the Klinefelter Syndrome," *The Lancet* 1, no. 7075 (1959): 709–10.

52. Renata Laxova, "Lionel Sharples Penrose, 1898–1972: A Personal Memoir in Celebration of the Centenary of his Birth," *Genetics* 150, no. 4 (1998): 1333–40, see esp. 1340.

53. Fiona Alice Miller, "Dermatoglyphics and the Persistence of 'Mongolism': Networks of Technology, Disease and Discipline," *Social Studies of Science* 33, no. 1 (2003): 75–94. In 1961, *The Lancet* published a call, signed by numerous eminent scientists, to eliminate the term *mongolism*. G. Allen, C. E. Benda, J. A. Böök, C. O. Carter, C. E. Ford, E. H. Y. Chu, et al., "Mongolism," *The Lancet* 277, no. 7180 (1961): 775. Despite this call, the term was still employed in the 1960s and 1970s.

54. On the history of fingerprints, see Simon Cole, *Suspect Identities: A History of Fingerprinting and Criminal Identification* (Cambridge, MA: Harvard University Press, 2001); Chandak Sengoopta, *Imprint of the Raj: How Fingerprinting Was Born in Colonial India* (London: Macmillan, 2003).

55. Kristine Bonnevie, "Studies on Papillary Patterns of Human Fingers," *Journal of Genetics* 15, no. 1 (1924): 1–111.

56. Harold Cummins and Charles Midlo, "Palmar and Plantar Epidermal Ridge Configurations (Dermatoglyphics) in European-Americans," *American Journal of Physical Anthropology* 9, no. 4 (1926): 471–502; Wladimir Wertelecky and Chris Plato, "Preface," in *Dermatoglyphics—Fifty Years Later*, ed. Wladimir Wertelecky and Chris Plato, Birth Defects, Original Articles Series, XV, no. 6 (1979): xxi–xxii.

57. Cummins and Midlo's book on methods to study dermatoglyphs became a reference tool for researchers in this domain. Harold Cummins and Charles Midlo, *Finger Prints, Palms and Soles: An Introduction to Dermatoglyphics* (Philadelphia: Blakiston, 1943).

58. David Rife, "Dr. Harold Cummins and Dermatoglyphics," in *Dermatoglyphics— Fifty Years Later*, 1–4; George Widney, "Harold Cummins: Memories of People Who Knew Him," in *Dermatoglyphics—Fifty Years Later*, 5–9.

59. Harold Cummins, "Dermatoglyphic Stigmata in Mongoloid Imbeciles," *The Anatomical Record* 73, no. 4 (1939): 407–15.

60. Raymond Turpin and Jérôme Lejeune, "Etude dermatoglyphique de la paume des mongoliens et de leur parents et germains," *Semaine des Hopitaux de Paris* 176, no. 76 (1953): 3904–10; Raymond Turpin and Jérôme Lejeune, "Analogies entre les types dermatoglyphiques palmaires des simiens inferieurs et des enfants atteints de mongolisme," *Comptes Rendus de l'Académie des Sciences* 238, no. 13 (1954): 397; Raymond Turpin and Jérôme Lejeune, "Etude comparé des dermatoglyphes de la partie distale de la paume de la main chez l'homme normal, les enfants mongoliens et les simiens inferieurs," *Comptes Rendus de l'Académie des Sciences, Paris* 238, no. 3 (1954): 1149–50.

61. Irène A. Uchida, Klaus Patau, and David W. Smith, "Dermal Patterns of 18 and D1 Trisomics," *American Journal of Human Genetics* 14, no. 4 (1962): 345–52, see esp. 345. Later, Uchida and her collaborators showed a unique dermatoglyphic pattern in an individual with two X and two Y chromosomes (48, XXYY); Irène A. Uchida, James R. Miller, and Hubert C. Soltan, "Dermatoglyphics Associated with the XXYY Chromosome Complement," *American Journal of Human Genetics* 16, no. 3 (1964): 284–91.

62. Patau to Uchida, August 10, 1960; Patau to Uchida, September 14, 1960, Patau's papers. Patau encouraged Uchida to prepare a separate publication on dermal patterns of two cases of trisomy they had studied.

63. Uchida to Patau, April 22, 1962, Patau's papers.

64. Uchida to Patau, March 25, 1962, Patau's papers.

65. Uchida saw Lionel Penrose as a potential competitor. She wrote to Patau after a human genetics meeting at The Hague, expressing that she was worried that "Penrose and Holt might have beaten us to the punch at The Hague, but Jim Miller tells me that their papers didn't amount to much and all the other papers on dermatoglyphics were 'appalling.'" Uchida to Patau, October 16, 1963, Patau's papers.

66. Lionel Penrose, "The Creases on the Minimal Digit in Mongolism," *The Lancet* 218, no. 5637 (1931): 585–86; Lionel S. Penrose, "Familial Studies on Palmar Patterns in Relation to Mongolism," *Hereditas* 35, no. S1 (1949): 412–16; Lionel Penrose, "The Distal Triradius *t* on the Hands of Parents and Sibs of Mongol Imbeciles," *Annals of Human Genetics* 19, no. 1 (1954): 10–38.

67. Notebooks and materials on dermatoglyphs, 1960s and early 1970s. Lionel S. Penrose papers, UCL archive, files 94/1, 94/2, 94/3.

68. Penrose to Patau, November 29, 1961, Patau's papers.

69. Lionel Penrose, "Finger-Prints, Palms and Chromosomes," *Nature* 197 (1963): 933–38.

70. Ibid.

71. Lionel Penrose, "Finger-Print Pattern and the Sex Chromosomes," *The Lancet* 289, no. 7485 (1967): 298–300. Today, researchers discuss epigenetic modifications of hereditary traits.

72. John J. Mulvihill and David W. Smith, "The Genesis of Dermatoglyphics," *Journal of Pediatrics* 75, no. 4 (1969): 579–89; Georgy Popich and David Smith, "The Genesis and Significance of Digital and Palmar Hand Creases: Preliminary Report," *Journal of Pediatrics* 77, no. 6 (1970): 1017–23.

73. Fetal medicine experts who observe malformed hands usually attempt to assess whether the cause is mechanic (e.g., amniotic bands) or genetic.

74. See, for example, Harold Cummins to Penrose, August 8, 1966; Sarah Holt to Penrose, June 27, 1966, Penrose papers, UCL archive, file 94/3.

75. Wertelecky and Plato, "Preface," xxii.

76. Patau to Sheldon Reed, March 6, 1962, Patau's papers.

77. M. W. Steele and W. R. Breg, "Chromosome Analysis of Human Amniotic Fluid Cells," *The Lancet* 1, no. 7434 (1966): 383–385. On the early history of amniocentesis, see Cowan, *Heredity and Hope*, 71–116.

78. Henry Nadler, "Antenatal Detection of Hereditary Disorders," *Pediatrics* 42, no. 6 (1968): 912–18; Henry Nadler, "Prenatal Detection of Genetic Defects," *Journal of Pediatrics* 74, no. 1 (1969): 132–43; Eugene Hoyme, "Comment on Henry Nadler's 'Antenatal Detection of Hereditary Disorders,' " *Pediatrics* 20(suppl.) (1998): 247–48.

79. A. Milunsky, J. W. Littlefields, J. N. Kanner, E. H. Kolodny, V. E. Shich, and L. Atkins, "Prenatal Genetic Diagnosis," *New England Journal of Medicine* 283 (1970): part I, 1370–76; part II, 1441–48; part III, 1498–1505; Ronald Davidson and Mario C. Rattazzi, "Review: Prenatal Diagnosis of Genetic Disorders," *Clinical Chemistry* 18, no. 3 (1972): 179–87; David J. Brock, "Biochemical Studies on Amniotic Fluid Cells," in *Antenatal Diagnosis of Genetic Disease*, ed. A. E. H. Emery (Edinburgh: Churchill Livingstone, 1973), 82–112.

80. Christie and Zallen, *Genetic Testing*, 43–45.

81. C. H. Rodeck and S. Campbell, "Sampling Pure Fetal Blood by Fetoscopy in Second Trimester of Pregnancy," *British Medical Journal* 2, no. 6139 (1978): 728–30.

82. S. Gilgenkrantz and E. M. Rivera, "The History of Cytogenetics: Portraits of Some Pioneers," *Annales de Génétique* 46, no. 4 (2003): 433–42; Peter Harper, interview with André and Joëlle Boué, April 22, 2005, *Genetics and Medicine Historical Network*, https://genmedhist.eshg.org/fileadmin/content/website-layout/interviewees-attachments/Boue%20A%26J.pdf; "Witness Seminar: Histoire du DPN en France," http://anr-dpn.vjf.cnrs.fr/?q.node/62.

83. Abigail Lippman Hand and Clarke Fraser, "Genetic Counseling—the Post Counseling Period: II. Making Reproductive Choices," *American Journal of Medical Genetics* 4, no. 1 (1979): 73–87; Ruth Faden, Judith Chwalow, Kimberly Quaid, et al., "Prenatal Screening and Pregnant Women's Attitude towards the Abortion of Defective Fetuses," *American Journal of Public Health* 77, no. 3 (1987): 288–90; P. Donnai, N. Charles, and R. Harris, "Attitudes of Patients after 'Genetic' Termination of Pregnancy," *British Medical Journal* 282 (1981): 621–23.

84. Malcolm Ferguson-Smith, "Address at the Service of Thanksgiving for the Life of John Hilton Edwards," Oxford, England, April 19, 2008. Papers of Malcom Ferguson Smith, http://catalogue.wellcomelibrary.org/record=b2002902.

85. For example, in northern France, the gynecology service of Jean-Pierre Farriaux started to propose amniocentesis to older pregnant women who were treated in that service in the mid-1970s. J.-P. Farriaux, M. F. Peyrat, and M. Delacour, "Le diagnostique

prénatal précoce: La situation dans le Nord-Pas de Calais," *NPN Médecine* 5 (1985): 842–45.

86. J. Bang and A. Northeved, "A New Ultrasonic Method for Transabdominal Amniocentesis," *American Journal of Obstetrics and Gynecology* 114 (1972): 599–601.

87. M. A. Ferguson-Smith and M. E. Ferguson-Smith, "Screening for Fetal Chromosome Aberrations in Early Pregnancy," *Journal of Clinical Pathology* 29, suppl. 10 (1976): 165–76; Tabitha M. Powledge, "Prenatal Diagnosis: New Techniques, New Questions," *The Hastings Center Report* 9 (1979): 16–17. Powledge reports that amniocentesis expanded exponentially in the late 1970s and early 1980s. In 1979, professionals estimated that of the forty thousand amniocenteses performed in the United States from 1969 onward, fifteen thousand were performed in 1978.

88. See, for example, Ernest B. Hook, Philip K. Cross, Laird Jackson, Eugene Pergament, and Bruno Brambati, "Maternal Age-Specific Rates of 47, 21 and Other Cytogenetic Abnormalities Diagnosed in the First Trimester of Pregnancy in Chorionic Villus Biopsy Specimens: Comparison with Rates Expected from Observations at Amniocentesis," *American Journal of Human Genetics* 42 (1988): 797–807.

89. The sequential representation—first the introduction of tests for hereditary conditions, then amniocentesis for maternal age—is schematic. In some laboratories, diagnosis of hereditary conditions was introduced at the same time as the testing for aneuploidies. However, the initial goal of researchers who developed prenatal diagnosis was often the diagnosis of hereditary conditions. The less intellectually challenging diagnosis of Down syndrome interested gynecologists for the most part. Peter Harper, interview with Bernadette Modell, December 15, 2007, *Genetics and Medicine Historical Network*, https:// genmedhist.eshg.org/fileadmin/content/website-layout/interviewees-attachments /Modell%2C%20Bernadette.pdf.

90. Editorial, "Who's for Amniocentesis?," *The Lancet* 309 (1977): 986–87.

91. Joyce Bermel, "Update on Genetic Screening: Views on Early Diagnosis," *The Hastings Center Report* 13 (1983): 4.

92. See, for example, the November 1973 declaration of Keith Russell, president of the American College of Obstetricians and Gynecologists, quoted in Tabitha M. Powledge and Sharmon Sollitto, "Prenatal Diagnosis: The Past and the Future," *The Hastings Center Report* 4 (1974): 11–13, see esp. 13.

93. Powledge, "Prenatal Diagnosis."

94. US Department of Health, Education, and Welfare, *Antenatal Diagnosis*, NIH publication 79-1973 (Bethesda, MD: National Institutes of Health, 1979), 1–59.

95. Henry Nadler and Albert Gerbie, "Role of Amniocentesis in the Intra-uterine Diagnosis of Genetic Disorders," *New England Journal of Medicine* 282 (1970): 596–98. This study was based on the analysis of 162 procedures. The same year Nadler reported that in an enlarged series of 310 amniocenteses, they observed one spontaneous abortion and one neonatal death: the latter was probably not related to the invasive test. Henry Nadler, "Risks in Amniocentesis," in *Early Diagnosis of Human Genetic Defects: Scientific and Ethical Considerations*, ed. Maureen Harris (Bethesda, MD: National Institutes of Health, 1970), 129–37; discussion following Nadler's paper, ibid., 139–44.

96. James Neel, "Ethical Issues Resulting from Prenatal Diagnosis," in *Early Diagnosis of Human Genetic Defects*, 219–29, see esp. 223.

97. In the early 1970s, amniocentesis was conducted without ultrasound guidance; gynecologists who performed this test feared that they would harm the fetus with the sampling needle.

98. H. H. Allen, F. Sergovich, E. M. Stuart, J. Pozsonyi, and B. Murray, "Infants Undergoing Prenatal Diagnosis: A Preliminary Report," *American Journal of Obstetrics and Gynecology* 118 (1974): 310–13.

99. MacIntyre, "Discussion Following Nadler's 'Risks in Amniocentesis,'" in *Early Diagnosis of Human Genetic Defects*, 143.

100. Allan Barnes, "Fetal Indications for Therapeutic Abortion," *Annual Review of Medicine* 22 (1974): 133–44, see esp. 143. James Neel raised very early on the question of amniocentesis as generating a new kind of uncertainty: diagnosis of a condition that has a probability, but not certainty, of an undesirable outcome. Neel, "Ethical Issues Resulting from Prenatal Diagnosis," 224.

101. "Discussion Following Nadler's 'Risks in Amniocentesis,'" 139–48, see esp. 144. Such explicit endorsement of abortion for Down syndrome was rarely expressed later; it was voiced, however, in 2014 by biologist Richard Dawkins. Richard Dawkins, "'Immoral' Not to Abort if Foetus Has Down's Syndrome," *The Guardian*, August 21, 2014, https://www.theguardian.com/science/2014/aug/21/richard-dawkins-immoral-not-to-abort-a-downs-syndrome-foetus.

102. Barbara Culliton, "Amniocentesis: HEW Backs Tests for Prenatal Diagnosis of Disease," *Science* 190 (1975): 537–39. The press conference that announced that amniocentesis is safe was held at the National Institutes of Health on October 20, 1975. HEW is the United States Department of Health, Education, and Welfare (renamed the United States Department of Health and Human Services in 1979).

103. A. C. Turnbull, D. V. I. Fairweather, B. M. Hibbard, et al., "An Assessment of the Hazards of Amniocentesis: Report to the Medical Research Council by their Working Party on Amniocentesis," *British Journal of Obstetrics and Gynecology* 85, suppl. 2 (1978), see esp. 34–36.

104. Theodore Cooper, "Implication of the Amniocentesis Registry Findings," press summary, Public Health Service and National Institutes of Health, Bethesda, MD, October 20, 1975. Cooper presented this text at the conclusion of four years of study conducted by the Department of Health, Education, and Welfare on the safety of amniocentesis. The report on amniocentesis was sponsored by the National Institutes of Health and National Institute of Child Health and Human Development. Culliton, "Amniocentesis."

105. J. M. Old, R. H. Ward, M. Petrou, M. Karagözlu, B. Modell, and D. Weatherall, "First-Trimester Fetal Diagnosis for Haemoglobinopathies: Three Cases," *The Lancet* 2, no. 8313 (1982): 1413–16; Christie and Zallen, *Genetic Testing*, testimony of Bernadette Modell, 43–45.

106. Z. Kazy, I. Rozovsky, and V. A. Bakharev, "Chorion Biopsy in Early Pregnancy: A Method of Early Prenatal Diagnosis for Inherited Disorders," *Prenatal Diagnosis* 2, no. 1 (1982): 39–45; Christie and Zallen, eds., *Genetic Testing*, 47–48.

107. Andrew Hogan, "Set Adrift in the Prenatal Diagnostic Marketplace: Analyzing the Role of Users and Mediators in the History of a Medical Technology," *Technology and Culture* 54, no. 1 (2013): 62–89.

108. Jérôme Lejeune, "La mongolie, trisomie dégressive" (thèse d'agrégation de médecine, Medical Faculty, Paris University, 1960). The president of the jury was geneticist

Boris Ephrusi and the examiners were Dr. L'Héritier and Dr. Lamotte. The thesis presents the study of chromosomes of people with mongolism as performed exclusively by Lejeune, who successfully confirmed his initial hypothesis that "mongolism" is a chromosomal disorder. The thesis mentions Marthe Gautier's contribution to this study in only one sentence. The omission of Gautier's work may support her claim that she was strongly encouraged to leave Turpin's laboratory in order to favor Lejeune's career and secure his place as Turpin's heir. Gautier and Harper, "Fiftieth Anniversary of Trisomy 21: Returning to a Discovery." In 1960, by unwritten rules, a woman could not become a full professor in a French medical school.

109. Lejeune, "La mongolie, trisomie dégressive," 30–31.

110. Diane Paul and Jeffrey Brosco, *The PKU Paradox: A Short History of a Genetic Disease* (Baltimore: Johns Hopkins University Press, 2013).

111. Inaugural lecture of "genetics in medicine" delivered by professor Alan Emery, University of Edinburgh, April 29, 1968. Materials on genetics and medicine from the 1960s, 1970s, and 1980s focused on the introduction of clinical genetics in Britain related to the preparation of the Wellcome Witness Seminar, Wellcome Archives of Modern Medicine, File GC/255/A/39/9.

112. A cure for PKU was also an argument often employed by opponents of abortion for fetal indication. Thus, Jérôme Lejeune explained that "not so long ago physicians could have proposed to eliminate all the people with phenylketonuria. . . . This shows the absurdity of the logic that pretends to attribute the right to live according to the curability of a given condition, and therefore pretends to fight against disease by eliminating the sick." Jérôme Lejeune, ed., "Histoire naturelle des hommes," in *Au commencement, la vie, conferences inédites* (Paris: MAME, 2014), 31–50, see esp. 48.

113. Philip Reilly, "Genetic Screening Legislation," *Advances in Human Genetics* 5 (1975): 319–76; Paul and Brosco, *The PKU Paradox*.

114. Jeffrey Brosco and Diane Paul, "The Political History of PKU: Reflections on 50 Years of Newborn Screening," *Pediatrics* 132 (2013): 987–89, see esp. 988.

115. Kathryn DeRoche and Marilyn Welsh, "Twenty-Five Years of Research on Neurocognitive Outcomes in Early-Treated Phenylketonuria: Intelligence and Executive Function," *Developmental Neuropsychology* 33 (2008): 474–504; Simona Cappelletti, Giovanna Cotugno, Bianca M. Goffredo, et al., "Cognitive Findings and Behavior in Children and Adolescents with Phenylketonuria," *Journal of Developmental and Behavioral Pediatrics* 34 (2013): 392–98.

116. Barbara Burton and Lauren Leviton, "Reaching Out to the Lost Generation of Adults with Early-Treated Phenylketonuria (PKU)," *Molecular Genetics and Metabolism* 101 (2010): 146–48; Ashley Bone, Angela K. Kuehl, and Andrew F. Angelino, "Review: Neuropsychiatric Perspective of Phenylketonuria: Overview of Phenylketonuria and Its Neuropsychiatric Sequelae," *Psychosomatics* 53 (2012): 517–23.

117. Paul and Brosco, *The PKU Paradox*.

118. Yury Verlinsky, Svetlana Rechitsky, Oleg Verlinsky, Charles Strom, and Anver Kuliev, "Preimplantation Testing for Phenylketonuria," *Fertility and Sterility* 76 (2001): 346–49; Stuart Lavery, Dima Abdo, Mara Kotrotsou, Geoff Trew, Michalis Konstantinidis, and Dagan Wells, "Successful Live Birth Following Preimplantation Genetic Diagnosis for Phenylketonuria in Day 3 Embryos by Specific Mutation Analysis and Elective Single Embryo Transfer," *Journal of Inherited Metabolic Disorders Reports* 7 (2013): 49–54. Lavery

and his colleagues explain that preimplantation genetic diagnosis offers couples another reproductive choice besides prenatal diagnosis and selective abortion, hinting that the latter option might have be employed by some couples.

119. http://guide.hfea.gov.uk/pgd/ (accessed February 11, 2017).

120. J. Stern, "Biochemistry of Down syndrome," in *Cellular Organelles and Membranes in Mental Retardation*, ed. P. Benson (Edinburgh: Churchill Livingstone, 1971), 143–60; P. F. Benson, "RNA Synthesis by Down Syndrome Leucocytes," in *Cellular Organelles and Membranes in Mental Retardation*, 171–72.

121. Memorandum, Metabolic Group, April 1971. Wellcome Archives and Manuscripts Collection, Birth Defects Group of MRC, file PP/CED/B1/4.

122. Dent's application of October 1, 1973. Wellcome Archives and Manuscripts Collection, file PP/CED/B1/4.

123. Peter Coventry, "The Dynamics of Medical Genetics: The Development and Articulation of Clinical and Technical Services under the NHS, Especially at Manchester c. 1945–1979" (PhD diss., Manchester University, 2000), chapter 5.

124. In the early 1970s, Lejeune exercised pressures on young researchers who aspired to develop prenatal diagnosis in their laboratories. In the mid-1970s, however, he realized that this was not a realistic option. Joëlle Boué testified that Lejeune had invited her to teach at his cytology and cytogenetics course at the medical faculty of Paris, knowing that she would speak about prenatal diagnosis and selective abortion. He then left the room while she gave her talk. *Genetics and Medicine Historical Network*, Cardiff University. Peter Harper, interview with André and Joëlle Boué. Peter Harper, interview with Simone Gilgenkrantz, April 19, 2015, https://genmedhist.eshg.org/fileadmin/content/website-layout/interviewees-attachments/Gilgenkrantz.pdf. Lejeune died in 1994. The Jérôme Lejeune Foundation continues to finance research on mental disabilities—above all, Down syndrome—but also is involved in opposition to abortion and to research on embryos in France.

125. H. Galjaard, "Early Diagnosis and Prevention of Genetic Diseases: Molecules and the Obstetrician," in *Towards the Prevention of Fetal Malformations*, ed. J. B. Scrimgoeur (Edinburgh: Edinburgh University Press, 1978), 3–18.

126. Julia Bell, "Letter: On Rubella in Pregnancy," *British Medical Journal*, April 4, 1959, p. 1302. Bell answered to criticism of her early text on the same topic. Julia Bell, "On Rubella in Pregnancy," *British Medical Journal* 1, no. 5123 (1959): 686–89. Bell (1879–1979), a physician and geneticist, was a pioneer of human genetics in the United Kingdom.

127. Interview with Helen Brooke Taussig, conducted by Charles Janeway, August 1975. Family Planning Oral History Project, Schlesinger Library, Harvard University.

128. John Smith, "Implications of Antenatal Diagnosis," in *Antenatal Diagnosis of Genetic Disease*, ed. A. E. H. Emery (Edinburgh: Churchill Livingstone, 1973), 137–55, see esp. 153. This is the only such proposal I encountered on early prenatal diagnosis debates, but its apparent tolerance, like the apparent tolerance of a similar proposal of the elimination of severely disabled newborns made in 1970 in the context of the discussion of the fate of "low-grade feeble-minded" people, may point to a greater acceptance of ideas seen as inadmissible later. Roger Francis Tredgold and Kenneth Soddy, *Tredgold's Mental Retardation*, eleventh edition (London: Baillière, Tindall and Cassell, 1970), 27.

129. Helen Statham, "Prenatal Diagnosis of Fetal Abnormality: The Decision to Terminate the Pregnancy and Its Consequences," *Fetal and Maternal Medicine Review* 13 (2002): 213–47; Veronique Mirlesse, Frederique Perrotte, Francois Kieffer, and Isabelle Ville, "Women's Experience of Termination of Pregnancy for Fetal Anomaly: Effects of Socio-political Evolutions in France," *Prenatal Diagnosis* 31 (2011): 1021–28.

130. Peter Harper, interview with Bernadette Modell; Christie and Zallen, eds., *Genetic Testing*, testimony of Bernadette Modell, 43–45. Statham, "Prenatal Diagnosis of Fetal Abnormality."

131. Rayna Rapp, *Testing the Woman, Testing the Fetus: The Social Impact of Amniocentesis in America* (New York: Routledge, 2000).

132. On the history of genetic counseling in the United States, see Diane Paul, "From Eugenic to Medical Genetics," *Journal of Policy History* 9 (1997): 96–116; Alexandra Minna Stern, *Telling Genes: The Story of Genetic Counseling in America* (Baltimore: Johns Hopkins University Press, 2012); Devon Stillwell, " 'Pretty Pioneering-Spirited People': Genetic Counsellors, Gender Culture, and the Professional Evolution of a Feminised Health Field, 1947–1980," *Social History of Medicine* 28 (2015): 172–93; and on the beginning of genetic counseling in Canada, see Fiona Alice Miller, "A Blueprint for Defining Health: Making Medical Genetics in Canada" (PhD diss., York University, 2000), chap. 6. The professionalization of genetic counseling was not a universal development. In France, small-scale training of specialized genetic counselors only started in the early twenty-first century. In 2015, the majority of French pregnant women continue to receive information about prenatal testing from midwives, gynecologists, fetal medicine experts, and, in complicated cases, clinical geneticists.

133. Coventry, "The Dynamics of Medical Genetics," chapter 7; Isabelle Ville and Lynda Lotte, "Évolution des politiques publiques: handicap, périnatalité, avortement," in *Final Report of the ANR project-09-SSOC-026, Les enjeux du diagnostic prénatal dans la prévention des handicaps*, Paris, 2013. http://anr-dpn.vjf.cnrs.fr/.

134. Abigail Lippman Hand and Clarke Fraser, "Genetic Counseling—the Postcounseling Period: I. Parents' Perceptions of Uncertainty," *American Journal of Medical Genetics* 4 (1979): 51–79.

135. See, for example, M. J. Korenromp, H. R. Iedema-Kuiper, H. G. van Spijker, G. C. M. L. Christiaens, and J. Bergsma, "Termination of Pregnancy on Genetic Grounds: Coping with Grieving," *Journal of Psychosomatic Obstetrics and Gynecology* 13, no. 2 (1992): 93–105. In this sample, about half of "terminations on genetic grounds" were a consequence of the detection of structural malformations of the fetus with no known genetic component.

136. Dorothy Wertz and John Fletcher, "Ethical Issues in Prenatal Diagnosis," *Pediatric Annals* 18 (1989): 739–49; M. Renaud, L. Bouchard, O. Kremp, et al., "Is Selective Abortion for a Genetic Disease an Issue for the Medical Profession? A Comparative Study of Quebec and France," *Prenatal Diagnosis* 13 (1993): 691–706. Conversely, many observers doubted if genetic counselors could be "nondirective." Laurence Karp, "The Terrible Question," *American Journal of Medical Genetics* 14 (1983): 1–4; Angus Clarke, "Is Non-directive Genetic Counselling Possible?," *The Lancet* 338 (1991): 998–1000; Barbara Bernhardt, "Empirical Evidence That Genetic Counseling is Directive: Where Do We Go from Here?," *American Journal of Human Genetics* 60 (1997): 17–20.

137. Peter Harper, Lois Reynolds, and Elisabeth Tansey, eds., *Clinical Genetics in Britain: Origins and Development, Witness Seminar in Twentieth Century Medicine*, vol. 39 (London: The Wellcome Trust, 2010), 31–32. Harper added that Carter openly voiced eugenic views but seldom applied these eugenic convictions in his medical practice. On continuities between genetics and eugenics, see, for example, Paul, *Controlling Human Heredity, 1885 to Present,*

138. Dorothy Wertz and John Fletcher, "A Critique of Some Feminist Challenges to Prenatal Diagnosis," *Journal of Women and Health* 2 (1993): 173–88; Arthur Caplan, "Foreword," in *Prenatal Testing: A Sociological Perspective*, ed. Aliza Kolker and B. Meredith Burke (Westport, CT: Bergin and Garvey, 1988), xiii–xviii; Peter Harper, interview with Malcolm Ferguson-Smith, *Genetics and Medicine Historical Network*, https://genmedhist.eshg.org/fileadmin/content/website-layout/interviewees-attachments/Ferguson-Smith%2C%20Malcolm.pdf.

139. Robert Resta, "Defining and Redefining the Scope and Goals of Genetic Counseling," *American Journal of Medical Genetics* 142C (2006): 269–75. Despite technological developments, even today, a large proportion of people at risk of giving birth to an impaired child elect to remain childless. Susan Kelly, "Choosing Not to Choose: Reproductive Responses of Parents of Children with Genetic Conditions or Impairments," *Sociology of Health and Illness* 31 (2009): 81–97.

140. The principle of neutrality of genetic counselors adopted in Western Europe and North America is not a universal ideal. International comparisons revealed important disparities in regard to the desirable level of nondirectiveness of genetic counseling and its frequent absence in other parts the world. Dorothy Wertz and John Fletcher, "Attitudes of Genetic Counselors: A Multinational Survey," *American Journal of Human Genetics* 42 (1988): 592–600; Yael Hashiloni-Dolev displayed striking differences in the attitudes of genetic counselors in Germany and Israel. Yael Hashiloni-Dolev, *A Life (Un)worthy of Living: Reproductive Genetics in Israel and Germany* (Dordrecht: Springer, 2007).

141. Clare Williams, Priscilla Alderson, and Bobbie Farsides, "Is Nondirectiveness Possible within the Contexts of Antenatal Screening and Testing?," *Social Science and Medicine* 54 (2002): 339–47.

142. Robert Resta pointed to the contrast between the abundance of literature on what genetic counseling should be and the paucity of studies that look at what is really going on during genetic counseling sessions. Resta, "Defining and Redefining the Scope and Goals of Genetic Counseling."

143. Charles Bosk, *All God's Mistakes: Genetic Counseling in a Pediatric Hospital* (Chicago: University of Chicago Press, 1992). The book was published in the early 1990s but is based on observations made by Bosk in the late 1970s.

144. Ibid., 6.

145. Ibid., 11, 55, 158.

146. Ibid., 42–44, 50–52.

147. Ibid., 143.

148. Susan Markens, "'It Just Becomes Much More Complicated': Genetic Counselors' Views on Genetics and Prenatal Testing," *New Genetics and Society* 32 (2013): 302–21.

Chapter 3 · Human Malformations

1. Peter Coventry, "The Dynamics of Medical Genetics: The Development and Articulation of Clinical and Technical Services under the NHS, Especially at Manchester c. 1945–1979" (PhD diss., Manchester University, 2000), chap. 7; Isabelle Ville and Lynda Lotte, "Évolution des politiques publiques: handicap, périnatalité, avortement," in Final Report of the ANR project-09-SSOC-026. "Les enjeux du diagnostic prénatal dans la prévention des handicaps: l'usage des techniques entre progrès scientifiques et action publique," Paris, 2013. http://anr-dpn.vjf.cnrs.fr/. French cytogeneticist Joëlle Boué recalled that she and her colleagues performed abortions for chromosomal anomalies in France before the legalization of abortion. They always sent a letter to the French health ministry informing them of what they did and why. The ministry did not react to their letters, and they were never bothered. Peter Harper, interview with Andre and Joëlle Boué, *Genetics and Medicine Historical Network*, April 22, 2005, https://genmedhist.eshg.org/fileadmin/content/website-layout/interviewees-attachments/Boue%20A%26J.pdf.

2. Peter Coventry reported that some physicians in the United Kingdom resisted the legalization of abortion because they believed it would shift the decision about abortion to the pregnant woman and favor abortion for "frivolous" reasons. Coventry, "The Dynamics of Medical Genetics," chap. 7.

3. The postulated relationships between progressive policies, feminism, and abortion were not always linear and simple; for example, in the 1960s and 1970s the protection of fetal rights was seen as a progressive cause by some US activists, especially those who were Catholic. Daniel Williams, *Defenders of the Unborn: The Pro-life Movement before Roe v. Wade* (New York: Oxford University Press, 2016). In Germany, segments of the feminist movement continue to view the protection of the fetus/unborn child as a major feminist issue.

4. Tom Smith, "A Report: The Sexual Revolution?," *The Public Opinion Quarterly* 54 (1990): 415–35; Ilana Löwy, "Reproductive Revolutions," *Studies in History and Philosophy of Biological and Biomedical Sciences* 41, no. 4 (2010): 422–24.

5. Masae Kato, *Women's Rights? The Politics of Eugenic Abortion in Modern Japan* (Amsterdam: Amsterdam University Press, 2009), 43–45.

6. This argument was developed by Leslie Reagan. Leslie Reagan, *Dangerous Pregnancies: Mothers, Disabilities and Abortion in Modern America* (Berkeley: University of California Press, 2010).

7. William G. McBride, "Thalidomide and Congenital Abnormalities," *The Lancet* 278 (1961): 1358.

8. See, for example, S. P. Ward, "Thalidomide and Congenital Anomalies," *British Medical Journal* 2, no. 5305 (1962): 646–47; E. A. Rodin, L. A. Koller, and J. D. Taylor, "Association of Thalidomide (Kevadon) with Congenital Anomalies," *Canadian Medical Association Journal* 86 (1962): 744–46.

9. Interview with Helen Brooke Taussig, made by Charles Janeway, August 1975. Schlesinger Library, Cambridge, MA, Oral History of Family Planning Project.

10. Sunday Times Insight Team, *Suffer the Children: The Story of Thalidomide* (London: André Deutsch, 1979); Ann Dally, "Thalidomide: Was the Tragedy Preventable?," *The Lancet* 351 (1998): 1197–99.

11. "The Thalidomide Disaster," *Time Magazine*, August 10, 1962; "Mrs. Finkbine Undergoes Abortion in Sweden; Surgeon Asserts Unborn Child Was Deformed— Mother of 4 Took Thalidomide," *New York Times*, August 18, 1962.

12. "Thalidomide and Abortion," *Time Magazine*, December 21, 1962.

13. Jan Hoffman, "'Romper Room' Host on Her Abortion Case," *New York Times*, June 16, 1992.

14. The first report was on the induction of fetal malformations by the rubella virus made by an Australian pediatric ophthalmologist in 1941. Norman McAlister Gregg, "Congenital Cataract following German Measles in the Mother," *Transactions of the Ophthalmological Society of Australia* 3 (1941): 35–46.

15. Mary Sheridan, "Final Report of a Prospective Study of Children Whose Mothers Had Rubella in Early Pregnancy," *British Medical Journal* 2, no. 5408 (1964): 536–39; Franklin Neva, Charles Alford, and Thomas Weller, "Emerging Perspective of Rubella," *Bacteriological Reviews* 28 (1964): 444–51.

16. Such a diagnosis was difficult in the 1980s, too. A famous French case in which a child was accorded compensation for a "prejudice of being born" was a judgment in favor of a mother who was mistakenly told in 1982 that she did not have rubella when she was pregnant and who then gave birth to a severely handicapped child. Quentin Mameri, Emmanuelle Fillion, and Bénédicte Champenois, "Le juge et le diagnostic prénatal depuis la loi du 4 mars 2002," *ALTER, European Journal of Disability Research* 9 (2015): 331–53.

17. Gregg's 1941 report on links between the rubella virus and birth defects immediately received wide coverage in Australia, including in newspapers. It reception abroad, however, was slower, perhaps because of the strong belief in the hereditary origins of birth defects. P. M. Dunn, "Perinatal Lessons from the Past: Sir Norman Gregg, ChM, MC, of Sydney (1892–1966) and Rubella Embryopathy," *Archives of Disease in Childhood: Fetal and Neonatal Edition* 92 (2007): F513–F514.

18. Julia Bell, "On Rubella in Pregnancy," *British Medical Journal* 1, no. 5123 (1959): 686–88, see esp. 686.

19. Julia Bell, "Correspondence," *British Medical Journal* 1, no. 5132 (1959): 1302.

20. B. H. Brock, "Correspondence," *British Medical Journal* 1, no. 5129 (1959): 1117.

21. Bell, "On Rubella in Pregnancy," 686.

22. Linda Greenhouse and Reva Siegel, eds., *Before Roe v. Wade: Voices That Shaped the Abortion Debate before the Supreme Court Ruling* (New York: Kaplan Publishing, 2010).

23. Rachel Benson Gold, "Lessons from before Roe: Will Past Be Prologue?," *The Guttmacher Report on Public Policy* 6 (March 2003): 8–12.

24. Greenhouse and Siegel, *Before Roe v. Wade*, 63–67.

25. Ville and Lotte, "Évolution des politiques publiques: handicap, périnatalité, avortement." On the integration of a future child into a family, see Luc Boltansky, *The Foetal Condition: A Sociology of Engendering and Abortion* (Cambridge: Polity Press, 2013).

26. Agence de la Biomedicine, "Tableau CPDPN-2a: Indications et termes des attestations delivrés en vue d'une IMG pour motif foetal en 2012," https://www.agence -biomedecine.fr/annexes/bilan2015/donnees/diag-prenat/01-diag_prenat/synthese.htm (accessed March 23, 2016).

27. Michel Foucault, *Naissance de la clinique: une archéologie du regard médical* (Paris: Presses Universitaires de France, 1963), xix. English translation, *The Birth of the Clinic:*

An Archaeology of Medical Perception, trans. A. M. Sheridan Smith (New York: Pantheon Books, 1973).

28. Lorraine Daston and Peter Galison, *Objectivity* (New York: Zone Books, 2007).

29. Ludwik Fleck, *Genesis and Development of a Scientific Fact*, trans. Fred Bradley and Thaddeus Trenn (Chicago: University of Chicago Press, 1979).

30. Josef Warkany, "The Medical Profession and Congenital Defects, 1900–1979," *Teratology* 20 (1979): 201–204.

31. Dally, "Thalidomide"; Aryn Martin and Kelly Holloway, "'Something There Is That Doesn't Love a Wall': Histories of the Placental Barrier," *Studies in History and Philosophy of Biological and Biomedical Sciences* 47 (2014): 300–10.

32. Rachel Carson, *Silent Spring* (New York: Houghton Mifflin, 1962).

33. On Warkany, see Robert Brent, "Biography of Josef Warkany," *Teratology* 25 (1982): 137–44; Wladimir Wertelecki, "Of Dreaming on Solid Ground and Silent Triumph of One Man: A Story about Josef Warkany," *American Journal of Medical Genetics* 33 (1989): 522–36; Bruce Lambert, "Dr. Josef Warkany, 90, Pioneer in Study of Prenatal Health Dies," *New York Times*, June 25, 1992.

34. Josef Warkany, "The Medical Profession and Congenital Malformations, 1900–1979," *Teratology*, 20 (1979): 201–204.

35. Josef Warkany, Berry Monroe, and Betty Sutherland, "Intrauterine Growth Retardation," *American Journal of Diseases of Children* 102 (1961): 249–79. Intrauterine growth delay is one of the main causes of fetal demise during pregnancy and of birth defects.

36. Josef Warkany and D. M. Hubbard, "Mercury in Urine of Children with Acrodynia," *The Lancet* 251 (1948): 829–30; Josef Warkany, "Acrodynia—Post Mortem of a Disease," *The American Journal of Diseases of Childhood* 112 (1966): 147–52. Warkany's conclusions were immediately accepted in the United States but not in the United Kingdom, because British doctors who attempted to repeat his studies did not find important differences in the presence of mercury in the urine of affected and unaffected children. This had happened, Warkany argued later, because mercury-laden teething powders were so popular the United Kingdom that there were practically no "normal controls."

37. Robert Miller, "Josef Warkany," *The Journal of Pediatrics* 126 (1995): 669–72.

38. Robert Brent, "Comments on the History of Teratology," *Teratology* 20 (1979): 199–200; James Wilson and Josef Warkany, "The History of Organized Teratology in North America," *Teratology* 31 (1985): 285–96.

39. David Smith, "Dysmorphology (Teratology)," *Journal of Pediatrics* 69 (1966): 1150–69; T. Shepard, "Obituary: David W. Smith, 1926–1981," *Teratology* 24 (1981): 111–12.

40. In 1966, when Smith moved from Wisconsin to the University of Seattle, he had already named his department "dysmorphology."

41. See, for example, K. Patau, D. W. Smith, E. Therman, S. L. Inhorn, and H. P. Wagner, "Multiple Congenital Anomaly Caused by an Extra Autosome," *The Lancet* 275 (1960): 790–93.

42. David Smith, "Classification, Nomenclature and Naming of Morphological Defects," *Journal of Pediatrics* 87 (1975): 162–64; David Smith, "An Approach to Clinical Dysmorphology," *Journal of Pediatrics* 91 (1977): 690–92.

43. Smith, "Dysmorphology (Teratology)"; Smith, "An Approach to Clinical Dysmorphology." Meningomyelocele, a type of spina bifida, is an incomplete closure of the neural tube and is closely related to anencephaly (the absence of a major portion of

the brain). These two malformations originate from similar defects of neural tube development.

44. P. Lemoine, P. H. Harousseau, J. B. Borteyru, and J. C. Menuet, "Les enfants de parents alcooliques: Anomalies observées, à propos de 127 cas," *Ouest Medical* 21 (1968): 476–82.

45. K. L. Jones, D. W. Smith, C. N. Ulleland, and A. P. Streissguth, "Pattern of Malformation in Offspring of Chronic Alcoholic Mothers," *The Lancet* 305 (1973): 1267–71. Deleterious effects of alcohol are amplified by other factors linked to the low socioeconomic status of women who gave birth to FAS children. Ernst Abel and John Hannigan, "Maternal Risk Factors in Fetal Alcohol Syndrome: Provocative and Permissive Influences," *Neurotoxicology and Teratology* 17 (1995): 445–62.

46. David Smith, *Recognizable Patterns of Human Malformation: Genetic, Embryologic and Clinical Aspects* (Philadelphia: Saunders, 1970). After Smith's death in 1981, the book was edited by his collaborator, Kenneth Jones, and became *Smith's Recognizable Patterns of Human Malformation.*

47. Alexander Schaffer, "Foreword," in *Recognizable Patterns of Human Malformation,* first edition.

48. Victor McKusick, "Review: Recognizable Patterns of Human Malformation: Genetic, Embryologic, and Clinical Aspects," American Journal of Human Genetics 23 (1971): 327. On Victor McKusick's role in the development of clinical genetics, see Susan Lindee, *Moments of Truth in Genetic Medicine* (Baltimore: Johns Hopkins University Press, 2005).

49. Victor McKusick, *Mendelian Inheritance in Man: Catalogs of Autosomal Dominant, Autosomal Recessive, and X-Linked Phenotypes* (Baltimore: Johns Hopkins University Press, 1966); Robert Gorlin and Jens Pindborg, *Syndromes of the Head and Neck* (New York: McGraw Hill, 1964); Josef Warkany, *Congenital Malformations: Notes and Comments* (Chicago: Year Book Medical Publishers, 1971). Despite the word *notes* in Warkany's book's title, the book had 1,309 pages.

50. Andrew Hogan, "The 'Morbid Anatomy' of the Human Genome: Tracing the Observational and Representational Approaches of Postwar Genetics and Biomedicine," *Medical History* 58 (2014): 315–36.

51. The fourth edition of this book was published in 1988, the fifth edition in 1997, and the sixth in 2007.

52. Kenneth Jones, Marilyn Crandall Jones, and Miguel Del Campo, *Smith's Recognizable Patterns of Human Malformation* (Philadelphia: Elsevier Saunders, 2013). Anomalies produced by external teratogens were gathered in a single chapter on environmental agents (728–51).

53. Recent editions of *Smith's Recognizable Patterns of Human Malformation* also contain photographs of newborns and fetuses, and the book is often used by fetal medicine experts.

54. Alice Domurat Dreger commented on the effects of "masking" the eyes of people with physical deformations or diseases in some medical books. Alice Domurat Dreger, "Jarred Bodies: Thoughts on the Display of Unusual Anatomies," *Perspectives in Biology and Medicine* 43 (2000): 161–72. Only a few photographs in *Recognizable Patterns of Human Malformation* represent individuals whose eyes are covered with a black band; all the other photographed subjects (usually babies or children) look into the camera and are presented as distinct individuals, not "specimens."

55. David Smith, *Recognizable Patterns of Human Deformation: Identification and Management of Mechanical Effects on Morphogenesis* (Philadelphia: Saunders, 1981).

56. John Graham, *Smith's Recognizable Patterns of Human Deformation* (Philadelphia: Elsevier Saunders, 2007), ix. Graham, like Jones, the editor of *Smith's Recognizable Patterns of Human Malformation*, was Smith's collaborator.

57. Ibid., 40.

58. McKusick, "Foreword," in *Syndromes of the Head and Neck*, vii.

59. Ibid.

60. David Milner, "Preface," in *Self-Assessment Picture Tests in Pediatrics*, ed. David Milner (London: Mosby-Wolfe, 1994).

61. Robert Brent, "Protecting the Public from Teratogenic and Mutagenic Hazards," *Journal of Clinical Pharmacology* 12 (1972): 61–70.

62. Sheila Sheppard, "Richard Worthington Smithells, 1924–2002," *Birth Defects Research* (Part A) 85 (2009): 252–53.

63. Jennie Kline, Zena Stein, and Mervyn Susser, *Conception to Birth: Epidemiology of Prenatal Development* (Oxford: Oxford University Press, 1989), 305–37.

64. Ian Leck and E. L. M. Milnar, "Short-Term Changes in the Incidence of Malformations," *British Journal of Preventive and Social Medicine* 17 (1963): 1–12; C. R. Lowe, "Congenital Malformations and the Problem of Their Control," *British Medical Journal* 2, no. 5824 (1972): 515–20.

65. John Meaney, "Introduction: Birth Defects Surveillance in the United States," *Teratology* 64 (2001): S1–S2; Thomas Shepard, Mason Barr, Robert Bent, et al., "History of the Teratological Society," *Teratology* 62 (2000): 301–12.

66. Larry Edmonds, Peter Layde, Levy James, William Flynt, David Erickson, and Godfrey Oakley, "Congenital Malformation Surveillance: Two American Systems," *International Journal of Epidemiology* 10 (1981): 247–52; M. F. Lechat, P. De Waals, and J. A. C. Waterhall, "European Economic Community Concerted Action on Congenital Anomalies: The EUROCAT Project," in *Prevention of Physical and Mental Congenital Defects, Part B*, ed. Maurice Marois (New York: Alan Liss, 1985), 11–15; Neil Holtzman and Muin Khoury, "Monitoring for Congenital Malformations," *Annual Review of Public Health* 7 (1986): 237–66.

67. J. W. Flynt and S. Hay, "International Clearinghouse for Birth Defects Monitoring System," *Contributions to Epidemiology and Biostatistics* 1 (1979): 44–52.

68. M. F. Lechat and H. Dolk, "Registries of Congenital Anomalies," *Environmental Health Perspectives* 101, suppl. 2 (1993): 153–57; http://www.eurocat-network.eu/pagecontent .aspx?tree=ABOUTUS/WhatIsEUROCAT#History (accessed March 23, 2016).

69. Bengt Kallen, "Search for Teratogenic Risks with the Aid of Malformation Registries," *Teratology* 35 (1987): 47–52.

70. Sonja Rasmussen, David Erickson, Susan Reef, and Danielle Ross, "Teratology: From Science to Birth Defects Prevention," *Birth Defects Research* (Part A) 85 (2009): 82–92.

71. Ian Leck, "The Etiology of Human Malformations: Insights from Epidemiology," *Teratology* 5 (1972): 301–14.

72. Lorenzo D. Botto, Elisabeth Robert-Gnansia, Csaba Siffel, John Harris, Barry Borman, and Pierpaolo Mastroiacovo, "Fostering International Collaboration in Birth Defects Research and Prevention: A Perspective from the International Clearinghouse

for Birth Defects Surveillance and Research," *American Journal of Public Health* 96 (2006): 774–80.

73. Muin Khoury, "Contribution of Epidemiology to the Study of Birth Defects in Humans," *Teratology* 52 (1995): 186–89.

74. Eduardo E. Castilla and Ieda M. Orioli, "ECLAMC: The Latin-American Collaborative Study of Congenital Malformations," *Community Genetics* 7 (2004): 76–94.

75. F. A. Poletta, J. A. Gili, and E. E. Castilla, "Latin American Collaborative Study of Congenital Malformations (ECLAMC): A Model for Health Collaborative Studies," *Public Health Genomics* 17 (2014): 61–67.

76. Robert Brent, "The Causes and Prevention of Human Birth Defects: What Have We Learned in the Past 50 Years?," *Congenital Anomalies* 41 (2001): 3–21; Sonja Rasmussen, "Human Teratogen Update 2011: Can We Ensure Safety during Pregnancy?," *Birth Defects Research* 94, no. 3 (2012): 123–28; Patricia Donahoe, Kristin Noonan, and Kasper Lage, "Genetic Tools and Algorithms for Gene Discovery in Major Congenital Anomalies," *Birth Defects Research* 85, no. 1 (2009): 6–12.

77. Rosalind Pollack Petchesky, "Fetal Images: The Power of Visual Culture in the Politics of Reproduction," *Feminist Studies* 13 (1987): 263–92; Sarah Franklin, "Fetal Fascinations: New Dimensions to the Medical-Scientific Construction of Fetal Personhood," in *Off-Centre: Feminism and Cultural Studies*, ed. Sarah Franklin, Celia Lury, and Jackie Stacey (London: HarperCollins, 1991), 190–205; Barbara Duden, *Disembodying Women: Perspectives on Pregnancy and the Unborn* (Cambridge, MA: Harvard University Press, 1993); Karen Newman, *Fetal Positions: Individualism, Science, Visuality* (Stanford, CA: Stanford University Press, 1996); Janelle Taylor, *The Public Life of the Fetal Sonogram: Technology, Consumption and the Politics of Reproduction* (New Brunswick, NJ: Rutgers University Press, 2008).

78. On the history of obstetrical ultrasound, see Elisabeth Tansey and Dafne Christie, eds., *Looking at the Unborn: Historical Aspects of Obstetrical Ultrasound*, Wellcome Witness to Twentieth-Century Medicine, vol. 5 (London: Wellcome Institute for the History of Medicine, 2000); Malcolm Nicolson and John Fleming, *Imaging and Imagining the Fetus: The Development of Obstetric Ultrasound* (Baltimore: Johns Hopkins University Press, 2013). See also Ann Oakley, *The Captured Womb: A History of the Medical Care of Pregnant Women* (Oxford: Blackwell, 1984), 155–71; Stuart Blume, *Insight and Industry: On the Dynamic of Technological Change in Medicine* (Cambridge, MA: MIT Press, 1992), 74–118.

79. Ian Donald, "Ultrasonic in Diagnosis (Sonar)," *Proceedings of the Royal Society of Medicine* 62 (1969): 442–46; Ian Donald, "Apologia: How and Why Medical Sonar Developed," *Annals of the Royal College of Surgeons of England* 54 (1974): 132–40.

80. Ibid., 5.

81. Tansey and Christie, eds., *Looking at the Unborn*, 54–56.

82. Bernard Ewigman, James Crane, Frederic Frigoletto, Michael LeFevre, Raymond Bain, Donald McNellis, and the RADIUS Study Group, "Effect of Ultrasound Screening on Perinatal Outcome," *New England Journal of Medicine* 329 (1993): 821–27, see esp. 821.

83. French pioneer of ultrasound Roger Bessis recalled that he and his colleagues found the conclusion of the RADIUS trial to be absurd, as their own practice displayed the great utility of obstetrical ultrasound. Witness seminar, Histoire du DPN en France (History of prenatal diagnosis in France). http://anr-dpn.vjf.cnrs.fr/?q1/4node/62 (accessed February 16, 2017).

84. José (Johanna) Van Dijck, *The Transparent Body: A Cultural Analysis of Medical Imaging* (Seattle: University of Washington Press, 2005), 100–17; Susan Erikson, "Fetal Views: Histories and Habits of Looking at the Fetus in Germany," *Journal of Medical Humanities* 28 (2007): 187–212; Eva Sänger, "Obstetrical Care as a Matter of Time: Ultrasound Screening, Temporality and Prevention," *History and Philosophy of Life Sciences* 37 (2015): 105–20.

85. Luc Gourand, "Le choix des mots en échographie prénatale," *Journal de Pédiatrie et de Puériculture* 10 (1997): 466–69.

86. Peter Harper, interview with Michael Braitser, March 1, 2005; Peter Harper, interview with Dian Donnai, February 6, 2007, *Genetics and Medicine Historical Network*, https://genmedhist.eshg.org/fileadmin/content/website-layout/interviewees-attachments/Donnai%2C%20Dian.pdf (accessed March 23, 2016).

87. Examples of such pathology clubs were the British Pathology subcommittee of the Clinical Cancer Research Committee, later renamed the Consultant Panel in Morbid Histology, which met regularly from 1945 to 1970 to discuss difficult cases in cancer diagnosis and agree on nomenclature (Wellcome Archives of Modern Medicine, Archives of British Empire Cancer Campaign, series SA/CRC: Clinics, pathology, research, box 35; box 38), or the Columbia University–based Arthur Purdy Stout Society of surgical pathologists, active from 1957 on (Columbia University Health Sciences Library, Archives and Special Collections, The Arthur Purdy Stout Society of Surgical Pathologists papers).

88. On the role of "slide sessions" in dysmorphology clinics, see Alison Shaw, Joanna Latimer, Paul Atkinson, and Katie Featherstone, "Surveying 'Slides': Clinical Perception and Clinical Judgment in the Construction of a Genetic Diagnosis," *New Genetics and Society* 22 (2003): 3–19, and on the history of microscope slides, see Ilana Löwy, "Microscope Slides: Reassessing a Neglected Historical Resource," *History and Philosophy of Life Sciences* 35, no. 3 (2013): 309–318.

89. Letter of John Burn to Dian Donnai, November 17, 1982, Wellcome Archives, Modern Medicine Collection, Peter Harper papers, CG/225A/39/9. More than half the slips for the November 1982 meetings were handwritten; the others were typed. The slips were glued together on paper sheets and photocopied.

90. Documents from dysmorphology club meeting, May and June 1981, Wellcome Archives, Modern Medicine Collection, Peter Harper papers, CG/225A/39/9. Joanna Latimer and Karen-Sue Taussig made detailed studies of practices of dysmorphologists and clinical geneticists, respectively, in the United Kingdom and the Netherlands. Karen-Sue Taussig, *Ordinary Genomes: Science, Citizenship and Genetic Identities* (Durham, NC: Duke University Press, 2009); Joanna Latimer, *The Gene, the Clinics and the Family* (London: Routledge, 2013).

91. Today, the journal *Birth Defects* is published in three parts. Part A is dedicated to clinical and molecular teratology, part B to developmental and reproductive toxicology, and part C to embryos today.

92. V. Cormier-Daire, "Approche clinique de l'enfant dysmorphique," *Archives de Pédiatrie* 8 suppl. 2 (2001): 382–84; M. Lipson, "Common Neonatal Syndromes," *Seminars in Fetal and Neonatal Medicine* 10 (2005): 221–31; S. Odent, L. Pasquier, C. de la Rochebrochard, H. Journel, and L. Lazaro, "Le retard mental syndromique," *Archives de Pédiatrie* 15 (2008): 705–707.

93. Jones, *Smith's Recognizable Patterns of Human Malformation*, seventh edition.

94. R. Robyr, J. P. Bernard, J. Roume, and Y. Ville, "Familial Diseases Revealed by a Fetal Anomaly," *Prenatal Diagnosis* 26 (2006): 1124–34.

95. Latimer, *The Gene, the Clinics and the Family*, 181–82.

96. On the nineteenth-century roots of pathological practices, see, for example, Cay-Rüdiger Prüll and John Woodward, eds., *Pathology in the 19th and 20th Centuries: The Relationship between Theory and Practice* (Sheffield, UK: European Association for the History of Medicine and Health Publications, 1998).

97. Michel Foucault, *La naisssance de la Clinique* (Paris: Presses Universitaires de France, 1963). English translation: *The Birth of the Clinic: An Archaeology of Medical Perception*, trans. A. Sheridan (London: Tavistock, 1973); Erwin Ackerknecht, *Medicine at the Paris Hospital, 1794–1848* (Baltimore: Johns Hopkins University Press, 1967).

98. "Ouvrez quelques cadavres: vous verrez aussitôt disparaître l'obscurité que la seule observation n'avait pu dissiper," in *Anatomie générale*, ed. Xavier Bichat (Paris: Brosson, Gabon et Cie, 1801), xcix, quoted by Michel Foucault, *Naissance de la Clinique*, 149. Foucault dedicates a chapter, "Open a Few Cadavers," to Bichat's pathology lessons.

99. The examination of fetal and newborn bodies played a key role in criminal investigations on issues such as illegal abortion and infanticide. On the history of midwives' involvement in criminal investigations, see, for example, Silvia De Renzi, "The Risks of Childbirth: Physicians, Finance, and Women's Death in the Law Courts of Seventeenth-Century Rome," *Bulletin of the History of Medicine* 84 (2010): 549–77; Cathy McClive, "Blood and Expertise: The Trials of the Female Medical Expert in the Ancien-Régime Courtroom," *Bulletin of the History of Medicine* 82 (2008): 86–108.

100. Claude Bernard, *An Introduction to the Study of Experimental Medicine*, trans. Henry Coopley Greene (New York: Schuman, 1949). Quoted in Andrew Cunningham and Perry Williams, eds., *The Laboratory Revolution in Medicine* (Cambridge: Cambridge University Press, 2002), 295.

101. Jones, Crandall Jones, and Del Campo, *Smith's Recognizable Patterns of Human Malformation*, 869–93.

102. Stefan Timmermans, *Postmortem: How Medical Examiners Explain Suspicious Deaths* (Chicago: University of Chicago Press, 2006).

103. Jacalyn Duffin, *To See with a Better Eye: A Life of R. T. H. Laennec* (Princeton, NJ: Princeton University Press, 1998).

104. Bernike Pasveer, "The Knowledge of Shadows: The Introduction of X-ray Images in Medicine," *Sociology of Health and Illness* 11 (1989): 360–81.

105. See, for example, Nick Hopwood, "'Giving Body' to Embryos: Modeling, Mechanism, and the Microtome in Nineteenth-Century Anatomy," *Isis* 90 (1999): 462–96; Lynn Morgan, *Icons of Life: A Cultural History of Human Embryos* (Berkeley: University of California Press, 2009); Salim Al-Gailani, "Teratology in the Clinics: Monsters, Obstetrics and the Making of an Antenatal Life in Edinburgh c. 1900" (PhD diss., University of Cambridge, 2012).

106. Robert Woods, *Death before Birth: Fetal Health and Mortality in Historical Perspective* (Oxford: Oxford University Press, 2009), 152–88.

107. P. M. Dunn, "Dr. Edith Potter (1901–1993) of Chicago: Pioneer in Perinatal Pathology," *Archives of Diseases of Children: Fetal and Neonatal Edition* 92 (2007): F419–F420.

108. Edith L. Potter and Fred L. Adair, *Fetal and Neonatal Death* (Chicago: University of Chicago Press, 1939).

109. Edith L. Potter and Fred L. Adair, *Fetal and Neonatal Death*, second edition (Chicago: University of Chicago Press, 1948). On the role of blood transfusion, sulpha drugs, and antibiotics in the decrease of maternal and newborn mortality, see Irvine Loudon, *Death in Childbirth: An International Study of Maternal Care and Maternal Mortality, 1800–1950* (Oxford: Oxford University Press, 1992).

110. Potter and Adair, *Fetal and Neonatal Death* (1948), 47–62.

111. Edith Potter, *Pathology of the Fetus and the Newborn* (Chicago: The Year Book Press, 1952).

112. Potter, *Pathology of the Fetus and the Newborn*, ix-xi. In the 1960s, with the development of genetic investigations, many cases of early miscarriage were attributed to chromosomal anomalies of the fetus.

113. Potter, *Pathology of the Fetus and the Newborn*, 140. Potter mainly studied fetal deaths that occurred beyond the twentieth week of pregnancy; miscarriages/abortions that occurred earlier frequently did not produce an "analysable fetus."

114. J. Edgar Morrison, *Fetal and Neonatal Pathology* (London: Butterworth, 1952), 21–22.

115. Ibid., 23.

116. See, for example, Peter Harper's interview with André and Joëlle Boué, https://genmedhist.eshg.org/fileadmin/content/website-layout/interviewees-attachments/Boue%20A%26J.pdf. In the 1960s and 1970s, the Boués grounded their studies of human chromosomal anomalies in miscarried and aborted fetuses.

117. John Opitz, "Foreword," in *Embryo and Fetal Pathology*, ed. Enid Gilbert-Barness and Diane Debich-Spicer (New York: Cambridge University Press, 2004), ix–xii. Enid Gilbert-Barness edited a posthumous edition of *Potter's Pathology of the Fetus and the Newborn* (St. Louis, MO: Mosby, 1997) and of *Potter's Atlas of Fetal and Infant Pathology* (St. Louis, MO: Mosby, 1998).

Chapter 4 · From Prenatal Diagnosis to Prenatal Screening

1. Zena Stein and Mervyn Susser, "The Preventability of Down's Syndrome," *HSMHA Health Reports* 86, no. 7 (1971): 650–58, see esp. 650.

2. Ibid., 658.

3. Zena Stein, Mervyn Susser, and Andrea Guterman, "Screening Programme for Prevention of Down's Syndrome," *The Lancet* 30 no. 7798 (1973): 305–10, see esp. 305.

4. Ibid., 308.

5. Ibid., 309. Zena Stein and Mervyn Susser were strongly committed to public health goals and in the 1960s became leading experts of the new area of "social epidemiology," which examined the social underpinning of inequality in health. Mervyn Susser, together with William Watson, was the author of the pioneering study *Sociology in Medicine* (Oxford: Oxford University Press, 1962).

6. Mervyn Susser and Zena Stein, "Prenatal Nutrition and Subsequent Development," paper presented at the conference of the Epidemiology of Prematurity, NICHD, Washington, DC, November 1976. Reproduced in Mervyn Susser, *Epidemiology, Health and Society: Selected Papers* (Oxford: Oxford University Press, 1987), 278–88.

7. Mervyn Susser, "A Backward Glance at Intervention and Care for Mental Retardation: An Introduction," in *Deficience mentale chez les jeunes*, ed. M. Manciaux and S. Tomkiewicz (Paris: Editions INSERM, 1981), 193–96.

8. Stein, Susser, and Guterman, "Screening Programme for Prevention of Down's Syndrome," 309.

9. US Department of Health, Education, and Welfare, *Antenatal Diagnosis*, NIH publication 79-1973 (Bethesda, MD: National Institutes of Health, 1979).

10. On the application of obstetrical ultrasound in the 1970s, see Stuart Blume, *Insight and Industry: On the Dynamic of Technological Change in Medicine* (Cambridge, MA: MIT Press, 1992).

11. Terrance Swanson, "Economics of Mongolism," *Annals of New York Academy of Science* 171 (1970): 679–82.

12. Ibid.

13. Philip Welch, "Genetic Screening by Amniocentesis: The Current Status," *Nova Scotia Medical Bulletin* 53 (1973): 115–16.

14. Ronald Conley and Aubrey Milunsky, "The Economics of Prenatal Genetic Diagnosis," in *The Prevention of Genetic Disorders and Mental Retardation*, ed. Aubrey Milunsky (Philadelphia: W. B. Saunders, 1975), 442–55.

15. M. Mikkelsen, G. Nielsen, and E. Rasmussen, "Cost Effectiveness of Antenatal Screening for Chromosome Abnormalities," in *Towards the Prevention of Fetal Malformations*, ed. J. B. Scrimgeour (Edinburgh: Edinburgh University Press, 1978), 209–16.

16. Berenike Cohen, Abraham Lilienfeld, and Arnold Sigler, "Some Epidemiological Aspects of Mongolism: A Review," *American Journal of Public Health* 50 (1963): 223–36; Ernest Hook and Geraldine Chambers, "Estimated Rates of Down Syndrome in Live Births by One Year Maternal Age Intervals for Mothers Aged 20–49 in a New York State Study: Implication of the Risk Figures for Genetic Counseling and Cost-Benefit Analysis of Prenatal Diagnosis Programs," *Birth Defects, Original Article Series* 13, no. 3A (1977): 123–41.

17. John Thompson and Wendy Greenfield, "Rights and Responsibilities of the Insurer," in *Genetics and the Law*, ed. Aubrey Milunsky and George Annas (New York: Plenum Press, 1975), 289–94; Jessica Davis, "Genetic Services Economics: Metropolitan New York Experience with Health Care Insurance Programs," in *Service and Education in Medical Genetics*, ed. Ian Porte and Ernest Hook (New York: Academic Press, 1979), 69–73.

18. Sue Mittenthal, "Amniocentesis: On the Increase," *New York Times*, August 22, 1984.

19. Ernest Hook and Agneta Lindsjo, "Down Syndrome in Live Births by Single Year Maternal Age Intervals in a Swedish Study: Comparison with Results from a New York State Study," *American Journal of Human Genetics* 30 (1978): 19–27.

20. Robert Resta, "Historical Aspects of Genetic Counseling: Why Was Maternal Age 35 Chosen as the Cut-Off for Offering Amniocentesis?," *Medicina nei Secoli* 14 (2002): 783–811.

21. US Department of Health, Education, and Welfare, *Antenatal Diagnosis*, I-135-I-162.

22. Helen Volodkevich and Carl Huether, "Causes of Low Utilisation of Amniocentesis by Women of Advanced Maternal Age," *Social Biology* 28 (1981): 176–86.

23. Aliza Kolker and Meredith Burke, "Afterword," in *Prenatal Diagnosis: A Sociological Perspective*, ed. Aliza Kolker and Meredith Burke, second edition (Westport, CT: Bergin and Garveley, 1998), 201–24, see esp. 204–205.

24. Trevor Sheldon and John Simpson, "Appraisal of a New Scheme for Prenatal Screening for Down's Syndrome," *British Medical Journal* 302 (1991): 1133–36.

25. David Brock and Roger Sutcliffe, "Alpha-Fetoprotein in the Antenatal Diagnosis of Anencephaly and Spina Bifida," *The Lancet* 300 (1972): 197–99.

26. David Brock, A. E. Bolton, and J. M. Monaghan, "Prenatal Diagnosis of Anencephaly through Maternal Serum Alpha-Fetoprotein Measurement," *The Lancet* 302 (1973): 923–24; David Brock, "Alphafetoprotein and Neural Tube Defects," *Journal of Clinical Pathology* 29, suppl. 10 (1976): 157–64.

27. C. R. Lowe, "Congenital Malformations and the Problem of their Control," *British Medical Journal* 2, no. 5825 (1972): 515–20, see esp. 519.

28. Sir John Brotherton, "Implications of Antenatal Screening for the Health Service," in *Towards the Prevention of Fetal Malformations*, ed. J. B. Scrimgoeur (Edinburgh: Edinburgh University Press, 1978), 247–57.

29. UK collaborative study on AFP in relation to neural tube defects, "Maternal Serum-Alpha-Fetoprotein Measurement in Antenatal Screening for Anencephaly and Spina Bifida in Early Pregnancy," *The Lancet* 309 (1977): 1323–32. See also Peter Coventry, "The Dynamics of Medical Genetics: The Development and Articulation of Clinical and Technical Services under the NHS, Especially at Manchester c. 1945–1979" (PhD diss., Manchester University, 2000), chap. 7.

30. Malcolm A. Ferguson-Smith, "Report of the Clinical Genetic Society Working Party on Prenatal Diagnosis in Relation to Genetic Counseling," *Bulletin of the Eugenic Society London* 10, suppl. 3 (1978): 3–32.

31. Gina Bari Kolata, "Mass Screening for Neural Tube Defects," *The Hastings Center Report* 10 (1980): 8–10, see esp. 8; T. D. Rogers, "Wrongful Life and Wrongful Birth: Medical Malpractice in Genetic Counselling and Prenatal Testing," *Southern California Law Review* 33 (1982): 713–25; Kolker and Burke, *Prenatal Diagnosis: A Sociological Perspective*, 3–6.

32. Kolata, "Mass Screening for Neural Tube Defects"; Nancy Press and C. H. Browner, "Risk, Autonomy, and Responsibility: Informed Consent for Prenatal Testing," *Hastings Center Report* 25 (1995): S9–S12.

33. Joyce Bermel, "An FDA Approved Kit," *Hastings Center Report* 13 (1983): 3–4.

34. Robert Steinbrook, "In California, Voluntary Mass Prenatal Screening," *Hastings Center Report* 16 (1986): 5–7.

35. H. S. Cuckle, N. J. Wald, and R. H. Lindenbaum, "Maternal Serum Alpha-Fetoprotein Measurements: A Screening for Down Syndrome," *The Lancet* 323 (1984): 926–29; D. J. Brock, "Maternal Serum Alpha-Fetoprotein as Screening Test for Down Syndrome," *The Lancet* 323 (1984): 1292–93; R. Harris and T. Andrews, "Prenatal Screening for Down's Syndrome," *Archives of Disease in Childhood* 63 (1988): 705–706.

36. Nancy Rose and Michael Mennuti, "Maternal Serum Screening for Neural Tube Defects and Fetal Chromosome Abnormalities," *Western Journal of Medicine* 159 (1983): 312–17; Nicolas Wald, Howard S. Cuckle, James W. Densem, et al., "Maternal Serum Screening for Down's Syndrome in Early Pregnancy," *British Medical Journal* 297 (1988): 883–87.

37. D. A. Aitken, E. M. Wallace, J. A. Crossley, et al., "Dimeric Inhibin A as a Marker for Down's Syndrome in Early Pregnancy," *New England Journal of Medicine* 334 (1996): 1231–36; L. Breimer, "First Trimester Biochemical Screening for Trisomy 21: The Role of Free Beta-hCG and Pregnancy Associated Plasma Protein A," *Annals of Clinical Biochemistry* 32 (1995): 233–34.

38. Sheldon and Simpson, "Appraisal of a New Scheme for Prenatal Screening for Down's Syndrome," 302.

39. Witness seminar, "History of Prenatal Diagnosis in France," http://anr-dpn.vjf .cnrs.fr/?q1/4node/62.

40. Carine Vassy, "How Prenatal Diagnosis Became Acceptable in France," *Trends in Biotechnology* 23 (2005): 246–49; Carine Vassy, "From a Genetic Innovation to Mass Health Programmes: The Diffusion of Down's Syndrome Prenatal Screening and Diagnostic Techniques in France," *Social Science and Medicine* 63 (2006): 2041–51.

41. Kolker and Burke, *Prenatal Testing*.

42. Monoclonal antibodies were central to the development of mass-diffused serum tests for the risk of a fetal anomaly. On the history of monoclonal antibodies, see Alberto Cambrosio and Peter Keating, *Exquisite Specificity: The Monoclonal Antibody Revolution* (New York: Oxford University Press, 1995); Lara Marks, *The Lock and Key of Medicine: Monoclonal Antibodies and the Transformation of Health Care* (New Haven, CT: Yale University Press, 2015).

43. Glenn Palomaki, Linda Bradley, Geraldine McDowell, and the Working Group of American College of Medical Genetics, "Technical Standards and Guidelines: Prenatal Screening for Down Syndrome," *Genetics in Medicine* 7 (2005): 344–54; Jacob Canick, "Prenatal Screening for Trisomy 21: Recent Advances and Guidelines," *Clinical Chemistry and Laboratory Medicine* 50 (2012): 1003–1008.

44. C. H. Roddeck, "New Developments in Prenatal Diagnosis," in *Development in Human Reproduction and Their Eugenic and Ethical Implications*, ed. Cedric Carter (London: Academic Press, 1983), 177–86; Rodney Harris and A. P. Read, "Review: New Uncertainties in Prenatal Screening for Neural Tube Effects," *British Medical Journal* 282 (1981): 1416–18.

45. Malcolm A. Ferguson-Smith and M. E. Ferguson-Smith, "Problems of Prenatal Diagnosis," in *Development in Human Reproduction and Their Eugenic and Ethical Implications*, 187–204, see esp. 203.

46. Roddeck, "New Developments in Prenatal Diagnosis," 180.

47. W. J. Watson, N. C. Chescheir, V. L. Katz, and J. W. Seeds, "The Role of Ultrasound in Evaluation of Patients with Elevated Maternal Serum Alpha-Fetoprotein: A Review," *Obstetrics and Gynecology* 78 (1991): 123–28.

48. André Boué, Francine Muller, Michel Briard, and Joëlle Boué, "Interest of Biology in the Management of Pregnancies Where a Fetal Malformation Has Been Detected by Ultrasonography," *Fetal Therapy* 3 (1988): 14–23; Beatrice Blondel, Virginie Ringa, and Gerald Breart, "The Use of Ultrasound Examinations, Intrapartum Fetal Heart Rate Monitoring and Beta-Mimetic Drugs in France," *British Journal of Obstetrics and Gynecology* 96 (1989): 44–55; Francine Muller, "Diagnostic prénatal des défauts de fermeture du tube neural," *Journal de Pédiatrie et de Puericulture* 8 (1991): 448–51.

49. The transformation of a fetus into a patient was also favored by the rise of fetal surgery. Monica Casper, *The Making of the Unborn Patient: A Social Anatomy of Fetal*

Surgery (New Brunswick, NJ: Rutgers University Press, 1998); Deborah Blizzard, *Looking Within: A Sociocultural Examination of Fetoscopy* (Cambridge, MA: MIT Press, 2007).

50. Jacques Abramowicz, "Ultrasound in Obstetrics and Gynecology: Is This Hot Technology Too Hot?," *Journal of Ultrasound in Medicine* 21 (2002): 1327–33; Danica Marinac-Dabic, Cara Krulewitch, and Roscoe Moore Jr., "The Safety of Prenatal Ultrasound Exposure in Human Studies," *Epidemiology* 13, suppl. 3 (2002): S19–S22; Steinar Westin and Leif Bakketeig, "Unnecessary Use of Ultrasound in Pregnancy Should Be Avoided: Probably Safe, but New Evidence Suggests Caution," *Scandinavian Journal of Primary Health Care* 21 (2003): 65–67. For the chronology of technical advances in obstetrical ultrasound, see J. M. Carrera, "Editorial: Fetal Sonography—the First 40 Years," *The Ultrasound Review of Obstetrics and Gynecology* 4 (2004): 141–47.

51. Beryl Benacerraf, V. A. Barss, and L. A. Laboda, "A Sonographic Sign for the Detection in the Second Trimester of the Fetus with Down's Syndrome," *American Journal of Obstetrics and Gynecology* 151 (1985): 1078–79; Bryann Bromley, Thomas Shipp, and Beryl R. Benacerraf, "Genetic Sonogram Scoring Index: Accuracy and Clinical Utility," *Journal of Ultrasound Medicine* 18 (1999): 523–28.

52. Bryann Bromley, Ellice Lieberman, Thomas Shipp, and Beryl Benacerraf, "The Genetic Sonogram: A Method of Risk Assessment for Down Syndrome in the Second Trimester," *Journal of Ultrasound Medicine* 21 (2002): 1087–96; Thomas Shipp and Beryl Benacerraf, "Second Trimester Ultrasound Screening for Chromosomal Abnormalities," *Prenatal Diagnosis* 22 (2002): 296–307; Beryl Benacerraf, "The History of the Second-Trimester Sonographic Markers for Detecting Fetal Down Syndrome, and Their Current Role in Obstetric Practice," *Prenatal Diagnosis* 30 (2010): 344–52.

53. A. S. Nadel, J. K. Green, L. B. Holmes, F. D. Frigoletto, and B. R. Benacerraf, "Absence of Need for Amniocentesis in Patients with Elevated Levels of Maternal Serum Alpha-Fetoprotein and Normal Ultrasonographic Examinations," *New England Journal of Medicine* 323 (1990): 557–61; Michael G. Pinette, John Garrett, Anthony Salvo, Jacquelyn Blackstone, Sheila Pinette, Nancy Boutin, and Angelina Cartin, "Normal Midtrimester (17–20 Weeks) Genetic Sonogram Decreases Amniocentesis Rate in a High-Risk Population," *Journal of Ultrasound Medicine* 20 (2001): 639–44.

54. Beryl Benacerraf, "Who Should Be Performing Fetal Ultrasound," *Ultrasound in Obstetrics and Gynecology* 3 (1993): 1–2.

55. K. H. Nicolaides, G. Azar, D. Byrne, et al., "Fetal Nuchal Translucency: Ultrasound Screening for Chromosomal Defects in the First Semester of Pregnancy," *British Medical Journal* 304 (1992): 867–69; M. Agathokleo Chaveeva, L. C. Y. Poon, P. Kosinski, and K. H. Nicolaides, "Meta-analysis of Second-Trimester Markers for Trisomy 21," *Ultrasound in Obstetrics and Gynecology* 41 (2013): 247–61.

56. R. Maymon, A. L. Zimerman, Z. Weinraub, A. Herman, and H. Cuckle, "Correlation between Nuchal Translucency and Nuchal Skin-Fold Measurements in Down Syndrome and Unaffected Fetuses," *Ultrasound in Obstetrics and Gynecology* 32 (2008): 501–505.

57. K. H. Nicolaides, G. Azar, D. Byrne, et al., "Fetal Nuchal Translucency: Ultrasound Screening for Chromosomal Defects in the First Semester of Pregnancy," *British Medical Journal* 304 (1992): 867–69.

58. Some gynecologists claim that, in their hands, invasive tests are much safer than reported in national or regional databases. Cumulative data, they argue, are meaningless,

because they represent an average between centers with excellent results and those with poor results.

59. For example, N. J. Wald, L. George, J. W. Densem, K. Petterson, and the International Prenatal Screening Research Group, "Serum Screening for Down's Syndrome between 8 and 14 Weeks of Pregnancy," *British Journal of Obstetrics and Gynecology* 103 (1996): 407–12; Howard Cuckle, "Rational Down Syndrome Screening Policy," *American Journal of Public Health* 88 (1998): 558–59; N. J. Wald and A. K. Hackshaw, "Combining Ultrasound and Biochemistry in First-Trimester Screening for Down's Syndrome," *Prenatal Diagnosis* 17 (1997): 821–29; R. Mangione, N. Fries, P. Godard, M. Fontanges, G. Haddad, V. Mirlesse, and the Collège français d'échographie foetale, "Outcome of Fetuses with Malformations Revealed by Echography during the First Trimester," *Journal de Gynécologie Obstétrique et Biologie de la Reproduction* 37 (2008): 154–62; K. H. Nicolaides, "Screening for Fetal Aneuploidies at 11 to 13 Weeks," *Prenatal Diagnosis* 3, no. 1 (2011): 7–15.

60. Romain Favre, "En quoi le niveau de connaissance médicale et la position de médecins respectent-ilts ou non le consentement des patientes dans le cadre de dépistage de la Trisomie 21" (PhD diss., University of Paris Descartes, 2007).

61. Klaus Hoeyer and Linda Hogle, "Informed Consent: The Politics of Intent and Practice in Medical Research Ethics," *Annual Review of Anthropology* 43 (2014): 347–62, see esp. 347.

62. Kolker and Burke added that the show's producers recognized that they had exaggerated the character's intellectual capacities. Kolker and Burke, *Prenatal Testing*, 216.

63. Ibid., 216–17.

64. This section follows only state-sponsored Down syndrome screening programs introduced in countries that have some form of national health insurance. Comparison of the implementation of prenatal screening in Europe is summarized in Patricia Boyd and Ester Game, *Special Report: Prenatal Screening Policies in Europe, 2010* (Ulster: EUROCAT Central Registry, 2011).

65. The concept of local biology was introduced by anthropologist Margaret Lock. Margaret Lock, "The Tempering of Medical Anthropology: Troubling Natural Categories," *Medical Anthropology Quarterly* 15 (2001): 478–92.

66. J. Caby, "Depistage anténatal des malformations," *Journal de Pédiatrie et de Puériculture* 5 (1989): 320–22; Francoise Muller and André Boué, "Dépistage des patientes à risque accru de trisomie 21 fœtale: étude prospective portant sur 10.000 cas," *Journal de Pédiatrie et de Puériculture* 4 (1991): 209–15; J. Goujard, S. Aymé, C. Stoll, and C. de Vigan, "Impact du diagnostic anténatal: Approche épidémiologique," *Journal de Pédiatrie et de Puériculture* 9 (1996): 464–69.

67. Yves Dumez, "Principes de dépistage au cours d'une grossesse à priori normale," *Journal de Pédiatrie et de Puériculture* 18 (2005): 277–84.

68. Babak Khoshnood, Catherine De Vigan, Véronique Vodovar, Gérard Bréart, François Goffinet, and Béatrice Blondel, "Advances in Medical Technology and Creation of Disparities: The Case of Down Syndrome," *American Journal of Public Health* 96 (2006): 2139–44.

69. Journal Officiel, République Française, "Arrêté du 23 Juin 2009: Les règles de bonnes pratiqes en matière de dépistage et de diagnostic prénatals avec utilisation des marqueurs sériques maternels de la trisomie 21,"

70. Vassy, "From a Genetic Innovation to Mass Health Programmes"; Dumez, "Principes de dépistage au cours d'une grossesse à priori normale."

71. Agence de la Biomédicine, "Tableau CPDPN5: Grossesses poursuivies malgré une pathologie foetale qui aurait pu faire autoriser une IMG et issues de ces grossesses en 2010," http://anr-dpn.vjf.cnrs.fr/sites/default/files/ABM%20CPDPN%202010.pdf. Marc Dommergues, Laurent Mandelbrot, Dominique Mahieu-Caputo, et al., "Termination of Pregnancy following Prenatal Diagnosis in France: How Severe Are the Foetal Anomalies?," *Prenatal Diagnosis* 30 (2010): 531–39. Data on terminating a pregnancy for Down syndrome after a "positive" prenatal diagnosis, Dommergues and his colleagues argue, are similar in all the surveyed European countries. Important differences in the number of abortions for Down syndrome generally reflect differences in the uptake of screening and testing for this condition.

72. On the development of prenatal diagnosis in France, see Lynda Lotte and Isabelle Ville, "Les politiques de prévention des handicaps de la naissance en France: perspective historique," in Final Report, ANR grant DPN-HP, ANR-09-SSOC-026, Paris, 2013.

73. Khoshnood, De Vigan, Vodovar, Bréart, Goffinet, and Blondel, "Advances in Medical Technology and Creation of Disparities," 2143.

74. Vassy, "From a Genetic Innovation to Mass Health Programmes."

75. On the history of prenatal diagnosis in the United Kingdom, see Coventry, "The Dynamics of Medical Genetics."

76. Clare Williams, Jane Sandall, Gillian Lewando-Hundt, Bob Heyman, Kevin Spencer, and Rachel Grellier, "Women as Moral Pioneers? Experiences of First Trimester Antenatal Screening," *Social Science and Medicine* 61 (2005): 1983–92.

77. UK government, *Abortion Statistics, England and Wales: 2013*, https://www.gov.uk/government/uploads/system/uploads/attachment_data/file/319460/Abortion_Statistics__England_and_Wales_2013.pdf (accessed March 23, 2016); Agence de la Biomédicine, Tableau CPDPN2a: Indications et termes des attestations délivrées en vue d'une IMG pour motif fœtal en 2012, http://www.agence-biomedecine.fr/annexes/bilan2013/donnees/diag-prenat/02-centres/telechargement/TCPDPN2a.gif (accessed March 23, 2016).

78. Olivier Cayla and Yan Thomas, *Le droit de ne pas naître: A propos de l'affaire Perrouche* (Paris: Gallimard, 2002).

79. Jepson told her story in her autobiography: Joanna Jepson, *A Lot Like Eve: Fashion, Faith and Fig Leaves* (London: Bloomsbury, 2015). Newspaper reports about Jepson's accusation do not provide details on the nature of the defect of the aborted fetus. Jaw and palate malformations have highly variable degrees of severity; some may be linked with additional structural and/or genetic problems.

80. Lyn Chitty, "Prenatal Screening for Chromosome Abnormalities," *British Medical Bulletin* 54 (1998): 839–56; Howard Cuckle, "Rational Down Syndrome Screening Policy," *American Journal of Public Health* 884 (1998): 558–59; B. Thilaganathan, "First-Trimester Nuchal Translucency and Maternal Serum Biochemical Screening for Down's Syndrome: A Happy Union?," *Ultrasound in Obstetrics and Gynecology* 13, no. 4 (1999): 229–30.

81. Judith Budd, Elizabeth Draper, Robyn Lotto, Laura Berry, and Lucy Smith, "Socioeconomic Inequalities in Pregnancy Outcome Associated with Down Syndrome: A Population-Based Study," *Archives of Disease in Childhood: Fetal and Neonatal Edition* 100 (2015): 400–404.

82. NHS National Screening Committee, *Screening Tests For You And Your Baby*, leaflet, 2012.

83. Carine Vassy, Sophia Rosman, and Bénédicte Rousseau, "From Policy Making to Service Use: Down's Syndrome Antenatal Screening in England, France and the Netherlands," *Social Science and Medicine* 106 (2014): 67–74, see esp. 72.

84. Clare Williams, Priscilla Alderson, and Bobbie Farsides, "What Constitutes 'Balanced' Information in the Practitioners' Portrayals of Down's Syndrome?," *Midwifery* 18 (2002): 230–37; Gareth Martin Thomas, "An Elephant in the Consultation Room? Configuring Down Syndrome in British Antenatal Care," *Medical Anthropology Quarterly* 30, no. 2 (2016): 238–58.

85. Nete Schwennesen, Mette Nordahl Svendsen, and Lene Koch, "Beyond Informed Choice: Prenatal Risk Assessment, Decision-Making and Trust," *Clinical Ethics* 5 (2010): 207–16; Nete Schwennsen, "Practicing Informed Choice: Inquiries into the Redistribution of Life, Risk and Relations of Responsibility in Prenatal Decision Making and Knowledge Production" (PhD diss., University of Copenhagen, 2011); Nete Schwennesen and Lene Koch, "Representing and Intervening: 'Doing' Good Care in First Trimester Prenatal Knowledge Production and Decision-Making," *Sociology of Health and Illness* 34 (2012): 283–98. On the contrast between logic of choice and logic of care, see Annemarie Mol, *The Logic of Care: Health and the Problem of Patient Choice* (New York: Routledge, 2008).

86. Mianna Meskus, "Governing Risk through Informed Choice: Prenatal Testing in Welfarist Maternity Care," in *Contested Categories: Life Sciences in Society*, ed. Susanne Bauer and Ayo Wahlberg (Farnham: Ashgate, 2012), 49–68.

87. Stephan Hau, "Is There One Way of Looking at Ethical Dilemmas in Different Cultures?," in *Ethical Dilemmas in Prenatal Diagnosis*, ed. Tamara Fischmann and Elisabeth Hildt (Dordrecht: Springer, 2011), 191–203.

88. Schwennesen, Nordahl Svendsen, and Koch, "Beyond Informed Choice," 208.

89. Neeltje Crombag, Ynke Vellinga, Sandra Kluijfhout, et al., "Explaining Variation in Down's Syndrome Screening Uptake: Comparing the Netherlands with England and Denmark Using Documentary Analysis and Expert Stakeholder Interviews," *BMC Health Services Research* 14 (2014): 437. The links between the uptake of diagnostic tests and their reimbursement by health insurance companies may be more complex. In countries where there is strong support for prenatal testing (e.g., Israel, Vietnam) or, alternatively, where women are afraid of negative pregnancy outcomes, women may be willing to pay out of pocket for many such tests. Tsipy Ivry, "The Ultrasonic Picture Show and the Politics of Threatened Life," *Medical Anthropology Quarterly* 23 (2009): 189–211; Yael Hashiloni-Dolev, "Between Mothers, Fetuses and Society: Reproductive Genetics in the Israeli-Jewish Context," *Nashim* 12 (2006): 129–50; Tine Gammeltoft, "Sonography and Sociality: Obstetrical Ultrasound Imaging in Urban Vietnam," *Medical Anthropology Quarterly* 21 (2007): 133–53.

90. Vassy, Rosman, and Rousseau, "From Policy Making to Service Use."

91. Sophia Rosman, "Down Syndrome Screening Information in Midwifery Practices in the Netherlands: Strategies to Integrate Biomedical Information," *Health* 20 (2016): 94–109. Some Dutch gynecologists are favorable to the extension of prenatal screening for Down syndrome and see the low uptake of such screening as problematic. Melanie Engels, Shama Bhola, Jos Twisk, Marinou Blankstein, and John van

Vugt, "Evaluation of the Introduction of the National Down Syndrome Screening Program in the Netherlands: Age-Related Uptake of Prenatal Screening and Invasive Diagnostic Testing," *European Journal of Obstetrics, Gynecology and Reproductive Biology* 174 (2014): 59–63. In the Netherlands, too, parents of children with Down syndrome face, on average, a greater amount of stress and lowered health-related quality of life. Jan Pieter Marchal, Heleen Maurice-Stam, Janneke Hatzmann, Paul van Trotsenburg, and Martha A. Grootenhuis, "Health Related Quality of Life in Parents of Six- to Eight-Year-Old Children with Down Syndrome," *Research in Developmental Disabilities* 34 (2013): 4239–247.

92. Magdalena Radkowska-Walkowicz, "Potyczki z technologią: Badania prenatalne w ujęciu antropologicznym" [Grappling with technology: Prenatal tests in an anthropological approach], in *Etnografie Biomedycyny* [Ethnographies of biomedicine], ed. Magdalena Radkowska-Walkowicz and Hubert Wierciński (Warsaw: Zakład Antropologii Kulturowej, 2014), 175–90.

93. Polish physicians can, in principle, legally perform an abortion for a fetal indication, but it is extremely difficult for a woman to obtain such an abortion in a public hospital because of the pressure on health professionals willing to provide abortions in the public sector, among other reasons. Joanna Mishtal, "Matters of 'Conscience': The Politics of Reproductive Healthcare in Poland," *Medical Anthropology Quarterly* 23 (2009): 161–83.

94. Schwennesen, Nordahl Svendsen, and Koch, "Beyond Informed Choice"; Schwennesen and Koch, "Representing and Intervening."

95. Elly Teman, Tsipy Ivry, and Barbara Bernhardt, "Pregnancy as a Proclamation of Faith: Ultra-Orthodox Jewish Women Navigating the Uncertainty of Pregnancy and Prenatal Diagnosis," *American Journal of Medical Genetics*, part A 155 (2010): 69–80; Rhoda Ann Kanaaneh, *Birthing the Nation: Strategies of Palestinian Women in Israel* (Berkeley: University of California Press, 2002), 206–28.

96. Michal Sagi, Vardiella Meiner, Nurith Reshef, Judith Dagan, and Joel Zlotogora, "Prenatal Diagnosis of Sex Chromosome Aneuploidy: Possible Reasons for High Rates of Pregnancy Termination," *Prenatal Diagnosis* 21 (2001): 461–65.

97. Yael Hashiloni-Dolev, *A Life (Un)worthy of Living: Reproductive Genetics in Israel and Germany* (Dordrecht: Springer, 2007); Yael Hashiloni-Dolev and Aviad Raz, "Between Social Hypocrisy and Social Responsibility: Professional Views of Eugenics, Disability and Repro-genetics in Germany and Israel," *New Genetics and Society* 29 (2010): 87–102.

98. Yael Hashiloni-Dolev and Noga Weiner, "New Reproductive Technologies, Genetic Counselling and the Standing of the Fetus: Views from Germany and Israel," *Sociology of Health and Illness* 30 (2008): 1055–69.

99. German women share a negative view of abortion for nonlethal fetal conditions; this may account for a somewhat lower uptake in prenatal screening in Germany. Conversely, when faced with a "positive" prenatal diagnosis, German women's decisions are not very different from the decisions of women in other Western European countries: the great majority elect to terminate the pregnancy. Susan L. Erikson, "Post-Diagnostic Abortion in Germany: Reproduction Gone Awry, Again?," *Social Science and Medicine* 56 (2003): 1987–2001.

100. Hashiloni-Dolev and Weiner, "New Reproductive Technologies."

101. Ivry, "The Ultrasonic Picture Show and the Politics of Threatened Life." On Vietnamese women's view of pregnancy as fraught with danger, see Gammeltoft, "Sonography and Sociality."

102. Ibid., 204.

103. Ibid., 207.

104. Dutch, German, and Japanese women are more likely to stay home or work part time only when their children are young than French, Danish, or Israeli women. European Commission, *Female Labour Market Participation*, 2012 data, http://ec.europa .eu/europe2020/pdf/themes/2015/labour_market_participation_women_20151126.pdf (accessed March 23, 2016). On Japan and Israel, see Tsipy Ivry, *Embodying Culture: Pregnancy in Japan and Israel* (New Brunswick, NJ: Rutgers University Press, 2010). An additional important element may be the availability and quality of collective resources for people with Down syndrome, especially those with more severe physical and intellectual impairments.

105. Kristin Luker, *Abortion and Politics of Motherhood* (Berkeley: University of California Press, 1984).

106. In the United States, testing for Down syndrome and other fetal anomalies is often justified by parents' wish to prepare for the birth of a "special needs" child, an argument fully accepted by opponents of selective abortion of trisomic fetuses. As genetic counselor Robert Resta has pointed out, there are very few studies that support—or examine—claims about the advantage of being prepared for the birth of a trisomic child. Robert Resta, "1193 to 4," *The DNA Exchange* blog, September 21, 2015, https:// thednaexchange.com/2015/09/21/1193-to-4/.

Chapter 5 · Sex Chromosome Aneuploidies

1. Henry Turner, "A Syndrome of Infantilism, Congenital Webbed Neck and Cubitus Valgus," *Endocrinology* 23 (1938): 566–74.

2. On the history of sex hormones, see Nelly Oudshoorn, *Beyond the Natural Body: An Archeology of Sex Hormones* (London: Routledge, 1994).

3. Johns Hopkins urologist Hugh Young described surgical methods employed in the interwar era for "correcting" atypical sexual organs, especially male. Hugh Young, *Genital Abnormalities: Hermaphroditism and Related Adrenal Diseases* (Baltimore: Williams and Wilkins Company, 1937).

4. Fuller Albright and Reed Ellsworth, *Uncharted Seas* (Portland, OR: Kalmia Press, 1990), 3. Albright, probably in collaboration with Ellsworth, wrote this text in the 1930s but never published it; it was rediscovered among Albright's papers.

5. Interview with Dr. Henry Turner, conducted by Dr. R. Palmer Howard in 1969. Reproduced in G. Bradley Schaefer and Harris D. Riley, "Tribute to Henry H. Turner, MD (1892–1970): A Pioneer Endocrinologist," *Endocrinologist* 14, no. 4 (2004): 179–84, see esp. 182.

6. In 1937, Hugh Young described the key role of hormones in producing atypical genital organs. Young, *Genital Abnormalities*, 585–615. Young, a professor of urology at Johns Hopkins University, displayed a high degree of tolerance toward atypical anatomy and unorthodox sexual behavior. Conversely, he was also strongly in favor of surgical "correction" of inborn defects of the development of sexual organs.

7. Fuller Albright, Patricia Smith, and Russell Fraser, "A Syndrome Characterized by Primary Ovarian Insufficiency and Decreased Stature: Report of 11 Cases with a Digression on Hormonal Control of Axillary and Pubic Hair," *American Journal of Medical Sciences* 204 (1942): 625–48. On patients as active participants in pioneering endocrinological research, see Renée Fox, *Experiment Perilous: Physicians and Patients Facing the Unknown* (Glencoe, IL: Free Press, 1959).

8. A letter from Fuller Albright to Harry Klinefelter of March 5, 1948, provides a detailed description of the quantification of regrowth of axillary hair in patients. Fuller Albright papers, Francis A. Countway Library of Medicine, Center for the History of Medicine, Albright, Fuller, 1900–1969. Papers, 1904–1964, Countway, H MS c72; see also the testimony of R. Palmer Howard in Schaffer and Riley, "Tribute to Henry H. Turner, MD (1892–1970)," 182.

9. "Symposium on Genetic Disorders of the Endocrine Glands." Anne Pappenheimer Forbes personal and professional papers, 1930–1991. H MS c180. Harvard Medical Library, Francis A. Countway Library of Medicine, Boston, Mass., Box 5, folder 48. The symposium was part of the 150th anniversary meeting of Massachusetts General Hospital, January 31, 1961; the manuscript is an uncorrected transcription of talks given at this symposium. Albright was alive in 1961 but was aphasic and totally incapacitated as a result of a stroke. "Kay" participated in this event.

10. Otto Ullrich, "Turner's Syndrome and Status Bonnevie-Ullrich: A Synthesis of Animal Phenogenetics and Clinical Observations on a Typical Complex of Developmental Anomalies," *American Journal of Human Genetics* 1 (1949): 179–202. The mutant my/my mice originated in stock produced by Clarence Little from an inbreed line of X-ray–irradiated mice. On Little and the production of inbreed mice, see Karen Rader, *Making Mice: Standardizing Animals for American Biomedical Research, 1900–1955* (Princeton, NJ: Princeton University Press, 2004).

11. Ullrich, "Turner's Syndrome and Status Bonnevie-Ullrich," 179.

12. See, for example, Alex Russell and G. I. M. Swyer, "Congenital Ovarian Aplasia with Minimal Evidence of Ullrich-Turner Syndrome," *Proceedings of the Royal Society of Medicine* 45 (1952): 596–98; J. B. Barlow and S. E. Levin, "The Symmetrical Form of the Status Bonnevie-Ullrich (Turner's syndrome)," *British Medical Journal* 1, no. 4918 (1955): 890–93. When this syndrome was defined as a chromosomal anomaly, the majority of researchers adopted the name Turner syndrome.

13. W. P. U. Jackson, "Turner Syndrome in the Female: Congenital Agonadism Combined with Developmental Abnormalities," *British Medical Journal* 2, no. 4932 (1953): 368–71; R. Sougin-Mibashan and W. P. U. Jackson, "Turner Syndrome in the Male," *British Medical Journal* 2, no. 4832 (1953): 371–72.

14. Harry Klinefelter, Edward Reifenstein, and Fuller Albright, "Syndrome Characterized by Gynecomastia, Aspermatogenesis without A-Leydigism, and Increased Secretion of Follicle-Stimulating Hormone," *Journal of Clinical Endocrinology* 2 (1942): 615–27. This study paralleled Albright's study of TS. Albright, Smith, and Fraser, "A Syndrome Characterized by Primary Ovarian Insufficiency and Decreased Stature."

15. Klinefelter initially had difficulties securing funds for his stay in Boston; he finally received a Johns Hopkins traveling scholarship. Despite Albright's initial lack of enthusiasm to receive Klinefelter in his already-crowded laboratory, the two became

good friends, and Albright had a high opinion of Klinefelter's abilities. Correspondence, Klinefelter-Albright, 1940–1956, in Fuller Albright papers, 1940–1956, Francis A. Countway Library of Medicine, Center for the History of Medicine, Countway, H MS c72, box 2, folder 57. Klinefelter's fellowship, he learned later, was a donation by his cousin and mentor, Dr. Walter Baetjer; Harry Klinefelter, "Klinefelter Syndrome: Historical Background and Development," *Southern Medical Journal* 79 (1986): 1089–93, see esp. 1089. In 1942, Klinefelter returned to Johns Hopkins; he was mobilized in 1943. After his demobilization, he returned to Baltimore, where he opened a private practice as an endocrinologist; he also collaborated with Johns Hopkins Hospital's endocrinology division. Lynn Loriaux, "Harry F. Klinefelter, 1912–1990," *Endocrinologist* 19 (2009): 1–4.

16. "Symposium on Genetic Disorders of the Endocrine Glands," Anne Pappenheimer Forbes papers, Countway Library.

17. Klinefelter, Reifenstein, and Albright, "Syndrome Characterized by Gynecomastia."

18. Harry Klinefelter's testimony, in "Symposium on Genetic Disorders of the Endocrine Glands," Anne Pappenheimer Forbes papers, Countway Library.

19. Klinefelter himself believed that this was unfair and that this syndrome should be included among the many diseases described by Albright; he was merely a junior researcher in Albright's laboratory. Klinefelter to Albright, September 25, 1956, Fuller Albright papers, 1940–1956, Francis A. Countway Library of Medicine, Center for the History of Medicine, Countway, H MS c72, box 2, folder 57 (henceforth, correspondence, Klinefelter-Albright); Klinefelter, "Klinefelter Syndrome."

20. See, for example, E. D. William, Eric Engel, and Anna P. Forbes, "Thyroiditis and Gonadal Agenesis," *New England Journal of Medicine* 270 (1964): 805–10; K. Zuppinger, E. Engel, A. P. Forbes, L. Mantooth, and J. Claffey, "Klinefelter's Syndrome: A Clinical and Cytogenetic Study in Twenty-Four Cases," *Acta Endocrinological (Copenhagen)* 54, suppl. 113 (1967): 5–17.

21. C. G. Heller and W. O. Nelson, "Hyalinization of Seminiferous Tubules Associated with Normal or Failing Leyding-Cell Function: Discussion of Relationships to Eunuchoidism, Gynecomastia, Elevated Gonadotrophins, Depressed 17-Ketosteroids, and Estrogens," *Journal of Clinical Endocrinology* 5 (1945): 1–12; F. A. de Balze, R. E. Manoni, F. C. Arriga, and J. Irazu, "Klinefelter's Syndrome: Histo-physiological Basis for a Pathogenic Interpretation," *Proceedings of the Royal Society of Medicine* 46 (1953): 1081–82. Gynecomastia was rapidly eliminated as an obligatory component of KS.

22. Schaffer and Riley, "Tribute to Henry H. Turner, MD (1892–1970)," 182; Klinefelter's testimony, in "Symposium on Genetic Disorders of the Endocrine Glands," Anne Pappenheimer Forbes papers, Countway Library.

23. Doggrel (author unknown) to Murray Barr by Bill Dafoe, February 19, 1953, after Barr's presentation of sex chromatin at the Academy of Medicine, Toronto. Quoted in Fiona Alice Miller, "Your True and Proper Gender: The Barr Body as a Good Enough Science of Sex," *Studies in the History and Philosophy of Biological and Biomedical Sciences* 37 (2006): 459–83, see esp. 459.

24. The origins of the term *gender* in the endocrinology department at Johns Hopkins were studied by Sandra Eder. Sandra Eder, "The Birth of Gender: Clinical Encounters with Hermaphroditic Children at Johns Hopkins (1940–1956)" (PhD diss., Johns Hopkins University, 2011).

25. Murray L. Barr and Ewart G. Bertram, "A Morphological Distinction between Neurons of the Male and the Female, and the Behaviour of the Nuclear Satellite during Accelerated Nucleoprotein Synthesis," *Nature* 163 (1949): 676–77.

26. Murray L. Barr, "Cytogenetics: Some Reminiscences," *BioEssays* 9 (1988): 79–83; Fiona Alice Miller, "A Blueprint for Defining Health: Making Medical Genetics in Canada, 1935–1975" (PhD diss., York University, 2000); Miller, "Your True and Proper Gender."

27. Peter Harper, *First Years of Human Chromosomes: The Beginnings of Human Cytogenetics* (Bloxham: Scion Publishing, 2006), 18–22.

28. K. L. Moore, M. A. Graham, and M. L. Barr, "The Detection of Chromosomal Sex in Hermaphrodites from Skin Biopsy," *Surgery, Gynecology and Obstetrics* 96 (1953): 641–48.

29. Melvin Grumbach, Judson Van Wyk, and Lawson Wilkins, "Chromosomal Sex in Gonadal Dysgenesis (Ovarian Agenesis): Relation to Male Pseudohermaphroditism and Theories of Human Sex Differentiation," *Journal of Clinical Endocrinology and Metabolism* 15 (1955): 1162–63. The redefinition of TS as a male pseudohermaphroditism led to the replacement of the older term *ovarian dysgenesis* by the nongendered term *gonadal dysgenesis*.

30. In the mid-1950s, KS was perceived as a variant of sex inversion and was redefined as a disorder characterized by the "enuchoid body," infertility and a female-type chromosomal pattern. The absence of a female-type chromatin was seen as an indication that the patient does not have KS. W. O. Nelson, "Sex Differences in Human Nuclei with Particular Reference to the Ketosteroid Gonad Agenesis and Other Types of Hermaphrodites," *Acta Endocrinologica* 23 (1956): 227–45.

31. Earl Plunkett and Murray Barr, "Testicular Dysgenesis Affecting the Seminiferous Tubules Principally, with Chromatin Positive Nuclei," *The Lancet* 268 (1956): 853–56; Murray Barr, "Dysgenesis of the Seminiferous Tubes," *British Journal of Urology* 29 (1957): 251–57; Miller, *A Blueprint for Defining Health*, 163–78.

32. Eder, *The Birth of Gender*; Sandra Eder, "The Volatility of Sex: Intersexuality and Clinical Practice in the 1950s," *Gender and History* 22 (2010): 692–707; Sandra Eder, "From 'Following the Push of Nature' to 'Restoring One's Proper Sex'—Cortisone and Sex at Johns Hopkins's Pediatric Endocrinology Clinic," *Endeavor* 36, no. 2 (2012): 69–76.

33. Lawson Wilkins, R. A. Lewis, R. Klein, and E. Rosenberg, "Suppression of Androgen Secretion by Cortisone in a Case of Congenital Adrenal Hyperplasia," *Bulletin of the Johns Hopkins Hospital* 86 (1950): 249–52.

34. John Money, "Hermaphroditism, Gender and Precocity in Hyperadrenocorticism: Psychological Findings," *Bulletin of the Johns Hopkins Hospital* 96 (1955): 253–64; John Money, Joan G. Hampson, and John L. Hampson, "Imprinting and the Establishment of a Gender Role," *Archives of Neurology and Psychiatry* 77 (1957): 333–36.

35. Later, Money (with Anke Ehrhardt) argued that while CAH girls socialized in the feminine gender role were for the most part closer to girls than to boys, some developed "intermediary" psychological profiles and maintained interest in boy's games and interests. John Money and Anke E. Ehrhardt, *Man and Woman, Boy and Girl: The Differentiation of Dimorphism of Gender Identity from Conception to Maturity* (Baltimore: Johns Hopkins University Press, 1972).

36. Johns Hopkins endocrinologists Howard Jones and William Scott argued that physicians should disregard the "true" biological nature of people with TS and KS, and provide treatments (estrogen therapy in TS; testosterone therapy and, when necessary, mastectomy in KS) that will help people with these conditions have fulfilling lives in the sex in which they were socialized. Howard W. Jones and William Wallace Scott, *Hermaphroditism, Genital Anomalies and Related Endocrine Disorders* (Baltimore: Williams and Wilkins Company, 1958), 63–90. KS and TS were included, together with cases of "true" hermaphroditism (the simultaneous presence of male and female sex glands or a mixed gland, ovotestis), in the book's section titled "Intersexuality and Chromosomal Discrepancy."

37. Melvin Grumbach, J. J. van Wyk, and Lawson Wilkins, "Chromosomal Sex in Gonadal Dysgenesis (Ovarian Agenesis): Relationships to Male Pseudohermaphroditism and Theories of Human Sex Differentiation," *Journal of Clinical Endocrinology and Metabolism* 15 (1955): 1161–93, see esp. 1189. See also Barr, "Human Cytogenetics"; Miller, "Your True and Proper Gender." Barr was not entirely comfortable with the definition of TS and KS patients as biological males and biological females, respectively, and proposed more neutral descriptions, such as "chromatin negative" and "chromatin positive" people. Barr, "Human Cytogenetics," 81.

38. John Money, Joan G. Hampson, and John L. Hampson, "Hermaphroditism: Recommendations concerning Assignment of Sex, Change of Sex and Psychological Management," *Bulletin of the Johns Hopkins Hospital* 97 (1955): 284–300; John Money, Joan G. Hampson, and John L. Hampson, "Sexual Incongruities and Psychopathology: The Evidence of Human Hermaphroditism," *Bulletin of the Johns Hopkins Hospital* 98 (1956): 45–57.

39. John Money, Joan G. Hampson, and John L. Hampson, "The Syndrome of Gonadal Agenesis (Ovarian Agenesis) and Male Chromosomal Pattern in Girls and Women: Psychological Studies," *Bulletin of the Johns Hopkins Hospital* 97 (1955): 207–26.

40. Ibid., 224.

41. M. A. Ferguson-Smith, B. Lennox, W. S. Mack, and J. S. Stewart, "Klinefelter Syndrome: Frequency and Testicular Morphology in Relation to Nuclear Sex," *The Lancet* 270 (1957): 167–69.

42. Murray Barr, "Dysgenesis of the Seminiferous Tubules," *British Journal of Urology* 29 (1957): 251–57, see esp. 255.

43. Money, Hampson, and Hampson, "The Syndrome of Gonadal Agenesis (Ovarian Agenesis) and Male Chromosomal Pattern in Girls and Women."

44. Mathilde Danon and Leo Sachs, "Sex Chromosomes and Human Sexual Development," *The Lancet* 270 (1957): 20–25, see esp. 25.

45. Paul Polani, W. F. Hunter, and Bernard Lennox, "Chromosomal Sex in Turner's Syndrome with Coarctation of the Aorta," *The Lancet* 267 (1954): 120–21; Paul E. Polanyi, M. H. Lessof, and P. M. F. Bishop, "Color Blindness in 'Ovarian Agenesis' (Gonadal Dysplasia)," *The Lancet* 268 (1956): 118–20. The title of the second article placed the previous definition of TS as ovarian agenesis in quotation marks: TS individuals were redefined as biological males and therefore could not have "ovarian agenesis," only gonadal dysplasia. On genetic studies of TS and KS in the late 1950s, see Peter Harper, *First Years of Human Chromosomes: The Beginnings of Human Cytogenetics* (Oxford: Scion, 2006), 79–86.

46. Danon and Sachs, "Sex Chromosomes and Human Sexual Development," 22; Miller, "Your True and Proper Gender."

47. Harper, *First Years of Human Chromosomes*. Peter Harper interview with Professor Paul Polanyi, November 12, 2003, *Genetics and Medicine Historical Network*, https://genmedhist.eshg.org/fileadmin/content/website-layout/interviewees-attachments/Polani%2C%20Paul.pdf. Daphne Christie and Doris Zallen, eds., *Genetic Testing*, Witness Seminar in Twentieth-Century Medicine (London: Wellcome Trust, 2002).

48. Charles E. Ford, K. W. Jones, Peter E. Polani, Carlos C. de Almeida, and J. H. Briggs, "A Sex Chromosome Anomaly in a Case of Gonadal Dysgenesis (Turner's Syndrome)," *The Lancet* 273 (1959): 711–13; Patricia A. Jacobs and J. A. Strong, "A Case of Human Intersexuality Showing a Possible XXY Sex Determining Mechanism," *Nature* 183 (1959): 302–303; Monica de Paula Jung, Maria Helena Cabral de Almeida Cardoso, Maria Auxiliadora Monteiro Villar, and Juan Clinton Llerena Jr., "Revisiting Establishment of the Etiology of Turner Syndrome," *Manguinhos* 16 (2009): 361–76.

49. Patricia Jacobs, A. G. Baikie, W. M. Court Brown, T. N. MacGregor, and N. MacLean, "Evidence for the Existence of the Human 'Super Female,'" *The Lancet* 2, no. 7100 (1959): 423–24.

50. See, for example, David Carr, Murray Barr, and Earl Plunkett, "Probable XXYY Sex Determining Mechanism in a Mentally Defective Male with Klinefelter's Syndrome," *Canadian Medical Association Journal* 84 (1961): 873–78; David Carr, Murray Barr, and Earl Plunkett, "An XXXX Sex Chromosome Complex in Two Mentally Defective Females," *Canadian Medical Association Journal* 84 (1961): 131–38; J. R. Ellis, O. J. Miller, L. S. Penrose, and G. E. B Scott, "A Male with XXYY Chromosomes," *Annals of Human Genetics* 25 (1961): 145–51; Murray Barr, David Carr, J. Pozsonyi, et al., "The XXXXY Chromosome Abnormality," *Canadian Medical Association Journal* 87 (1962): 891–901; Irène Uchida, James R. Miller, and Hubert C. Soltan, "Dermatoglyphics Associated with the XXYY Chromosome Complement," *American Journal of Human Genetics* 16 (1964): 284–91.

51. Paul Polani, "The Chromosomes in Ovarian Dysgenesis, Klinefelter's Syndrome, and Translocation Mongolism," *Association for Research in Nervous and Mental Disease* 5 (1962): 78–86; Malcolm Ferguson-Smith, "Chromosome Studies in Klinefelter's Syndrome," *Proceedings of the Royal Society of Medicine* 56 (1963): 557–58.

52. Mary Lyon, "Gene Action in the Mammalian X Chromosome of the Mouse (*Mus musculus L*)," *Nature* 190 (1961): 372–73; Mary Lyon, "Some Milestones in the History of X-Chromosome Inactivation," *Annual Review of Genetics* 26 (1992): 17–28.

53. Interview with Turner in Schaffer and Riley, "Tribute to Henry H. Turner, MD (1892–1970)."

54. Polani, "The Chromosomes in Ovarian Dysgenesis."

55. Women with TS are, as a rule, infertile, but there were a few reports of pregnancy in TS women. Mosaic TS women have fertility problems but some can conceive; their children are at an increased risk of TS and other chromosomal anomalies. David Wasserman and Adrienne Asch, "Reproductive Medicine and Turner Syndrome: Ethical Issues," *Fertility and Sterility* 98 (2012): 792–96.

56. Henry L. Nadler, "Antenatal Detection of Hereditary Disorders," *Pediatrics* 42 (1968): 912–18.

57. Peter Coventry, "The Dynamics of Medical Genetics: The Development and Articulation of Clinical and Technical Services under the NHS, especially at Manchester, c. 1945–1979" (PhD diss., University of Manchester, 2000), chap. 6.

58. Shirley Ratcliffe, "Psychological Investigations of Children with Sex Chromosome Anomalies," Shirley Ratcliffe papers, PP/SRA, Wellcome Collection of Modern Medicine, File PP/SRA/A/1/1. For more on Ratcliffe's studies, see Soraya de Chadarevian, "Putting Human Genetics on a Solid Basis: Chromosome Research, 1950s–1970s," in *Human Heredity in the Twentieth Century*, ed. Bernd Gausemeier, Staffan Müller-Wille, and Edmund Ramsden (London: Pickering and Chatto, 2013), 141–52, see esp. 149–51.

59. Shirley Ratcliffe and D. G. Axworthy, "What Is to Be Done with the XYY Fetus," *British Medical Journal* 2, no. 6191 (1979): 672.

60. Shirley Ratcliffe, "Long-Term Outcome in Children with Sex Chromosome Abnormalities," *Archives of Diseases of Childhood* 80 (1999): 192–95.

61. Ibid.

62. Patricia Jacobs, Muriel Brunton, and Marie Melville, "Aggressive Behaviour, Mental Subnormality and the XYY Male," *Nature* 208 (1965): 1351–52. Jacobs and her co-authors started their text by pointing to "abnormal" behavior in KS men: "It is well known that one percent of males in institutions for the mentally subnormal are chromatin positive and that the majority of those have an XXY sex chromosome constitution." Ibid., 1351.

63. Peter Harper, interview with Professor Patricia Jacobs, February 13, 2004, *Genetics and Medicine Historical Network*, https://genmedhist.eshg.org/fileadmin/content/website-layout/interviewees-attachments/Jacobs%2C%20Pat.pdf. Jacobs recognized that because sex chromosome aneuploidies were studied mainly in prisons and psychiatric hospitals, the frequency of these conditions in the general population and their consequences are not known: see, for example, D. G. Harden and Patricia Jacobs, "Cytogenetics of Abnormal Sexual Development in Men," *British Medical Bulletin* 17 (1961): 206–12. Jacobs nevertheless believed that her 1965 data were not an artefact.

64. Howard W. Jones and William Wallace Scott, *Hermaphroditism, Genital Anomalies and Related Endocrine Disorders*, second edition (Baltimore: Williams and Wilkins Company, 1971), 190–92.

65. Ernest B. Hook and Kristine M. Healy, "Height and Seriousness of Crime in XYY Men," *Journal of Medical Genetics* 14 (1977): 10–12. Hook also found that the XYY karyotype is more prevalent among US whites. Ernest B. Hook, "Racial Differentials in the Prevalence Rates of Males with Sex Chromosome Abnormalities (XXY, XYY) in Security Settings in the United States," *American Journal of Human Genetics* 26 (1974): 504–11.

66. Jan-Dieter Murken, *The XYY Syndrome and Klinefelter Syndrome: Investigations into Epidemiology, Clinical Picture, Psychology, Behavior and Genetics* (Stuttgart: Georg Thieme Publisher, 1973). Murken strongly refuted generalizations about XXY and XYY men. The studied samples, he argued, were too small to make a valid conclusion about the behavior of people with these conditions.

67. James Neel, "Ethical Issues Resulting from Prenatal Diagnosis," in *Early Diagnosis and Human Genetic Defects: Scientific and Ethical Considerations*, ed. Maureen Harris (Bethesda, MD: National Institutes of Health, 1970), 219–29, see esp. 224.

68. Critics of Walzer and Gerald's study did not discuss the inclusion of XXY boys in that study, perhaps because in some cases KS induces "visible" anomalies such as gynecomastia.

69. Jon Beckwith, Dirk Elseviers, Luigi Gorini, Chuck Mandansky, Leslie Csonka, Jonathan King, Wayne H. Davis, and Michael Mage, "Harvard XYY Study," *Science* 187 (1975): 298.

70. Barbara J. Culliton, "XYY: Harvard Researcher under Fire Stops Newborn Screening," *Science* 188 (1975): 1284–85.

71. Critiques of the Harvard experiment declared that "since there is no XYY syndrome and no possible therapy for a non-existing syndrome, no benefit can accrue to the family." Beckwith, Elseviers, Gorini, Mandansky, Csonka, King, Davis, and Mage, "Harvard XYY Study." Walzer claimed that while talk about the "criminal chromosome" is nonsense, there were indications that XYY males may have reading problems and other learning disabilities. Early diagnosis of this condition will therefore favor more efficient remedial interventions. Culliton, "XYY."

72. John Hamerton, "Human Population Cytogenetics: Dilemmas and Problems," *American Journal of Human Genetics* 28 (1976): 107–22; John L. Hamerton, "Ethical Considerations in Newborn Chromosome Screening Programs," in *Sex Chromosome Aneuploidies: Prospective Studies on Children*, ed. Arthur Robinson, Herbert A. Lubs, and Daniel Bergsma (New York: Alan R. Liss, 1976), 267–78.

73. Ernest B. Hook, "Geneticophobia and the Implications of Screening for the XYY Genotype in Newborn Infants," in *Genetics and the Law*, ed. Aubrey Milunsky and George Annas (New York: Plenum Press, 1975), 73–86. Hook argued that there is convincing proof of the association of the XYY genotype with deviance. He attributed this association to a greater difficulty of XYY men to cope with stress. Ernst B. Hook, "Letter to the Editors," *Science* 189 (1975): 1040–41.

74. Aubrey Milunsky, *Know Your Genes: Crucial Information about Hereditary Disorders and Your Personal Risks and Options* (Middlesex: Penguin Books, 1977), 58.

75. Ratcliffe and Axworthy, "What Is to Be Done with the XYY Fetus?," 192.

76. Ratcliffe, "Long-Term Outcomes in Children with Sex Chromosome Abnormalities."

77. Shirley Ratcliffe and Natalie Paul, eds., *Prospective Studies on Children with Sex Chromosome Aneuploidy* (New York: Alan R. Liss, 1986).

78. Stanley Walzer, Antony Bashir, John M. Graham, Annette Sibert, Nicholas Lange, Michale DeNapoli, and Julius Richmond, "Behavioral Development of Boys with X Chromosome Aneuploidy: Impact of Reactive Style on the Educational Intervention for Learning Deficits," in *Prospective Studies on Children with Sex Chromosome Aneuploidy*, 1–21.

79. Some researchers proposed to replace the ethically problematic screening of newborns for sex chromosome aneuploidy with a less problematic screening of consenting adults. Loretta Kopelman, "Ethical Controversies in Medical Research: The Case of XYY Screening," *Perspectives in Biology and Medicine* 21 (1978): 196–204.

80. Usually, TS was not discussed in that context because this condition produces recognizable physical signs. On parents' and specialists' conviction that an early diagnosis of autism is important to improve outcomes, see, for example, Martine Lappé, "Taking Care: Anticipation, Extraction and the Politics of Temporality in Autism Science," *BioSocieties* 9 (2014): 304–28.

81. However, some experts argue that such a consensus was not grounded in reliable evaluations of long-term efficacy of early interventions. Amy S. Herlihy, Robert I. McLachlan, Lynn Gillam, Megan L. Cock, Veronica Collins, and Jane L. Halliday, "The Psychosocial Impact of Klinefelter Syndrome and Factors Influencing Quality of Life," *Genetics in Medicine* 13 (2011): 632–42.

82. C. A. Bondy, "Care of Girls and Women with Turner Syndrome: A Guideline of the Turner Syndrome Study Group," *Journal of Clinical Endocrinology and Metabolism* 92 (2007): 10–25.

83. N. Baena, C. De Vigan, E. Cariati, M. Clementi, C. Stoll, M. R. Caballin, and M. Giuitart, "Turner Syndrome: Evaluation of Prenatal Diagnosis in 19 European Registries," *American Journal of Medical Genetics* 129A (2004): 16–20; N. P. Iyer, D. F. Tucker, S. H. Roberts, M. Moselhi, M. Morgan, and J. W. Matthes, "Outcome of Fetuses with Turner Syndrome: A 10-Year Congenital Anomaly Register Based Study," *Journal of Maternal, Fetal and Neonatal Medicine* 25 (2012): 68–73.

84. Jean-Luc Brun, Flore Gangbo, Zon Qi Wen, Katia Galant, Laurence Tain, Brigitte Maugey-Laulom, Denis Roux, Raphaelle Mangione, Jacques Horovitz, and Robert Saura, "Prenatal Diagnosis and Management of Sex Chromosome Aneuploidy: A Report on 98 Cases," *Prenatal Diagnosis* 24 (2004): 213–18; Hanan A. Hamamy and Sophie Dahoun, "Parental Decisions Following the Prenatal Diagnosis of Sex Chromosome Abnormalities," *European Journal of Obstetrics and Gynecology and Reproductive Biology* 116 (2004): 58–62; Brian L. Shaffer, Aaron B. Caughey, and Mary E. Norton, "Variation in the Decision to Terminate Pregnancy in the Setting of Fetal Aneuploidy," *Prenatal Diagnosis* 26 (2006): 667–71. A cystic hygroma is a collection of fluid-filled sacs (cysts), often in the head or neck region. It develops as a result of a malformation in the lymphatic system and is strongly correlated with the presence of chromosomal anomalies.

85. Wasserman and Asch, "Reproductive Medicine and Turner Syndrome." Wasserman and Asch's view that abortion for TS is always grounded in an irrational fear may be oversimplified. In many cases, TS diagnosis is linked with the presence of a severe hygroma (accumulation of liquid behind a fetus' neck), often associated with other important fetal anomalies. The clinical meaning of a moderate hygroma, especially when detected early in pregnancy, is less clear.

86. Rayna Rapp, "Amniocentesis in Sociocultural Perspective," *Journal of Genetic Counseling* 2, no. 3 (1993): 183–96.

87. Shaffer, Caughey, and Norton, "Variation in the Decision to Terminate Pregnancy in the Setting of Fetal Aneuploidy"; P. Boyd, M. Loanne, B. Koshnood, and H. Dolk for EUROCAT Working Group, "Sex Chromosome Trisomies in Europe: Prevalence, Prenatal Detection and Outcome of Pregnancy," *European Journal of Human Genetics* 19 (2011): 231–34; Arthur Robinson, Mary Linden, and Bruce Bender, "Prenatal Diagnosis of Sex Chromosome Anomalies," in *Genetic Disorders and the Fetus: Diagnosis, Prevention and Treatment*, ed. Aubrey Milunsky (Baltimore: Johns Hopkins University Press, 2008), 249–85.

88. http://www.invs.sante.fr/Dossiers-thematiques/Maladies-chroniques-et-traum atismes/Malformations-congenitales-et-anomalies-chromosomiques/Donnees (accessed March 23, 2016). The percentage of pregnancy terminations for TS in France decreased slightly between the 1980s and the 2010s, a development that was attributed to better genetic counseling for women who received a diagnosis of fetal TS as well as the differ-

entiation between full and mosaic TS. N. Gruchy, F. Vialard, E. Blondel, et al., "Pregnancy Outcomes of Prenatally Diagnosed Turner Syndrome: A French Multicenter Retrospective Study Including a Series of 975 Cases," *Prenatal Diagnosis* 34 (2014): 1–6.

89. A Danish survey revealed that a majority of KS men in Copenhagen were unaware of their condition. A. Bojesen, S. Juul, and C. H. Gravholt, "Prenatal and Postnatal Prevalence of Klinefelter Syndrome: A National Registry Study," *Journal of Clinical Endocrinology and Metabolism* 88 (2003): 622–26.

90. Amy S. Herlihy, Robert I. McLachlan, Lynn Gillam, Megan L. Cock, Veronica Collins, and Jane L. Halliday, "The Psychosocial Impact of Klinefelter Syndrome and Factors Influencing Quality of Life," *Genetics in Medicine* 13 (2011): 632–42.

91. For example, a 2012 publication proposed that treatment with testosterone in young KS boys improves their cognitive abilities, an argument for early detection and early hormonal treatment of this condition. Carole Samango-Sprouse, Teresa Sadeghin, Francine L. Mitchell, Teresa Dixon, Emily Stapleton, Madison Kingery, and Andrea Gropman, "Positive Effects of Short Course Androgen Therapy on the Neurodevelopmental Outcome in Boys with 47,XXY Syndrome at 36 and 72 Months of Age," *American Journal of Medical Genetics* 161A (2013): 501–8.

92. Ian Whitmarsh, Arlene Davis, Debra Skinner, and Donald Bailey, "A Place for Genetic Uncertainty: Parents Valuing an Unknown in the Meaning of Disease," *Social Sciences and Medicine* 65 (2007): 1082–93.

93. M. J. Goetz, E. C. Johnstone, and S. G. Ratcliffe, "Criminality and Antisocial Behaviour in Unselected Men with Sex Chromosome Abnormalities," *Psychological Medicine* 29 (1999): 953–62; Ratcliffe, "Long-Term Outcome in Children of Sex Chromosome Abnormalities."

94. See, for example, Judith L. Ross, Martha P. D. Zeger, Harvey Kushner, Andrew R. Zinn, and David P. Roeltgen, "An Extra X or Y Chromosome: Contrasting the Cognitive and Motor Phenotypes in Childhood in Boys with 47,XYY Syndrome or 47,XXY (Klinefelter Syndrome)," *Deviation and Disability Research Review* 15 (2009): 309–17; Herlihy, McLachlan, Gillam, Cock, Collins, and Halliday, "The Psychosocial Impact of Klinefelter Syndrome and Factors Influencing Quality of Life."

95. Pascale Nivelle, "Francis Heaulme et Didier Gentil aux assises de la Dordogne pour le meurtre d'un appelé," *Liberation*, April 9, 1997; Jean-François Abgrall, "Francis Heaulme n'éprouve ni sentiments ni remords," *Le Point*, March 21, 2013; "Francis Heaulme: psychologie d'un tueur," *France Inter*, August 4, 2014. http://www.franceinter.fr/depeche-francis-heaulme-psychologie-dun-tueur (accessed February 23, 2017).

96. Herlihy, McLachlan, Gillam, Cock, Collins, and Halliday, "The Psychosocial Impact of Klinefelter Syndrome and Factors Influencing Quality of Life."

97. Amy Herlihy and Lynn Gillam, "Thinking Outside the Square: Considering Gender in Klinefelter Syndrome and 47, XXY," *International Journal of Andrology* 34 (2011): e348–e349.

98. Hilgo Bruining, Hanna Swaab, Martien Kas, and Herman van Engeland, "Psychiatric Characteristics in a Self-selected Sample of Boys with Klinefelter Syndrome," *Pediatrics* 123 (2009): 865–70; Martin Cederlöf, Agnes Ohlsson Gotby, Henrik Larsson, et al., "Klinefelter Syndrome and Risk of Psychosis, Autism and ADHD," *Journal of Psychiatric Research* 48 (2014): 128–30; David S. Hong and Allan L. Reiss, "Review: Cognitive and Neurological Aspects of Sex Chromosome Aneuploidies," *Lancet Neurology* 13

(2014): 306–18. These studies point to a four- to sixfold greater risk of psychiatric disorders in individuals with sex chromosome aneuploidy.

99. Linda Blum, *Raising Generation Rx: Mothering Kids with Invisible Disabilities in the Age of Inequality* (New York: New York University Press, 2015).

100. In France, for example, after fourteen weeks of pregnancy, an abortion has to be approved by a pluridisciplinary ethical committee; in some hospitals, such committees nearly always approve an abortion for KS, and in others, they often refuse it. In Israel, the women diagnosed with a KS fetus frequently opt for termination, a decision often encouraged by genetic counselors. Michal Sagi, Vardiella Meiner, Nurith Reshef, Judith Dagan, and Joel Zlotogora, "Prenatal Diagnosis of Sex Chromosome Aneuploidy: Possible Reasons for High Rates of Pregnancy Termination," *Prenatal Diagnosis* 21 (2001): 461–65; Yael Hashiloni-Dolev, "Genetic Counseling for Sex Chromosome Anomalies (SCAs) in Israel and Germany: Assessing Medical Risks according to the Importance of Fertility in Two Cultures," *Medical Anthropology Quarterly* 20 (2006): 469–86. Israeli genetic counselors interrogated by Hashiloni-Dolev and by Sagi and her colleagues do not mention the risk of psychiatric problems in individuals with KS: data on such a risk are relatively recent.

101. A diagnosis of KS before or immediately after birth, one may argue, compromises the child's right to an open future. Joseph Millum, "The Foundation of the Child's Right to an Open Future," *Journal of Social Philosophy* 45 (2014): 522–38.

102. Charles Rosenberg, "The Tyranny of Diagnosis: Specific Entities and Individual Experience," *Milbank Quarterly* 80 (2002): 237–60; Lochlann Jain, "Living in Prognosis: Toward an Elegiac Politics," *Representations* 98 (2007): 77–92.

103. Michael Greene, "Screening for Trisomies in Circulating DNA," *New England Journal of Medicine* 370 (2014): 874–75; Mary Norton, Bo Jacobson, Geeta Swamy, et al., "Cell-Free DNA Analysis for Noninvasive Examination of Trisomy," *New England Journal of Medicine* 372 (2015): 1589–97.

Chapter 6 · Prenatal Diagnosis and New Genomic Approaches

1. Susan Lindee, *Moments of Truth in Genetic Medicine* (Baltimore: Johns Hopkins University Press, 2005); Soraya de Chadarevian, "Mutations in the Nuclear Age," in *Making Mutations: Objects, Practices, Contexts*, ed. Luis Campos and Alexander von Schwerin (Berlin: Max Plank Institute for the History of Science, 2010), 179–88; María Jesús Santesmases, "Size and the Centromere: Translocations and Visual Cultures in Early Human Genetics," in *Making Mutations: Objects, Practices, Contexts*, 189–208.

2. Jérôme Lejeune's laboratory in Paris was one of the main sites of development of the banding technique.

3. Andrew Hogan, "The 'Morbid Anatomy' of the Human Genome: Tracing the Observational and Representational Approaches of Postwar Genetics and Biomedicine," *Medical History* 58 (2014): 315–36; Andrew Hogan, *Life Histories of Genetic Diseases* (Baltimore: Johns Hopkins University Press, 2016).

4. Andrew Hogan, "Locating Genetic Disease: The Impact of Clinical Nosology on Biomedical Conceptions of the Human Genome (1966–1990)," *New Genetics and Society* 32 (2013): 78–96.

5. Multiplex litigation-dependent probe amplification (MPLA) is a variation of the polymerase chain reaction. The rapid amplification of a selected DNA segment allows

experts to quickly check, for example, whether a parent has an anomaly already identified in a child or a fetus.

6. D. Pinkel, J. Langedent, C. Collins, J. Fuscoe, R. Sergraves, J. Lucas, and J. Gray, "Fluorescence In Situ Hybridization with Human Chromosome-Specific Libraries: Detection of Trisomy 21 and Translocations of Chromosome 4," *Proceedings of the National Academy of Science (USA)* 85 (1988): 9128–41; Daniel Navon, "Genomic Designation: How Genetics Can Delineate New, Phenotypically Diffuse Medical Categories," *Social Studies of Science* 41 (2011): 203–26.

7. L. G. Shaffer, C. D. Kashork, R. Saleki, E. Rorem, K. Sundin, B. C. Baliff, and B. A. Bejjani, "Target Genomic Microarray Analysis for Identification of Chromosome Abnormalities in 1500 Consecutive Clinical Cases," *Journal of Pediatrics* 149 (2006): 98–102.

8. Joanna Latimer, *The Gene, the Clinics and the Family* (London: Routledge, 2013). Karen-Sue Taussig made a similar observation in a Dutch clinic. Karen-Sue Taussig, *Ordinary Genomes: Science, Citizenship and Genetic Identities* (Durham, NC: Duke University Press, 2009).

9. See, for example, C. Shaw-Smith, R. Redon, L. Rickman, M. Rio, L. Willatt, H. Fiegler, H. Firth, D. Sanlaville, R. Winter, L. Colleaux, M. Bobrow, and N. P. Carter, "Microarray Based Comparative Genomic Hybridisation (Array-CGH) Detects Submicroscopic Chromosomal Deletions and Duplications in Patients with Learning Disability / Mental Retardation and Dysmorphic Features," *Journal of Medical Genetics* 41 (2004): 241–48; Leigh Anne Flore and Jeff Milunsky, "Updates in the Genetic Evaluation of the Child with Global Developmental Delay or Intellectual Disability," *Seminars in Pediatric Neurology* 19 (2012): 173–80.

10. http://www.rarechromo.org/html/home.asp (assessed February 24, 2017).

11. Kenneth Lyons Jones, Marilyn Crandall Jones, and Miguel Del Campo, *Smith's Recognizable Patterns of Human Malformation*, seventh edition (Philadelphia: Elsevier Saunders, 2013).

12. Jason Homsy, Samir Zaidi, Yufeng Shen, et al., "De Novo Mutations in Congenital Heart Disease with Neurodevelopmental and Other Congenital Anomalies," *Science* 350 (2015): 1262–66.

13. Ibid., 1266.

14. Shaw-Smith, Redon, Rickman, et al., "Microarray Based Comparative Genomic Features Hybridisation (Array-CGH) Detects Submicroscopic Chromosomal Deletions and Duplications."

15. Lisa G. Shaffer, on behalf of the American College of Medical Genetics' (ACMG) Professional Practice and Guidelines Committee, "American College of Medical Genetics Guideline on the Cytogenetic Evaluation of the Individual with Developmental Delay or Mental Retardation," *Genetics in Medicine* 7, no. 9 (2005): 650–54; Leigh and Milunsky, "Updates in the Genetic Evaluation of the Child with Global Developmental Delay or Intellectual Disability."

16. Daniel H. Geschwind and Matthew W. State, "Gene Hunting in Autism Spectrum Disorder: On the Path to Precision Medicine," *The Lancet Neurology*, April 17, 2015, http://dx.doi.org/10.1016/S1474-4422(15)00044-7.

17. Catalina Betancur, "Etiological Heterogeneity in Autism Spectrum Disorders: More Than 100 Genetic and Genomic Disorders and Still Counting," *Brain Research* 380 (2011): 42–77; Heather C. Mefford, Mark L. Batshaw, and Eric P. Hoffman, "Genomics,

Intellectual Disability, and Autism," *New England Journal of Medicine* 366 (2012): 733–43.

18. Charles E. Schwartz and Giovanni Neri, "Autism and Intellectual Disability: Two Sides of the Same Coin," *American Journal of Medical Genetics* 160C (2012): 89–90. This development may be linked with the expansion of the definition of autism from the 1970s and the inclusion in this category of children and adults previously diagnosed with "mental retardation." Gil Eyal with Brendan Hart, Emine Onculer, Neta Oren, and Natasha Rossi, *The Autism Matrix: The Social Origins of the Autism Epidemics* (Cambridge: Polity Press, 2010).

19. Robert Marion, "Autism Spectrum Disorders and the Geneticist: An Approach to the Family," *Exceptional Parent* 41 (2013): 33–36; Daniel Navon and Gil Eyal, "The Trading Zone of Autism Genetics: Examining the Intersection of Genomic and Psychiatric Classification," *BioSocieties* 9 (2014): 329–52.

20. Navon and Eyal, "The Trading Zone of Autism Genetics"; Navon, "Genomic Designation."

21. Brenda Finucane, "What's in a Name? Symptoms versus Causes in the Diagnostic Age," *Exceptional Parent* 35 (2005): 26–27; Joanna Latimer, "Diagnosis, Dysmorphology, and the Family: Knowledge, Motility, Choice," *Medical Anthropology* 26 (2007): 97–138; Navon, "Genomic Designation."

22. Pinkel, Collins, Fuscoe, Sergraves, Lucas, and Gray, "Fluorescence in situ Hybridization with Human Chromosome-Specific Libraries."

23. Bernadette Modell's testimony in *Genetic Testing*, ed. Daphne Christie and Doris Zallen, Witness Seminar in Twentieth-Century Medicine (London: The Wellcome Trust, 2002), 43–45.

24. S. Hillman, J. McMullan, D. Williams, R. Maher, and M. D. Kilby, "Microarray Comparative Genomic Hybridization in Prenatal Diagnosis: A Review," *Ultrasound Obstetrics and Gynecology* 40 (2012): 385–91.

25. On the history of the application of GGH to prenatal diagnosis, see Andrew Hogan, *Life Histories of Genetic Disease: Visibility and Prevention in Postwar Medical Genetics* (Baltimore: Johns Hopkins University Press, 2016).

26. Jonathan Callaway, Lisa Shaffer, Lynn Chitty, Jill Rosenfeld, and John Crolla, "The Clinical Utility of Microarray Technologies Applied to Prenatal Cytogenetics in the Presence of a Normal Conventional Karyotype: A Review of the Literature," *Prenatal Diagnosis* 33 (2013): 1119–23.

27. Ronald Wapner, Christa Lese Martin, Brynn Levy, et al., "Chromosomal Microarray versus Karyotyping for Prenatal Diagnosis," *New England Journal of Medicine* 367 (2012): 2176–84, see esp. 2182–83. CGH mainly detects rare conditions. Most chromosomal anomalies diagnosed before birth are aneuploidies, above all, Down syndrome.

28. ACOG (American College of Obstetricians and Gynecologists): Clinical Management Guidelines for Obstetricians—Gynecologists, "Invasive Prenatal Testing for Aneuploidy," *Obstetrics and Gynecology* 110 (2007): 1459–67.

29. European gynecologists may occasionally prescribe amniocentesis to a woman worried about the possibility of having an impaired child (e.g., because she already had a disabled child or lost a previous pregnancy), even in the absence of a formal indication for this test.

30. Naomi Nakata, Yuemei Wang, and Sucheta Bhatt, "Trends in Prenatal Screening and Diagnostic Testing among Women Referred for Advanced Maternal Age," *Prenatal Diagnosis* 30 (2010): 198–206.

31. Zena Stein, Mervyn Susser, and Andrea Guterman, "Screening Programme for Down Syndrome," *The Lancet* 301 (1973): 305–10.

32. Marian Reiff, Barbara A. Bernhardt, Surabhi Mulchandani, Danielle Soucier, Diana Cornell, Reed E. Pyeritz, and Nancy B. Spinner, "What Does It Mean? Uncertainties in Understanding Results of Chromosomal Microarray Testing," *Genetics in Medicine* 14 (2012): 250–58; Stefan Timmermans, "Trust in Standards: Transitioning Clinical Exome Sequencing from Bench to Bedside," *Social Studies of Science* 45 (2015): 77–99.

33. R. Robyr, J.-P. Bernard, J. Roume, and Y. Ville, "Familial Diseases Revealed by a Fetal Anomaly," *Prenatal Diagnosis* 26 (2006): 1224–34.

34. Stefan Timmermans and his colleagues recently argued that the epistemic uncertainty of variants of unknown significance is productive because it indicates future causality and suggests that genetic causes can explain clinical symptoms, even in cases in which it is not (yet) possible to locate known pathogenic variants. Stefan Timmermans, Caroline Tietbohl, and Eleni Skaperdas, "Narrating Uncertainty: Variants of Uncertain Significance (VUS) in Clinical Exome Sequencing," *BioSocieties* (2016): doi:10.1057/s41292-016-0020-5.

35. John A. Crolla, Ronald Wapner, and Jan M. M. Van Lith, "Controversies in Prenatal Diagnosis 3: Should Everyone Undergoing Invasive Testing Have a Microarray?," *Prenatal Diagnosis* 34, no. 1 (2014): 18–22; Barbara Bernhardt, Danielle Soucier, Karen Hanson, Melissa Savage, Laird Jackson, and Ronald J. Wapner, "Women's Experiences Receiving Abnormal Prenatal Chromosomal Microarray Testing Results," *Genetics in Medicine* 15 (2013): 139–45.

36. Reiff, Bernhardt, Mulchandani, Soucier, Cornell, Pyeritz, and Spinner, "What Does It Mean?"

37. On the potentially dramatic consequences of the imperfect detection of variants of unknown significance, see Robert Resta, "Everybody's Worst Nightmare," *The DNA Exchange* blog, March 6, 2016. https://thednaexchange.com/2016/03/06/everyones-worst-nightmare/. The ClinGen resource collects data on genetic variations in order to help clinical decisions. Heidi Rehm, Jonathan Berg, Lisa Brooks, Carlos Bustamante, James Evans, Melissa Landrum, David Ledbetter, Donna Maglott, Christa Lese Martin, Robert Nussbaum, Sharon Plon, Erin M. Ramos, Stephen Sherry, and Michael Watson for ClinGen, "ClinGen—the Clinical Genome Resource," *New England Journal of Medicine* 372 (2015): 2235–42.

38. Some experts use the term *noninvasive prenatal screening*, or NIPS, to stress the nondefinitive nature of results obtained with this approach. Today, however, the majority of publications employ the acronym NIPT.

39. M. H. Julius, T. Masuda, and L. A. Herzenberg, "Demonstration that Antigen-Binding Cells Are Precursors of Antibody-Producing Cells after Purification with a Fluorescence-Activated Cell Sorter," *Proceedings of the National Academy of Sciences, USA* 69, no. 7 (1972): 1934–38. On the history of FACS, see, for example, Alberto Cambrosio and Peter Keating, "A Matter of FACS: Constituting Novel Entities in Immunology," *Medical Anthropology Quarterly* 6 (1992): 362–84; Peter Keating and Alberto Cambrosio,

"Ours Is an Engineering Approach: Flow Cytometry and the Constitution of Human T-Cell Subsets," *Journal of the History of Biology* 27, no. 3 (1994): 449–79.

40. H. H. R. Hulett, W. A. Bonner, R. G. Sweet, and L. A. Herzenberg, "Development and Application of a Rapid Cell Sorter," *Clinical Chemistry* 19 (1973): 813–16, see esp. 816.

41. Diana Bianchi, "From Michael to Microarrays: 30 Years of Studying Fetal Cells and Nucleic Acids in Maternal Blood," *Prenatal Diagnosis* 30 (2010): 622–23.

42. Bianchi, "From Michael to Microarrays." Herzenberg's wife was 26 years old when she gave birth to a child with Down syndrome. This was perhaps additional motivation for him to look for a simple way to test all pregnant women, including those classified as being at "low risk" of giving birth to a child with Down syndrome.

43. Leonard Herzenberg, Diana Bianchi, Jim Schroder, Howard Cann, and Michael Iverson, "Fetal Cells in the Blood of Pregnant Women: Detection and Enrichment by Fluorescence-Activated Cell Sorting," *Proceedings of the National Academy of Sciences (USA)* 76 (1979): 1453–55. Herzenberg and Bianchi's affirmation that the goal of development of a noninvasive test for Down syndrome is early recognition of large numbers of abnormal fetuses that currently go to term before diagnosis (i.e., giving women the option to abort these fetuses) may be contrasted with Bianchi's recent argument that the main aim of the development of a noninvasive test for Down syndrome is to develop a cure for this condition. Faycal Guedj, Diana W. Bianchi, and Jean-Maurice Delabar, "Prenatal Treatment of Down Syndrome: A Reality?," *Current Opinions in Obstetrics and Gynecology* 26 (2014): 92–103.

44. Michael Iverson, Diana Bianchi, Howard Cann, and Leonard Herzenberg, "Detection and Isolation of Fetal Cells in Maternal Blood Using the Fluorescence-Activated Cell Sorter (FACS)," *Prenatal Diagnosis* 1, no. 1 (1981): 61–73.

45. J. Walknowska, F. A. Conte, and M. M. Grunbach, "Practical and Theoretical Implications of Fetal/Maternal Transfer," *The Lancet* 293 (1969): 1119–23.

46. Diana Bianchi, Gretchen K. Zickwolf, Weil Garry, et al., "Male Fetal Progenitor Cells Persist in Maternal Blood for as Long as 27 Years Postpartum," *Proceedings of the National Academy of Sciences, USA* 93 (1996): 705–708; Kirby Johnson, D. K. Zhen, and Diana Bianchi, "The Use of Fluorescence In Situ Hybridization on Paraffin-Embedded Tissue Sections for the Study of Microchimerism," *Biotechniques* 29 (2000): 1220–24.

47. Editorial, "Microchimerism and Autoimmune Disease," *New England Journal of Medicine* 338 (1998): 1223–25; Diana Bianchi, "Fetomaternal Cell Trafficking: A New Cause of Disease," *American Journal of Medical Genetics* 91 (2000): 22–28.

48. J. Lee Nelson, "Microchimerism: Expanding New Horizon in Human Health or Incidental Remnant of Pregnancy?," *The Lancet* 358, no. 9298 (2001): 2011–12.

49. Dennis Lo, Elena Lo, Neale Watson, Lisa Noakes, et al., "Two-Way Cell Traffic between Mother and Fetus: Biologic and Clinical Implications," *Blood* 88, no. 11 (1996): 4390–95. Interest in maternal-fetal microchimerism diminished in the early twenty-first century but did not disappear altogether. See, for example, Hilary Gammill, Kristina Adams Waldorf, Tessa Aydelotte, et al., "Pregnancy, Microchimerism, and the Maternal Grandmother," *PLoS ONE* 6, no. 8 (2011): e24101.

50. Diana Bianchi, Alan Flint, Mary Frances Pizzimenti, Joan Knoll, and Samuel Latt, "Isolation of Fetal DNA from Nucleated Erythrocytes in Maternal Blood," *Proceedings of the National Academy of Science, USA* 87 (1990): 3279–83.

51. D. W. Bianchi, J. L. Simpson, L. G. Jackson, et al., "Fetal Gender and Aneuploidy Detection Using Fetal Cells in Maternal Blood: Analysis of NIFTY I Data. National Institute of Child Health and Development Fetal Cell Isolation Study," *Prenatal Diagnosis* 22, no. 7 (2002): 609–15. The acronym NIFTY may be confusing, because it is also the name of noninvasive prenatal tests based in the analysis of circulating cfDNA produced by the Chinese biotechnology company BGI and first marketed in 2013.

52. Bianchi, Simpson, Jackson, et al., "Fetal Gender and Aneuploidy Detection Using Fetal Cells in Maternal Blood."

53. Bianchi, "From Michael to Microarrays."

54. In 2016, a Danish group reported on the success of isolating sufficient fetal cells from maternal circulation to make possible an accurate prenatal diagnosis. At the time of the publication, the results were not validated by large-scale trials. Steen Kølvraa, Ripudaman Singh, Elizabeth Normand, et al., "Genome-Wide Copy Number Analysis on DNA from Fetal Cells Isolated from the Blood of Pregnant Women," *Prenatal Diagnosis* 36 (2016): 1–8.

55. Antonio Farina and Diana Bianchi, "Fetal Cells in Maternal Blood as a Second Non-invasive Step for Fetal Down Syndrome Screening," *Prenatal Diagnosis* 18 (1998): 979–86.

56. Diana Bianchi, "Fetal DNA in Maternal Plasma: The Plot Thickens and the Placental Barrier Thins," *American Journal of Human Genetics* 62 (1998): 763–64.

57. On the radical shift in the perception of the placenta, see Aryn Martin and Kelly Holloway, " 'Something There Is That Doesn't Love a Wall': Histories of the Placental Barrier," *Studies in History and Philosophy of Biological and Biomedical Sciences* 47, part B (2014): 300–10, http://www.sciencedirect.com/science/journal/13698486.

58. A dynamic understanding of the relationship between fetal DNA and maternal circulation can recall the change in the understanding of the dynamic of multiplication of the HIV virus in the body in the late 1990s. In both cases, a radical shift in the perception of a biological phenomenon was made possible by the development of new technology for the study of nucleic acids, the polymerase chain reaction.

59. Bianchi, "From Michael to Microarrays," 623. A review published in 2011 still evoked the uncertain commercial future of cfDNA-based prenatal tests. Sinuhe Hahn, Olav Lapaire, Sevgi Tercanli, Varaprasad Kolla, and Irene Hösli, "Determination of Fetal Chromosome Aberrations from Fetal DNA in Maternal Blood: Has the Challenge Finally Been Met?," *Expert Reviews in Molecular Medicine* 13, no. e6 (2011): doi:10.1017/S1462399411001852.

60. Kevin Davies, "In Conversation: Tufts Geneticist Diana Bianchi on Noninvasive Prenatal Testing," *BioIT World*, November 5, 2012. www.bio-itworld.com/2012/11/05/tufts-geneticist-bianchi-noninvasive-prenatal-testing.html.

61. On Lo's trajectory, see Misia Landau, "Yuk-Ming Dennis Lo," *Clinical Chemistry* 58 (2012): 784–86; Zoe Corbyn, "Dennis Lo: Should Parents Be Told about a Disease Their Child Might Get?," *The Guardian*, September 3, 2013, https://www.theguardian.com/science/2013/sep/01/dennis-lo-prenatal-research-cancer; Y. M. Dennis Lo, "Noninvasive Prenatal Diagnosis: From Dream to Reality," *Clinical Chemistry* 61 (2015): 32–37.

62. Y. M. D. Lo, P. Patel, J. S. Wainscoat, M. Sampietro, M. D. G. Gillmer, and K. A. Fleming, "Prenatal Sex Determination by DNA Amplification from Maternal Peripheral Blood," *The Lancet* 334 (1989): 1363–65, see esp. 1365.

63. Y. M. D. Lo, P. J. Bowell, M. Selinger, et al. "Prenatal Determination of Fetal RhD Status by Analysis of Peripheral Blood of Rhesus Negative Mothers," *The Lancet* 341, no. 8853 (1993): 1147–48, see esp. 1148.

64. See, for example, M. Stroun, P. Anker, P. Maurice, J. Lyautey, C. Lederrey, and M. Beljanski, "Neoplastic Characteristics of the DNA Found in the Plasma of Cancer Patients," *Oncology* 46 (1989): 318–22; H. E. Mulcahy, D. T. Croke, and M. J. G. Farthing, "Cancer and Mutant DNA in Blood Plasma," *The Lancet* 348 (1996): 628–29.

65. Y. M. Dennis Lo, Noemi Corbetta, Paul Chamberlain, Vik Rai, Ian Sargent, Christopher Redman, and James Wainscoat, "Presence of Fetal DNA in Maternal Plasma and Serum," *The Lancet* 350 (1997): 485–87. For comment, see Bianchi, "Fetal DNA in Maternal Plasma."

66. Landau, "Yuk-Ming Dennis Lo"; Corbyn, "Dennis Lo"; Dennis Lo, "Noninvasive Prenatal Diagnosis."

67. Y. M. Dennis Lo, Magnus Hjelm, C. Fidler, et al., "Prenatal Diagnosis of Fetal Rh Status by Molecular Analysis of Maternal Plasma," *New England Journal of Medicine* 339 (1998): 1734–38.

68. Y. M. Dennis Lo, Tze K. Lau, Jun Zhang, Tse N. Leung, Allan M. Chang, Magnus Hjelm, Sarah Elmes, and Diana Bianchi, "Increased Fetal DNA Concentrations in the Plasma of Pregnant Women Carrying Fetuses with Trisomy 21," *Clinical Chemistry* 45 (1999): 1747–51.

69. Stephan C. Schuster, "Next-Generation Sequencing Transforms Today's Biology," *Nature Methods* 5 (2008): 16–18.

70. The development of next-generation sequencing also paved the way for diagnostic uses of free-circulating tumor DNA. See, for example, Mark Roschewski, Kieron Dunleavy, Stefania Pittaluga, et al., "Circulating Tumor DNA and CT Monitoring in Patients with Untreated Diffuse Large B-Cell Lymphoma: A Correlative Biomarker Study," *The Lancet Oncology* 16 (2015): 541–49.

71. H. Christina Fan, Yair J. Blumenfeld, Usha Chitkara, Louanne Hudgins, and Stephen R. Quake, "Noninvasive Diagnosis of Fetal Aneuploidy by Shotgun Sequencing DNA from Maternal Blood," *Proceedings of the National Academy of Sciences (USA)* 105 (2008): 16266–71; Rossa Chiu, Allen Chan, Yuan Gao, et al., "Noninvasive Prenatal Diagnosis of Fetal Chromosomal Aneuploidy by Massively Parallel Genomic Sequencing of DNA in Maternal Plasma," *Proceedings of the National Academy of Sciences (USA)* 105 (2008): 20458–63. The article of Lo's group (Rossa et al.) was published slightly later than the one of Quake's group, an important argument in the following patent wars.

72. Landau, "Yuk-Ming Dennis Lo," 784.

73. Some experts argued that, for technical reasons, the list of chromosomal anomalies detected by NIPT may remain relatively short. Kitty Lo, Evangelia Karampetsou, Christopher Lefkowitz, Fiona McKay, Sarah Mason, Melissa Hill, Vincent Plagnol, and Lyn Chitty, "Limited Clinical Utility of Non-invasive Prenatal Testing for Subchromosomal Abnormalities," *American Journal of Human Genetics* (2016): http://dx.doi.org/10 .1016/j.ajhg.2015.11.016.

74. G. E. Palomaki, E. M. Kloza, G. M. Lambert-Messerlian, et al., "DNA Sequencing of Maternal Plasma to Detect Down Syndrome: An International Clinical Validation Study," *Genetics in Medicine* 13 (2011): 913–20; M. Ehrich, C. Deciu, T. Zwiefelhofer, et al., "Noninvasive Detection of Fetal Trisomy 21 by Sequencing of DNA in Maternal Blood: A

Study in a Clinical Setting," *American Journal of Obstetrics and Gynecology* 204 (2011): 205–11.

75. G. E. Palomaki, C. Deciu, E. M. Kloza, et al., "DNA Sequencing of Maternal Plasma Reliably Identifies Trisomy 18 and Trisomy 13 as Well as Down Syndrome: An International Collaborative Study," *Genetics in Medicine* 14 (2012): 296–305.

76. Ashwin Agarwal, Lauren C. Sayres, Mildred K. Cho, Robert Cook-Deegan, and Subhashini Chandrasekharan, "Commercial Landscape of Noninvasive Prenatal Testing in the United States," *Prenatal Diagnosis* 33 (2013): 521–31.

77. Erika Check Hayden, "Fetal Tests Spur Legal Battle," *Nature* 486 (2012): 453–54; Anonymous, "Illumina and Sequenom Pool Noninvasive Prenatal Testing Intellectual Property and End Outstanding Patent Disputes," *Business Wire*, December 3, 2014, http://investor.illumina.com/phoenix.zhtml?c=121127&p=irol-newsArticle_print&ID=1994454.

78. Julia Karow, "NIPT Landscape Shifts in 2014 as Providers Transfer Technology, Plan IVDs," *Genome Web*, January 8, 2015, https://www.genomeweb.com/molecular-diagnostics/nipt-landscape-shifts-2014-providers-transfer-technology-plan-ivds; Mark Ratner, "Roche Swallows Ariosa, Grabs Slice of Prenatal Test Market," *Nature Biotechnology* 33 (2015): 113–14.

79. For a good explanation for why the information provided by NIPT producers, while not false, may be grossly misleading, see Katie Stoll, "NPIS Is Not Diagnostic—Convincing Our Patients and Convincing Ourselves," *The DNA Exchange* blog, July 11, 2013, http://thednaexchange.com/2013/07/11/guest-post-nips-is-not-diagnostic-convincing-our-patients-and-convincing-ourselves/. An editorial of *Scientific American* criticized in 2016 the low positive predictive value of NIPT. Editorial, "We Need More Proof That Prenatal Gene Screens Are Beneficial," *Scientific American*, February 1, 2016, https://www.scientificamerican.com/article/we-need-more-proof-that-prenatal-gene-screens-are-beneficial/.

80. Diana Bianchi, R. Lamar Parker, Jeffrey Wentworth, et al., for the CARE study group, "DNA Sequencing versus Standard Prenatal Aneuploidy Screening," *New England Journal of Medicine* 370 (2014): 799–808; Michael Greene, "Screening for Trisomies in Circulating DNA," *New England Journal of Medicine* 370 (2014): 874–75.

81. NIPT does not always yield reliable results. For example, this test is less efficient in overweight women. Eric Wang, Annette Batey, Craig Struble, Thomas Musci, Ken Song, and Arnold Oliphant, "Gestational Age and Maternal Weight Effects on Fetal Cell-Free DNA in Maternal Plasma," *Prenatal Diagnosis* 33 (2013): 662–66. In 2015, experts evaluated that about 1%–8% of tests (depending on the provider) returned without a test result. Lisa Demers and Stephanie Snow, "Guest Post: Sometimes It's Okay to Fail," *The DNA Exchange* blog, August 17, 2015, https://thednaexchange.com/2015/08/17/guest-post-sometimes-its-okay-to-fail/.

82. Mary Norton, Bo Jacobson, Geeta Swamy, et al., "Cell-Free DNA Analysis for Noninvasive Examination of Trisomy," *New England Journal of Medicine* 372 (2015): 1589–97.

83. These points are discussed, for example, in a background paper on NIPT published by the Nuffield Council on Bioethics. Vardit Ravitsky, "Noninvasive Prenatal Testing (NIPT): Identifying Key Clinical, Ethical, Social, Legal and Policy Issues," background paper, Nuffield Council on Bioethics, November 8, 2015. http://nuffieldbioethics.org/wp-content/uploads/NIPT-background-paper-8-Nov-2015-FINAL.pdf.

84. Erika Check Hayden, "Fetal Gene Screening Comes to the Market," *Nature* 478 (2011): 440.

85. A study conducted in Hong Kong concluded that the majority of women who underwent NIPT wished to be informed about a "positive" sex chromosome aneuploidy result. Tze Kin Lau, Mei Ki Chan, Pui Shan Salome Lo, et al., "Non-invasive Prenatal Screening of Fetal Sex Chromosomal Abnormalities: Perspective of Pregnant Women," *Journal of Maternal-Fetal and Neonatal Medicine* (2012): 2616–19. It is not excluded that women in other countries have different preferences.

86. Marc Dommergues, Laurent Mandelbrot, Dominique Mahieu-Caputo, Noel Boudjema, Isabelle Durand-Zaleski, and the ICI Group-Club de médecine fœtale, "Termination of Pregnancy Following Prenatal Diagnosis in France: How Severe Are the Foetal Anomalies?," *Prenatal Diagnosis* 30 (2010): 531–39.

87. Yanlin Wang, Yan Chen, Feng Tian, Jianguang Zhang, Zhuo Song, Yi Wu, Xu Han, Wenjing Hu, Duan Ma, David Cram, and Weiwei Cheng, "Maternal Mosaicism Is a Significant Contributor to Discordant Sex Chromosomal Aneuploidies Associated with Noninvasive Prenatal Testing," *Clinical Chemistry* 60 (2014): 1251–59. Since these women were pregnant, they might have had mosaic Turner syndrome.

88. C. Michael Osborne, Emily Hardisty, Patricia Devers, Kathleen Kaiser-Rogers, Melissa A. Hayden, William Goodnight, and Neeta L. Vora, "Discordant Noninvasive Prenatal Testing Results in a Patient Subsequently Diagnosed with Metastatic Disease," *Prenatal Diagnosis* 33 (2013): 1–3; Molika Ashford, "Patient's NIPT Cancer Dx Highlights Lack of Standards for Consent, Return of Secondary Findings," *Genome Web*, March 10, 2015, https://www.genomeweb.com/molecular-diagnostics/patients-nipt-cancer-dx-high lights-lack-standards-consent-return-secondary; Diana Bianchi, "Pregnancy: Prepare for Unexpected Prenatal Test Results," *Nature* 522, no. 7554 (2015): 29–30.

89. On the experience of a very early miscarriage, see Sally Han, "The Chemical Pregnancy: Technology, Mothering and the Making of a Reproductive Experience," *Journal of the Motherhood Initiative* 5 (2015): 42–53.

90. On women's reluctance to make their pregnancy public before the second trimester because of a high probability of first trimester pregnancy loss, see, for example, Zoe Williams, "With Miscarriage, There Are Many Routes to Shame," *The Guardian*, August 2, 2015, https://www.theguardian.com/commentisfree/2015/aug/02/social -media-miscarriage-mark-zuckerberg-pregnancy; Emily Jane Ross, " 'I Think It's Self-Preservation': Risk Perception and Secrecy in Early Pregnancy," *Health, Risk and Society* 17 (2015): 329–48.

91. This was, for example, the experience of the disability activist Chloe Atkins, who compared her measured reaction to the loss of one of her triplets produced by IVF in an early stage of pregnancy with her deep distress over the demise of one of the remaining fetuses in a much more advanced stage of pregnancy. Chloe Atkins, "The Choice of Two Mothers: Disability, Gender, Sexuality and Prenatal Testing," *Cultural Studies* 8 (2008): 106–29, see esp. 122–23. Conversely, some women are deeply distressed by an early pregnancy loss. Helen Statham, "Prenatal Diagnosis of Fetal Abnormality: The Decision to Terminate the Pregnancy and the Psychological Consequences," *Fetal and Maternal Medicine Review* 13 (2002): 213–47.

92. Patricia Taneja, Holly Snyder, Eileen de Feo, Kristina Kruglyak, Meredith Halks-Miller, Kirsten Curnow, and Sucheta Bhatt, "Noninvasive Prenatal Testing in the General

Obstetric Population: Clinical Performance and Counseling Considerations in over 85000 Cases," *Prenatal Diagnosis* 36 (2016): 237–43. This article was sponsored by Illumina.

93. Henry Greely and Jaime King evoked in 2010 the potential consequences of a shift toward an earlier diagnosis of fetal malformations, but, like many other scholars did, they mainly focused on the risks of "reproductive selection," especially of the child's sex. Henry Greely and Jaime King, "The Coming Revolution in Prenatal Genetic Testing," *AAA Professional Ethics Report* 23 (2010): 1–8, see esp. 3; Jaime King, "And Genetic Testing for All . . . The Coming Revolution in Non-invasive Prenatal Genetic Testing," *Rutgers Law Journal* 42 (2011): 599–658.

94. Pe'er Dar, Kirsten J. Curnow, Susan Gross, et al., "Clinical Experience and Follow-up with Large Scale Single-Nucleotide Polymorphism-Based Noninvasive Prenatal Aneuploidy Testing," *American Journal of Obstetrics and Gynecology* 211 (2014): 527.e1–527.e17. doi:10.1016/j.ajog.2014.08.006. It is not clear how representative this study is.

95. Erika Check Hayden, "Prenatal-Screening Companies Expand Scope of DNA Tests, but the Increasingly Accurate Analyses Carry the Ethical Dilemma of Uncertain Outcomes," *Nature* 507 (2014): 19; Davies, "Tufts Geneticist Diana Bianchi on Noninvasive Prenatal Testing."

96. Neeta Vora and Barbara O'Brien, "Correspondence," *Obstetrics and Gynecology* 124 (2014): 379–80.

97. In 2016, several groups affirmed that NIPT can reliably detect fetal copy number variants. R. Li, J. Wan, Y. Zhang, F. Fu, Y. Ou, X. Jing, J. Li, D. Li, and C. Liao, "Detection of Fetal Copy Number Variants by Non-invasive Prenatal Testing for Common Aneuploidies," *Ultrasound Obstetrics and Gynecology* 47 (2016): 53–57; Roy Lefkowitz, John Tynan, Tong Liu, Yijin Wu, Amin Mazloom, Eyad Almasri, Grant Hogg, Vach Angkachatchai, Chen Zhao, Daniel Grosu, Graham Mclennan, and Mathias Ehrich, "Clinical Validation of a Noninvasive Prenatal Test for Genome-Wide Detection of Fetal Copy Number Variants," *American Journal of Obstetrics and Gynecology* 215, no. 2 (2016): 227.e1–227.e16. The latter paper was written by scientists who work with Sequenom.

98. Davies, "Tufts Geneticist Diana Bianchi on Noninvasive Prenatal Testing."

99. Thomas Musci, Genevieve Fairbrother, Annette Batey, Jennifer Bruursema, Craig Struble, and Ken Song, "Non-invasive Prenatal Testing with Cell-Free DNA: US Physician Attitudes toward Implementation in Clinical Practice," *Prenatal Diagnosis* 33 (2013): 424–28; Lori Haymon, Eve Simi, Kelly Moyer, Sharon Aufox, and David Ouyang, "Clinical Implementation of Noninvasive Prenatal Testing among Maternal Fetal Medicine Specialists," *Prenatal Diagnosis* 34 (2014): 416–23.

100. Wybo Dondorp, G. C. M. Page-Christiaens, and Guido de Wert, "Genomic Futures of Prenatal Screening: Ethical Reflection," *Clinical Genetics* 89, no. 5 (2016): 531–38.

101. Taneja, Snyder, de Feo, Kruglyak, Halks-Miller, Curnow, and Bhatt, "Noninvasive Prenatal Testing in the General Obstetric Population."

102. Nanalyse, "Warning: The NIPT Growth Story May Be Ending," June 9, 2015, http://www.nanalyze.com/2015/06/warning-the-nipt-growth-story-may-be-ending/. The warning was relative: financial experts predicted the continuation of an increase in demand for NIPT, but also an increasingly competitive market, and therefore a slowdown of growth of producers' profits.

103. Neeta Vora and Barbara O'Brien, "Noninvasive Prenatal Testing for Microdeletion Syndromes and Expanded Trisomies: Proceed with Caution," *Obstetrics and Gynecology* 123 (2014): 1097–99. Sequenom scientists energetically defended their offer of tests for microdeletions, arguing that their studies displayed the efficacy of tests for microdeletions because they indicate a much higher than average probability of such deletions. Allan Bombard, Daniel Farkas, Thomas Monroe, and Juan Sebastian Sakdivar, "Correspondence," *Obstetrics and Gynecology* 124 (2014): 379.

104. Karow, "NIPT Landscape Shifts in 2014 as Providers Transfer Technology, Plan IVDs."

105. The biotechnology company BGI (Beijing Genomic Institute), founded in 1999 in Beijing, is located today in Shenzhen in the Guangdong province. It claims to be the greatest genomic science center in the world. Michael Specter, "The Gene Factory," *The New Yorker*, January 6, 2014, http://www.newyorker.com/magazine/2014/01/06/the-gene-factory.

106. Heather Skirton, Lesley Goldsmith, Leigh Jackson, Celine Lewis, and Lyn Chitty, "Offering Prenatal Diagnostic Tests: European Guidelines for Clinical Practice," *European Journal of Human Genetics* 22 (2014): 580–86.

107. Wybo Dondorp, Guido de Wert, Yvonne Bombard, et al., on behalf of the European Society of Human Genetics (ESHG) and the American Society of Human Genetics (ASHG), "Non-invasive Prenatal Testing for Aneuploidy and Beyond: Challenges of Responsible Innovation in Prenatal Screening," *European Journal of Human Genetics* 23, no. 11 (2015): 1438–50, see esp. 1444. On the child's right to an open future, see Joseph Millum, "The Foundation of the Child's Right to an Open Future," *Journal of Social Philosophy* 45 (2014): 522–38.

108. In 2016, national health systems in France and the United Kingdom negotiated with NIPT producers the replacement of serum screening for Down syndrome with NIPT, limited to the detection of major autosomal aneuploidies.

109. Megan Allyse, Mollie A Minear, Elisa Berson, Shilpa Sridhar, Margaret Rote, Anthony Hung, and Subhashini Chandrasekharan, "Non-invasive Prenatal Testing: A Review of International Implementation and Challenges," *International Journal of Women's Health* 7 (2015): 113–26, see esp. 119.

110. Illegal does not mean rare: In 2010, one in every five Brazilian women was reported to have had an abortion. It means, however, that only affluent women have access to safe abortions. Debora Diniz and Marcelo Medeiros, "Aborto no Brasil: uma pesquisa domiciliar com técnica de urna," *Ciencia e Saude Publica* 15, suppl. 1 (2010): 2105–12.

111. Jairnilson Paim, Claudia Travassos, Celia Almeida, Ligia Bahia, and James Macinko, "The Brazilian Health System: History, Advances, and Challenges," *The Lancet* 377, no. 9779 (2011): 1778–97.

112. C. Lewis, M. Hill, H. Skirton, and L. Chitty, "Non-invasive Prenatal Diagnosis for Fetal Sex Determination: Benefits and Disadvantages from the Service Users' Perspective," *European Journal of Human Genetics* 20 (2012): 1127–33.

113. Renata Moscolini Romão, José Eduardo Levi, Mário Henrique Burlacchini de Caravalho, et al., "Use of Cell-Free Fetal Nucleic Acids in Maternal Blood for Prenatal Diagnosis: The Reality of This Scenario in Brazil," *Revista de Associaao Medica Brasileira* 58 (2012): 615–19.

114. Dafne Dain Gandelman Horovitz, Victor Evangelista de Faria Ferraz, Sulamis Dain, and Antonia Paula Marques-de-Faria, "Genetic Services and Testing in Brazil," *Journal of Community Genetics* 4 (2013): 355–75.

115. Ricardo Senra, "'Aborto já é livre no Brasil: Proibir é punir quem não tem dinheiro,' diz Drauzio Varella," *BBC Brazil*, February 2, 2016, http://www.bbc.com/portuguese /noticias/2016/02/160201_drauzio_aborto_rs. On upper-class Brazilian women's access to abortion for fetal indications, see Véronique Mirlesse, "Diagnostic prénatal et médecine fœtale: Du cadre des pratiques à l'anticipation du handicap. Comparaison France–Brésil" (PhD diss., Université Paris Sud–Paris XI, 2014). In Argentina, too, NIPT is accessible only to upper-class women, as is access to illegal, but safe, abortion. Lucas Otañoa and Laura Igarzábal, "Noninvasive Prenatal Testing for Fetal Aneuploidy in Argentina," *AJOB Empirical Bioethics* 6 (2015): 111–14.

116. José Eduardo Levi, Silvano Wendel, Deise Tihe Takaoka, and Ciro Dresch Martinhago, "Determinação pré-natal do sexo fetal por meio da análise de DNA no plasma materno," *Revista Brasileira de Ginecologia e Obstetrícia* 25 (2003): 687–89; Ciro Dresch Martinhago, Ricardo Manoel de Oliveira, Maria do Carmo Tomitao Canas, et al., "Accuracy of Fetal Gender Determination in Maternal Plasma at 5 and 6 Weeks of Pregnancy," *Prenatal Diagnosis* 26 (2006): 1219–23.

117. Caroline Wright, Yinghui Wei, Julian Higgins, and Gurdeep Sagoo, "Noninvasive Prenatal Diagnostic Test Accuracy for Fetal Sex Using Cell-Free DNA: A Review and Meta-analysis," *BMC Research Notes* 5 (2012): 476–77.

118. Audrey R. Chapman and Peter A. Benn, "Noninvasive Early Sex Determination: A Few Benefits and Many Concerns," *Perspectives in Biology and Medicine* 56 (2013): 530–47. The use of ultrasound to select the "right" fetuses (i.e., male fetuses) is problematic not only in countries with a strong preference for sons, such as India or China, but also in migrant communities abroad. Sunita Puri, Vincanne Adams, Susan Ivey, and Robert D. Nachtigall, "'There Is Such a Thing as Too Many Daughters, but Not Too Many Sons': A Qualitative Study of Son Preference and Fetal Sex Selection among Indian Immigrants in the United States," *Social Science and Medicine* 72 (2011): 1169–76. Women pregnant with a female fetus diagnosed with congenital adrenal hyperplasia are treated with dexamethasone to prevent the "virilization" of the fetus' genital organs. Some researchers have criticized this treatment on ethical grounds. Alice Dreger, Ellen K. Feder, and Anne Tamar-Mattis, "Prenatal Dexamethasone for Congenital Adrenal Hyperplasia: An Ethics Canary in the Modern Medical Mine," *Bioethical Inquiry* 9 (2012): 277–94.

119. Ross, "'I Think It's Self-Preservation.'"

120. Lilian Krakowski Chazan described the importance of learning the fetal sex for their inclusion in the family narrative. Lilian Krakowski Chazan, "'É . . . tá grávida mesmo! E ele é lindo!' A construção de 'verdades' na ultra-sonografia obstétrica," *Manguinhos* 15 (2008): 99–116. Brazilian physicians also explained the popularity of tests that detect fetal sex early in pregnancy by the fact that such tests allow women to start shopping for their future child abroad, especially in Florida, a popular shopping outlet for upper-class Brazilians. This explanation seems to be widely accepted in Brazil, although it may be inaccurate.

121. On the globalization of NIPT, see Subhashini Chandrasekharan, Mollie A. Minear, Anthony Hung, and Megan Allyse, "Noninvasive Prenatal Testing Goes Global,"

Science Translational Medicine 6, no. 231 (2014): 231fs15, doi:10.1126/scitranslmed.3008704; Mollie Minear, Celine Lewis, Subarna Pradhan, and Subhashini Chandrasekharan, "Global Perspectives on Clinical Adoption of NIPT," *Prenatal Diagnosis* 35, no. 10 (2015): 959–67.

122. "Ariosa Diagnostics and Fleury Group Announce Offering of the Highly Accurate Harmony Prenatal Test in Brazil to Assess Risk for Chromosome Conditions in Singleton and Twin Pregnancies," *Ariosa Diagnostic News*, September 12, 2013, http://www.prnewswire.com/news-releases/ariosa-diagnostics-and-fleury-group-announce-offering-of-the-highly-accurate-harmony-prenatal-test-in-brazil-to-assess-risk-for-chromosome-conditions-in-singleton-and-twin-pregnancies-223453321.html; DASA Group to Provide Natera's Panorama Non-invasive Prenatal Test for Detection of Chromosomal Abnormalities, Such as Down Syndrome, from the Ninth Week of Gestation, *Business Wire*, August 8, 2013, http://www.businesswire.com/news/home/20130808005340/en/DASA-Group-Provide-Natera%E2%80%99s-Panorama%E2%84%A2-Non-Invasive-Prenatal.

123. Fábio Rossi, "Em busca do DNA perfeito," *O Globo*, February 23, 2012; Luna D'Alama, "Exame de sangue que vê síndrome de Down em feto chega ao Brasil," *O Globo*, January 23, 2013. Down syndrome is often presented in the Brazilian press and media as a difference, not a disability, with a strong focus on the blessings of having an "angel-child." Ana Cristina Bohrer Gilbert, *Vertice do impensável: um estudo de narrativas em síndrome de Down* (Rio de Janeiro: Editora Fiocruz, 2012).

124. These deletions are DiGeorge syndrome (22q11.3 deletion), cri du chat syndrome (5p deletion), 1p36 deletion syndrome, Angelman syndrome (maternal 15q11-13 deletion), and Prader-Willi syndrome (paternal 15q11-13 deletion).

125. "Bebe saudvel, gravidez tranquila, a partir de 9 semanes de gestacao," http://www.laboratoriogene.com.br/exames/nipt-teste-pre-natal-nao-invasivo-em-sangue-materno/. Laboratório Gene was founded by well-known Brazilian geneticist Sergio Pena.

126. Hayden, "Prenatal Screening Companies Expand the Scope of DNA Tests"; Davies, "Tufts Geneticist Diana Bianchi on Noninvasive Prenatal Testing."

127. The data were presented in a Natera leaflet intended for the Brazilian market. The estimates of frequency of the described syndromes vary according to sources and may be inaccurate, especially when dealing with very rare syndromes and those that, like DiGeorge syndrome, are not diagnosed in some mutation carriers.

128. A 2015 evaluation of tests for major chromosomal deletions found that positive predictive value (i.e., the chance that a woman who tests positive indeed carried an affected fetus) is low (less than 5%). Conversely, some experts estimate that, while imperfect, NIPT should be able to spot about 70% of fetuses with deletions. Ronald Wapner, Joshua Babiarz, Brynn Levy, Melissa Stosic, Bernhard Zimmermann, Styrmir Sigurjonsson, Nicholas Wayham, Allison Ryan, Milena Banjevic, Phil Lacroute, Jing Hu, Megan P. Hall, Zachary Demko, Asim Siddiqui, Matthew Rabinowitz, Susan Gross, Matthew Hill, and Peter Benn, "Expanding the Scope of Noninvasive Prenatal Testing: Detection of Fetal Microdeletion Syndromes," *American Journal of Obstetrics and Gynecology* 212 (2015): 332.e1-9.

129. On the origins of the nomenclature of chromosomal segments, see Hogan, "The 'Morbid Anatomy' of the Human Genome."

130. Wai Lun, Alan Fung, Nancy J. Butcher, Gregory Costain, et al., "Practical Guidelines for Managing Adults with 22q11.2 Deletion Syndrome," *Genetics in Medicine* 17 (2015): 599–609.

131. On the history of DiGeorge syndrome, see Hogan, *Life Histories of Genetic Diseases*, 147–77.

132. Daniel Navon and Uri Shwed, "The Chromosome 22q11.2 Deletion: From the Unification of Biomedical Fields to a New Kind of Genetic Condition," *Social Science and Medicine* 75 (2012): 1633–41.

133. P. J. Scambler, "The 22q11 Deletion Syndromes," *Human Molecular Genetics* 9 (2000): 2421–26; N. H. Robin and R. J. Shprintzen, "Defining the Clinical Spectrum of Deletion 22q11.2," *Journal of Pediatrics* 147 (2005): 90–96.

134. Rebecca Dimond, "Multiple Meanings of a Rare Genetic Syndrome: 22q11 Deletion Syndrome" (PhD diss., Cardiff University, 2011), 62–93.

135. Mary Umlauf, "22q11 Deletion Syndrome: A Mystery No More," *Exceptional Parent* 38 (2008): 26–28. The strong association of DiGeorge syndrome with psychiatric diseases is relatively new. It was not central to Dimond's observations of patients with 22q11 deletion syndrome in Cardiff (perhaps also because Dimond mainly observed children with this condition), and it does not appear, for example, in a Brazilian review on manifestations of 22q11.2 deletion. Társis Paiva Vieira, Ilária Cristina Sgardioli, and Vera Lúcia Gil-da-Silva-Lopes, "Genetics and Public Health: The Experience of a Reference Center for Diagnosis of 22q11.2 Deletion in Brazil and Suggestions for Implementing Genetic Testing," *Journal of Community Genetics* 4 (2013): 99–106.

136. Ludwik Fleck, *Genesis and Development of Scientific Fact* (Chicago: University of Chicago Press, 1979), 1–19.

137. R. J. Shprintzen, R. Goldberg, K. J. Golding-Kushner, and R. W. Marion, "Late-Onset Psychosis in the Velo-Cardio-Facial Syndrome," *American Journal of Medical Genetics* 42 (1992): 141–42; K. M. Antshel, A. Aneja, A. L. Strunge, et al., "Autistic Spectrum Disorders in Velo-Cardio Facial Syndrome (22q11.2 Deletion)," *Journal of Autism and Developmental Disorders* 37 (2007): 1776–86.

138. Alex Habel, Richard Herriot, Dinakantha Kumararatne, et al., "Towards a Safety Net for Management of 22q11.2 Deletion Syndrome: Guidelines for Our Times," *European Journal of Pediatrics* 173 (2014): 757–65.

139. Lun, Fung, Butcher, Costain, et al., "Practical Guidelines for Managing Adults with 22q11.2 Deletion Syndrome."

140. Nancy J. Butcher, Eva W. C. Chow, Gregory Costain, Dominique Karas, Andrew Hol, and Anne S. Bassett, "Functional Outcomes of Adults with 22q11.2 Deletion Syndrome," *Genetics in Medicine* 14 (2012): 836–43; Nicole Philip and Anne Bassett, "Cognitive, Behavioural and Psychiatric Phenotype in 22q11.2 Deletion Syndrome," *Behavioral Genetics* 41 (2011): 403–12; Nicole Martin, Marina Mikhaelian, Cheryl Cytrynbaum, Cheryl Shuman, David A. Chitayat, Rosanna Weksberg and Anne S. Bassett, "22q11.2 Deletion Syndrome: Attitudes towards Disclosing the Risk of Psychiatric Illness," *Journal of Genetic Counseling* 21 (2012): 825–34.

141. Laura Hercher and Georgette Bruenner, "Living with a Child at Risk for Psychotic Illness: The Experience of Parents Coping with 22q11 Deletion Syndrome: An Exploratory Study," *American Journal of Medical Genetics* 146A (2008): 2355–60; D. J. Karas, G. Costain, E. W. Chow and A. S. Bassett, "Perceived Burden and Neuropsychiatric Morbidities in

Adults with 22q11.2 Deletion Syndrome," *Journal of Intellectual Disability Research* 56 (2014): 198–210.

142. Anne-Claire Noël, Fanny Pelluard, Anne-Lise Delezoide, et al., "Fetal Phenotype Associated with the 22q11 Deletion," *American Journal of Medical Genetics* 164A (2014): 2724–31.

143. Florence Bretelle, Laura Beyer, Marie Christine Pellissier, et al., "Prenatal and Postnatal Diagnosis of 22q11.2 Deletion Syndrome," *European Journal of Medical Genetics* 53, no. 6 (2010): 367–70.

144. J. Besseau-Ayasse, C. Violle-Poirsier, A. Bazin, et al., "A French Collaborative Survey of 272 Fetuses with 22q11.2 Deletion: Ultrasound Findings, Fetal Autopsies and Pregnancy Outcomes," *Prenatal Diagnosis* 34 (2014): 424–30.

145. Anne Bassett, Gregory Costain, and Christian Marshall, "Neuropsychiatric Aspects of 22q11.2 Deletion Syndrome: Considerations in the Prenatal Setting," *Prenatal Diagnosis* 37, no. 1 (2016): 61–69. In France, a 10% risk of a severe intellectual disability is usually viewed by the pluridisciplinary committees that grant permission for the termination of pregnancy for a fetal indication as a cutoff point of a justification of such demand. Lynda Lotte and Isabelle Ville, "Les politiques de prévention des handicaps de la naissance en France: perspective historique," in final report, ANR grant DPN-HP, ANR-09-SSOC-026, Paris 2013.

146. Hayden, "Prenatal-Screening Companies Expand Scope of DNA Tests, but the Increasingly Accurate Analyses Carry the Ethical Dilemma of Uncertain Outcomes."

147. Gregory Costain, Donna McDonald McGinn, and Anne Bassett, "Prenatal Genetic Testing with Chromosomal Microarray Analysis Identifies Major Risk Variants for Schizophrenia and Other Later-Onset Disorders," *American Journal of Psychiatry* 170 (2013): 1498. doi:10.1176/appi.ajp.2013.13070880. The estimated positive predictive power of NIPT for DiGeorge syndrome was 5.3%. In addition, NIPT diagnosis of DiGeorge syndrome revealed in some cases an unsuspected maternal 22q11.2 mutation. Wapner, Babiarz, Levy, et al., "Expanding the Scope of Noninvasive Prenatal Testing."

148. Philip and Bassett, "Cognitive, Behavioural and Psychiatric Phenotype in 22q11.2 Deletion Syndrome"; R. Robyr, J.-P. Bernard, J. Roume, and Y. Ville, "Familial Diseases Revealed by a Fetal Anomaly," *Prenatal Diagnosis* 26 (2006): 1224–34.

149. Olivia Gordon, "Living with Down's Syndrome: 'He's Not a List of Characteristics. He's My Son,'" *The Guardian*, October 17, 2015, https://www.theguardian.com /society/2015/oct/17/living-with-downs-syndrome-hes-not-list-characteristics. In the United States, Down syndrome associations usually do not strongly reject prenatal testing for Down syndrome but focus on a strong opposition to selective abortion for this condition.

150. Jaime King, "Politics and Fetal Diagnostics Collide," *Nature* 491 (2012): 33–34.

151. French National Consultative Ethics Committee for Health and Life Sciences, Opinion No. 120, "Ethical Issues in Connection with the Development of Foetal Genetic Testing on Maternal Blood," April 25, 2013, http://www.ccne-ethique.fr/sites/default /files/publications/avis120vbeng.pdf.

152. There is a rich body of literature on the collaboration of patients in genetic research and the forms of "biosociality" it generates. See, for example, Paul Rabinow, "Artificiality and Enlightenment: From Sociobiology to Biosociality," in *Incorporations*, ed. Jonathan Crary and Sanford Kwinter (New York: Zone Books, 1992), 234–52; Rayna

Rapp, Deborah Heath, and Karen-Sue Taussig, "Geneological Dis-Ease: Where Hereditary Abnormality, Biomedical Explanation and Family Responsibility Meet," in *Relative
Values: Reconfiguring Kinship Studies*, ed. Susan McKinon and Sarah Franklin (Durham, NC: Duke University Press, 2001), 384–409; Lindee, *Moments of Truth in Genetic
Medicine*. In the United Kingdom, Unique supports individuals with rare chromosomal
disorders and their families: http://www.rarechromo.org/html/home.asp (accessed
March 23, 2016).

153. Daniel Navon, "Genetic Counseling, Activism and 'Genotype-First' Diagnosis of
Developmental Disorders," *Journal of Genetic Counseling* 21 (2012): 770–76.

154. Andrew Hogan, "Visualizing Carrier Status: Fragile X Syndrome and Genetic
Diagnosis since the 1940s," *Endeavor* 35, no. 2 (2012): 77–84; Navon, "Genomic Designation: How Genetics Can Delineate New, Phenotypically Diffuse Medical Categories";
Navon, "Genetic Counseling, Activism and 'Genotype-First' Diagnosis of Developmental Disorders."

155. See, for example, Peter Glasner, Paul Atkinson, and Helen Greenslade, eds., *New Genetics, New Social Formations* (New York: Routledge, 2007); Aviad Raz, *Community Genetics
and Genetic Alliances: Eugenics, Carrier Testing and Networks of Risk* (New York: Routledge,
2010). Chloe Silverman described tensions between genetic-centered activism of parents of
autistic children and other forms of activism. Chloe Silverman, *Understanding Autism: Parents, Doctors, and the History of a Disorder* (Princeton, NJ: Princeton University Press, 2012).

156. James Neel, "The Meaning of Empirical Risk Figures for Disease or Defect," in
Heredity and Counseling, ed. Helen Hammonds (New York: Paul B. Hoeber, 1959),
65–69.

157. Report, *Antenatal Diagnosis*, US Department of Health, Education and Welfare
(Bethesda, MD: NIH Publication No. 79-1973, 1979), 58.

158. The joined opinion of the European Society of Human Genetics (ESHG) and
the American Society of Human Genetics (ASHG) of 2015 mentions dilemmas that
may result from prenatal diagnosis of syndromes such as DiGeorge and Klinefelter
but, alternatively, presents the practical difficulty in providing appropriate genetic
counseling to all pregnant women diagnosed with such fetal anomalies as the main
reason for the recommendation to restrict NIPT to the detection of autosomal aneuploidies. Dondorp, de Wert, Bombard, et al., "Non-invasive Prenatal Testing for Aneuploidy and Beyond."

159. A recent linking of KS with a sixfold increase in the risk of developing autism
and a fourfold increase in the risk of developing schizophrenia or psychosis may increase the difficulties of children whose parents are aware of such a risk. Martin
Cederlöf, Agnes Ohlsson Gotby, Henrik Larsson, Eva Serlachius, Marcus Boman, Nik-
las Långström, Mikael Landén, and Paul Lichtenstein, "Klinefelter Syndrome and Risk
of Psychosis, Autism and ADHD," *Journal of Psychiatric Research* 48 (2014): 128–30.

160. Mark Evans and Joris Robert Vermeesch, "Current Controversies in Prenatal
Diagnosis 3: Industry Drives Innovation in Research and Clinical Application of Genetic
Prenatal Diagnosis and Screening," *Prenatal Diagnosis* 36, no. 13 (2016): 1172–77. Evans
and Vermeesch made this argument during their intervention at the 2016 International
Society for Prenatal Diagnosis meeting in Berlin, Germany.

161. Greely and King, "The Coming Revolution in Prenatal Genetic Testing"; Henry
Greely, "Get Ready for the Flood of Fetal Gene Screening," *Nature* 469 (2011): 289–91.

162. See, for example, Jacob O. Kitzman, Matthew W. Snyder, Mario Ventura, et al., "Noninvasive Whole-Genome Sequencing of a Human Fetus," *Science and Translational Medicine* 4, 137 (2012): 137ra76; Michael E. Talkowski, Zehra Ordulu, Vamsee Pillalamarri, et al., "Clinical Diagnosis by Whole-Genome Sequencing of a Prenatal Sample," *New England Journal of Medicine* 267 (2012): 2226–32; Matthew W. Snyder, LaVone E. Simmons, Jacob O. Kitzman, et al., "Noninvasive Fetal Genome Sequencing: A Primer," *Prenatal Diagnosis* 33 (2013): 1–8.

163. Greely, "Get Ready for the Flood of Fetal Gene Screening;" Greer Donley, Sara Chandros Hull, and Benjamin Berkman, "Prenatal Whole Genome Sequencing: Just Because We Can, Should We?," *Hastings Center Report* 42 (2012): 28–40; Ilana Yurkiewicz, Bruce Korf, and Lisa Soleymani Lehmann, "Prenatal Whole-Genome Sequencing—Is the Quest to Know a Fetus's Future Ethical?," *New England Journal of Medicine* 379 (2014): 195–97; Millum, "The Foundation of the Child's Right to an Open Future"; Dondorp, Page-Christiaens, and de Wert, "Genomic Futures of Prenatal Screening."

164. Angus Clarke, "Managing the Ethical Challenges of Next Generation Sequencing in Genomic Medicine," *British Medical Journal* 111 (2014): 17–28.

165. Bertrand Jordan, "En route vers l'enfant parfait," *Médecine/Sciences* 29 (2013): 5665–68. Lee Silver's book is *Remaking Eden: How Genetic Engineering and Cloning Will Transform the American Family* (New York: Avon Books, 1997). Jordan might have also mentioned Aldous Huxley's *Brave New World* (London: Chatto and Windus, 1932) or George Herbert Wells's *The Time Machine* (London: William Heinemann, 1895).

166. This point was summarized, for example, in Ravitsky, "Noninvasive Prenatal Testing (NIPT)."

167. Stoll, "NPIS Is Not Diagnostic"; Stoll, "NIPS and the Threat to Informed Decision Making."

168. Lyn Chitty and Mark Kroese, "Realising the Promise of Non-invasive Prenatal Testing," *British Medical Journal* (2015): doi:10.1136/bmj.h1792; Dondorp, de Wert, Bombard, et al., "Non-invasive Prenatal Testing for Aneuploidy and Beyond."

169. Paul Wenzel Geissler, "Public Secrets in Public Health: Knowing Not to Know While Making Scientific Knowledge," *American Ethnologist* 40 (2013): 13–34; Claire Marris, Catherine Jefferson, and Filippa Lentzos, "Negotiating the Dynamics of Uncomfortable Knowledge: The Case of Dual Use and Synthetic Biology," *Biosocieties* 9 (2014): 393–420.

170. A careful explanation of goals and limits of NIPT does not seem to diminish the anguish of pregnant women who face difficult decisions. Jessica Mozersky, "Hoping Someday Never Comes: Deferring Ethical Thinking about Noninvasive Prenatal Testing," *AJOB Empirical Bioethics* 6, no. 1 (2015): 31–41. Mozersky studied US women.

Conclusion • *Prenatal Diagnosis' Slippery Slopes, Imagined and Real*

1. Stephen Wilkinson, "Prenatal Screening, Reproductive Choice and Public Health," *Bioethics* 29 (2015): 26–35.

2. Wybo Dondorp and Jan Van Lith, "Editorial: Dynamics of Prenatal Screening: New Developments Challenging the Ethical Framework," *Bioethics* 29 (2015): ii–iv; Wybo Dondorp, Godelieve Page-Christiaens, and Guido de Wert, "Genomic Futures of Prenatal Screening: Ethical Reflection," *Clinical Genetics* 89, no. 5 (2016): 531–38.

3. Susan Markens, C. H. Browner, and Nancy Press, "Because of the Risks: How US Pregnant Women Account for Refusing Prenatal Screening," *Social Science and Medicine* 49 (1999): 359–69, see esp. 366.

4. Antina de Jong, Idit Maya, and Jan Van Lith, "Prenatal Screening: Current Practice, New Developments, Ethical Challenges," *Bioethics* 29 (2015): 1–8; Antina de Jong and Guido de Wert, "Prenatal Screening: An Ethical Agenda for the Near Future," *Bioethics* 29 (2015): 46–55.

5. The same is true for other diagnostic tests. Women who undergo yearly mammograms have a much higher chance of receiving false positive or borderline results than those tested every three years. And women who are told that they harbor abnormal cells in their breast tissue are more inclined to undergo preventive treatment than those informed about a higher statistical risk of breast cancer. Ilana Löwy, "Treating Health Risks or Putting Healthy Women at Risk: Controversies around Chemoprevention of Breast Cancer," in *Ways of Regulating Drugs in the 19th and 20th Centuries*, ed. Jean-Paul Gaudillière and Volker Hess (Houndmills, Basingstoke: Palgrave Macmillan, 2013), 206–27.

6. Jeremy Greene, *Prescribing by Numbers: Drugs and the Definition of Disease* (Baltimore: Johns Hopkins University Press, 2007); Ilana Löwy, *Preventive Strikes: Women, Precancer and Prophylactic Surgery* (Baltimore: Johns Hopkins University Press, 2009); Robert Aronowitz, *Risky Medicine: Our Quest to Cure Risk and Uncertainty* (Chicago: Chicago University Press, 2015).

7. David Armstrong, "Screening: Mapping Medicine's Temporal Spaces," *Sociology of Health and Illness* 34 (2012): 177–93.

8. Darren Schicle and Ruth Chadwick, "The Ethics of Screening: Is 'Screeningitis' an Incurable Disease?," *Journal of Medical Ethics* 20 (1994): 12–18.

9. Natalie Armstrong and Helen Eborall, "The Sociology of Medical Screening: Past, Present and Future," *Sociology of Health and Illness* 34 (2012): 161–76.

10. See, for example, H. Gilbert Welch, *Should I Be Tested for Cancer? Maybe Not and Here's Why* (Berkeley: University of California Press, 2006); H. Gilbert Welch, Lisa Schwartz, and Steven Woloshin, *Overdiagnosed: Making People Sick in the Pursuit of Health* (Boston, MA: Beacon Press, 2011); Stefan Timmermans and Mara Buchbinder, *Saving Babies? The Consequences of Newborn Genetic Screening* (Chicago: University of Chicago Press, 2013); Aronowitz, *Risky Medicine.*

11. Sara Dubow, *Ourselves Unborn: A History of the Fetus in Modern America* (Oxford: Oxford University Press, 2011).

12. Dondorp, Page-Christiaens, and de Wert, "Genomic Futures of Prenatal Screening."

13. J. M. Jørgensen, P. L. Hedley, M. Gjerris, and M. Christiansen, "Including Ethical Considerations in Models for First-Trimester Screening for Pre-eclampsia," *Reproductive Biomedicine Online* 28 (2014): 638–43; Wybo Dondorp, Guido de Wert, Yvonne Bombard, et al., "Non-invasive Prenatal Testing for Aneuploidy and Beyond: Challenges of Responsible Innovation in Prenatal Screening," *European Journal of Human Genetics* 23 (2015): 1438–50.

14. Rayna Rapp, *Testing Women, Testing the Fetus: The Social Impact of Amniocentesis in America* (New York: Routledge, 2000). Prenatal diagnosis' promoters may have an interest in maintaining an ambivalence about prenatal diagnosis' goals because it

weakens objections to prenatal diagnosis as an approach that aims, above all, to eliminate "imperfect" fetuses.

15. Thus, opponents of mammographic screening for breast cancer argue that its harm outweighs its benefits. See, for example, Nikola Biller-Andorno and Peter Jüni, "Abolishing Mammography Screening Programs? A View from the Swiss Medical Board," *New England Journal of Medicine* 370 (2014): 1965–67.

16. Judith McCoyd, "Pregnancy Interrupted: Loss of a Desired Pregnancy after Diagnosis of Fetal Anomaly," *Journal of Psychosomatic Obstetrics and Gynecology* 28 (2007): 37–48; Judith McCoyd, "'I'm Not a Saint': Burden Assessment as an Unrecognized Factor in Prenatal Decision Making," *Qualitative Health Research* 18 (2008): 1489–1500.

17. See, for example, Anne Kaasen, Anne Helbig, Ulrik Fredrik Malt, Tormod Naes, Hans Skari, and Guttorm Nils Haugen, "Acute Maternal Social Dysfunction, Health Perception and Psychological Distress after Ultrasonographic Detection of a Fetal Structural Anomaly," *BJOG: An International Journal of Obstetrics and Gynaecology* 117 (2010): 1127–38; Joanna Cole, Julie Moldenhauer, Kelsey Berer, Mark Carry, Haley Smith, Victoria Martino, Norma Rendon, and Lori Howell, "Identifying Expectant Parents at Risk of Psychological Distress in Response to a Confirmed Fetal Abnormality," *Archives of Women Mental Health* 19, no. 3 (2016): 443–53.

18. R. Robyr, J.-P. Bernard, J. Roume, and Y. Ville, "Familial Diseases Revealed by a Fetal Anomaly," *Prenatal Diagnosis* 26 (2006): 1224–34.

19. Marian Reiff, Barbara A. Bernhardt, Surabhi Mulchandani, Danielle Soucier, Diana Cornell, Reed E. Pyeritz, and Nancy B. Spinner, "'What Does It Mean?': Uncertainties in Understanding Results of Chromosomal Microarray Testing," *Genetics in Medicine* 14 (2012): 250–58.

20. Barbara Bernhardt, Danielle Soucier, Karen Hanson, Melissa Savage, Laird Jackson, and Ronald Wapner, "Women's Experiences Receiving Abnormal Prenatal Chromosomal Microarray Testing Results," *Genetics in Medicine* 15 (2013): 139–45. The authors of this and the precedent study (conducted by the same group) added that in order to limit women's stress and neutralize the "toxic" effects of some results (their term), it is important to provide careful pre- and post-test counseling, and educate health providers. Other specialists argued that uncertainty produced by prenatal use of microarrays is not different from the uncertainty generated by many other diagnostic tests and should not be an obstacle for the diffusion of this approach. Zornitza Stark, Lynn Gilliam, Susan Walker, and George McGillivray, "Ethical Controversies in Prenatal Microarray," *Current Opinion in Obstetrics and Gynecology* 25 (2013): 133–37.

21. Bernhardt, Soucier, Hanson, Savage, Jackson, and Wapner, "Women's Experiences Receiving Abnormal Prenatal Chromosomal Microarray Testing Results." Postnatal diagnosis of an anomaly can produce similar uncertainty and stress, which often are not eliminated by the (apparent) good health of the child. Rachel Grob, *Testing Baby: The Transformation of Newborn Screening, Parenting, and Policymaking* (New Brunswick, NJ: Rutgers University Press, 2011); Timmermans and Buchbinder, *Saving Babies?*

22. Reiff, Bernhardt, Mulchandani, Soucier, Cornell, Pyeritz, and Spinner, "'What Does It Mean?,'" 255. The phrase *patient in waiting* was coined by Stefan Timmermans and Mara Buchbinder in their discussion of the consequences of finding a genetic anomaly in a healthy-looking newborn. Stefan Timmermans and Mara Buchbinder, "Patients-in-Waiting: Living between Sickness and Health in the Genomics Era," *Jour-*

nal of Health and Social Behavior 51 (2010): 408–23. See also Rachel Grob, "Is My Sick Child Healthy? Is My Healthy Child Sick? Changing Parental Experiences of Cystic Fibrosis in the Age of Expanded Newborn Screening," *Social Science and Medicine* 67 (2008): 1056–64.

23. Melanie Watson, Sue Hall, Kate Langford, and Theresa Marteau, "Psychological Impact of the Detection of Soft Markers on Routine Ultrasound Scanning: A Pilot Study Investigating the Modifying Role of Information," *Prenatal Diagnosis* 22 (2002): 569–75.

24. Sylvie Viaux-Savelon, Marc Dommergues, Ouriel Rosenblum, Nicolas Bodeau, Elizabeth Aidane, Odile Philippon, Philippe Mazet, Claude Vibert-Guigue, Daniele Vauthier-Brouzes, Ruth Feldman, and David Cohen, "Prenatal Ultrasound Screening: False Positive Soft Markers May Alter Maternal Representations and Mother-Infant Interaction," *PloS ONE* 7, no. 1 (2012): e30935. This is the only study I found that investigated the consequences of false-positive results of obstetrical ultrasound.

25. Jane Fisher, "First-Trimester Screening: Dealing with the Fall-out," *Prenatal Diagnosis* 31 (2011): 46–49. ARC provides advice and support to women with a "positive" prenatal diagnosis during the pregnancy. Its aim is to support a woman's decision about her pregnancy's future, whatever it may be.

26. "Bebe saudvel, gravidez tranquila, a partir de 9 semanes de gestacao," http://www.laboratoriogene.com.br/blog/entenda-nossos-exames/teste-pre-natal-nao-invasivo-em-sangue-materno-nipt-panorama/. On the awareness of (some) women of the limited capacity of genetic studies to uncover fetal anomalies, see Rayna Rapp and Faye Ginsburg, "Fetal Reflections: Confessions of Two Feminist Anthropologists as Mutual Informants," in *Fetal Positions, Feminist Practices*, ed. Lynn Morgan and Meredith Michaels (Philadelphia: University of Pennsylvania Press, 1999), 279–95.

27. Anne Kerr, "Reproductive Genetics: From Choice to Ambivalence and Back Again," in *Handbook of Genetics and Society: Mapping the New Genomic Era*, ed. Paul Atkinson, Peter Glasner, and Margaret Lock (New York: Routledge, 2009), 59–76.

28. The phrase *new standards of care* is borrowed from Sharon Kaufman. Sharon Kaufman, Paul Mueller, Abigail Ottenberg, and Barbara Koenig, "Ironic Technology: Old Age and the Implantable Cardioverter Defibrillator in US Health Care," *Social Science and Medicine* 72 (2011): 6–14.

29. Troy Duster, *Backdoor to Eugenics* (New York: Routledge, 1990); Joan Rothschild, *The Dream of the Perfect Child* (Bloomington: Indiana University Press, 2005).

30. Diane Paul, *Controlling Human Heredity, 1865 to the Present* (Amherst, NY: Humanity Books, 1995).

31. Susan Lindee, "Human Genetics after the Bomb: Archives, Clinics, Proving Grounds and Board Rooms," *Studies in History and Philosophy of Biological and Biomedical Sciences* 55 (2016): 45–53.

32. Lene Koch, "The Meanings of Eugenics: Reflection on the Government of Genetic Knowledge in the Past and the Present," *Science in Context* 17, no. 3 (2004): 315–31, see esp. 318, 329.

33. Diane Paul, *The Politics of Heredity: Essays on Eugenics, Biomedicine and the Nature-Nurture Debate* (Albany: State University of New York Press, 1998), 97.

34. There is a rich historical body of literature on eugenics. In the context of prenatal diagnosis, especially useful studies are Paul, *Controlling Human Heredity, 1865 to the Present*; Paul, *The Politics of Heredity*; Nathaniel Comfort, *The Science of Human Perfection:*

How Genes Became the Heart of American Medicine (New Haven, CT: Yale University Press, 2012); Alexandra Minna Stern, *Telling Genes: The Story of Genetic Counseling in America* (Baltimore: Johns Hopkins University Press, 2012). On the (presumed) aspiration for perfect offspring, see Rothschild, *The Dream of the Perfect Child,* and on the aspiration to perfect human beings, see Silvia Camporesi, *From Bench to Bedside to Track and Field: The Context of Enhancement and Its Ethical Relevance* (Berkeley: University of California Press, 2014).

35. Rothschild, *The Dream of the Perfect Child.*

36. Arthur Caplan, "Foreword," in *Prenatal Testing: A Sociological Perspective,* ed. Aliza Kolker and B. Meredith Burke (Westport, CT: Bergin and Garvey, 1888), xiii-xviii.

37. Ibid., xiv–xv.

38. Aldous Huxley, *Brave New World* (London: Chatto and Windus, 1932).

39. The supposition that women will readily abort fetuses who do not correspond to their ideal "dream child" may recall the argument, advanced by opponents of the liberalization of abortion in the 1960s and early 1970s, that with the decriminalization of abortion, scores of women will have abortions for trivial reasons such as a wish not to spoil a planned vacation.

40. Evelyne Shuster, "Microarray Genetic Screening: A Prenatal Roadblock for Life?," *The Lancet* 369 (2007): 526–29.

41. Marc Dommergues, Laurent Mandelbrot, Dominique Mahieu-Caputo, Noel Boudjema, Isabelle Durand-Zaleski, and the ICI Group-Club de médecine foetale, "Termination of Pregnancy following Prenatal Diagnosis in France: How Severe Are the Foetal Anomalies?," *Prenatal Diagnosis* 30 (2010): 531–39. The percentage of pregnancy terminations following a "positive" prenatal diagnosis is relatively homogenous in all Western European countries: by contrast, the framing of prenatal diagnosis and the uptake of prenatal testing vary greatly. P. A. Boyd, C. Devigan, B. Khoshnood, M. Loane, E. Garne, H. Dolk, and the EUROCAT Working Group, "Survey of Prenatal Screening Policies in Europe for Structural Malformations and Chromosome Anomalies, and Their Impact on Detection and Termination Rates for Neural Tube Defects and Down Syndrome," *BJOG: An International Journal of Obstetrics and Gynaecology* 115 (2008): 689–96. In France, "voluntary termination of pregnancy" (IVG), decided by a woman alone, is possible only up to fourteen weeks, while a "medical termination of pregnancy" (IMG), for fetal or maternal indications, is possible until the end of the pregnancy, but the ethics committee of a hospital has to authorize such an intervention. Since a great majority of pregnancy terminations for fetal indications in France are performed (for the time being) after fourteen weeks and all CPPND decisions are recorded and tabulated, France has probably more accurate statistics of the causes of such interruptions than countries in which a woman can decide for herself to terminate a pregnancy up to twenty to twenty-four weeks of gestation.

42. The most contentious fetal impairment is the one that was at the origin of the large-scale diffusion of prenatal diagnosis: Down syndrome. Activists for this condition rightly stress that people with Down syndrome can live a fulfilling and content life, and that "high-functioning" people with Down syndrome can be semiautonomous. They tend, however, to underplay the fact that Down syndrome is not a single impairment but a spectrum with highly variable levels of physical and intellectual impairments, including severe ones. Joan Noble, "Natural History of Down's Syndrome: A Brief Review for Those Involved in Antenatal Screening," *Journal of Medical Screening* 5 (1998): 172–77.

43. The right to an abortion for a fetal indication is threatened in the United States in several conservative states that officially banned such an abortion. Today, such a ban has mainly symbolic value. It is in contradiction with the *Roe v. Wade* supreme court judgment and is therefore unconstitutional. Moreover, it is quasi-impossible today to show what a woman's intent is when she is seeking an abortion. However, it is not inconceivable that with a nomination of more conservative judges to the Supreme Court, *Roe v. Wade* will be overturned, or that a state will produce a registry of women diagnosed with fetal impairments and supervise the pregnancies of these women.

44. Such risks may include the end of a romantic relationship and subsequent economic and emotional hardship. An article on microcephaly induced by Zika epidemics in Pernambuco, Brazil, is titled, "Men Abandon Mothers of Babies with Microcephaly in Pernambuco." Felipe Resk, "Homens abandonam mães de bebês com microcefalia em PE," *Estado*, February 4, 2016, http://noticias.uol.com.br/saude/ultimas-noticias/estado/2016/02/04/homens-abandonam-maes-de-bebes-com-microcefalia-em-pe.htm.

45. Anna Quindlen, "Public and Private: A Public Matter," *New York Times*, June 17, 1992.

46. On the role of fear in the expansion of "risk / risky medicine," see Charles Rosenberg, "Managed Fear," *The Lancet* 373 (2009): 802–803; Aronowitz, *Risky Medicine*.

47. Tine Gammeltoft, *Haunting Images: A Cultural Account of Selective Reproduction in Vietnam* (Berkeley: University of California Press, 2014).

48. Bruno Latour, "Morality and Technology: The End of the Means," *Theory, Culture and Society* 19 (2002): 247–60, see esp. 252. Latour's argument resonates with the ideas of French philosophers of technology Gilbert Simondon and Michel Serres. Gilbert Simondon, *Du mode de l'existence des objets téchniques* (Paris: Aubier-Montaigne, 1969); Michel Serres, *Conversation on Science, Culture and Time* (Ann Arbor: University of Michigan Press, 1995). On the transformation of scientific facts through their circulation, see Ludwik Fleck, *Genesis and Development of a Scientific Fact*, trans. Fred Bradley and Thaddeus Trenn (Chicago: University of Chicago Press, 1979), 42.

49. Ilana Löwy, "'A River That Is Cutting Its Own Bed': The Serology of Syphilis between Laboratory Society and the Law," *Studies in History and Philosophy of Biological and Biomedical Sciences* 35, no. 3 (2004): 509–24.

50. Lester King, *Medical Thinking: A Historical Preface* (Princeton, NJ: Princeton University Press, 1982), 309.

51. A *feeder layer* is a layer of irradiated cells that makes the growth of other, more delicate cells in the test tube possible. This term was used by Franklin to describe the environment that makes possible the development of new biomedical technologies. Sarah Franklin, "Stem Cells R Us: Emergent Life Forms and the Global Biological," in *Global Assemblages*, ed. A. Ong and S. Collier (Malden, MA: Blackwell, 2005), 59–78.